T0313722

THE SMALLPOX REPORT

Vaccination and the Romantic Illness Narrative

FUSON WANG

The Smallpox Report

Vaccination and the Romantic Illness Narrative

UNIVERSITY OF TORONTO PRESS
Toronto Buffalo London

ISBN 978-1-4875-4659-5 (cloth)   ISBN 978-1-4875-4660-1 (EPUB)
ISBN 978-1-4875-4662-5 (PDF)

Library and Archives Canada Cataloguing in Publication

Title: The smallpox report : vaccination and the romantic illness narrative / Fuson Wang.
Names: Wang, Fuson, author.
Description: Includes bibliographical references and index.
Identifiers: Canadiana (print) 20220472211 | Canadiana (ebook) 20220472335 |
ISBN 9781487546595 (cloth) | ISBN 9781487546625 (PDF) |
ISBN 9781487546601 (EPUB)
Subjects: LCSH: English literature – 18th century – History and criticism. |
LCSH: Literature and medicine – England – History – 18th century. |
LCSH: Vaccination – England – History – 18th century. |
LCSH: Medicine in literature. | LCSH: Vaccination in literature. |
LCSH: Smallpox in literature. | LCSH: Diseases in literature. |
LCSH: Romanticism – England.
Classification: LCC PR448.M42 W36 2023 | DDC 820.9/3561–dc23

We wish to acknowledge the land on which the University of Toronto Press operates. This land is the traditional territory of the Wendat, the Anishnaabeg, the Haudenosaunee, the Métis, and the Mississaugas of the Credit First Nation.

This book has been published with the assistance of the University of California, Riverside.

University of Toronto Press acknowledges the financial support of the Government of Canada, the Canada Council for the Arts, and the Ontario Arts Council, an agency of the Government of Ontario, for its publishing activities.

 Canada Council
for the Arts
Conseil des Arts
du Canada

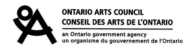 ONTARIO ARTS COUNCIL
CONSEIL DES ARTS DE L'ONTARIO
an Ontario government agency
un organisme du gouvernement de l'Ontario

Funded by the Financé par le
Government gouvernement
of Canada du Canada

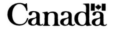 Canadä

Contents

List of Illustrations   vii

Acknowledgments   ix

Part One: Classification

Introduction   3
1 Wordsworth's Romantic Path to Biopower   38

Part Two: Experimentation

2 Darwin's Evolutionary Metaphor   59
3 Blake's Revolutionary Metaphor   86

Part Three: Interdisciplinarity

4 Keats and the End of Disease   123
5 Shelley and Romantic Immunity   152

Part Four: Modern Biopower

6 The Case of Sherlock Holmes   181
Conclusion   199

Notes   207

Works Cited   227

Index   241

Illustrations

Figure 1   "Edward Jenner" by James Northcote, 1803. 7

Figure 2   "VACCINATION against SMALL POX or Mercenary & Merciless spreaders of Death & Devastation driven out of society!" by Isaac Cruikshank, 1808. 9

Figure 3   Illustration of the right hand of Sarah Nelmes, Case XVI in Edward Jenner's *Inquiry into the Causes and Effects of the Variolæ Vaccinæ, Or Cow-Pox*, 1798. 15

Figure 4   Edward Jenner letter to William Clement, page three of four, 19 December 1807. 18

Figure 5   Edward Jenner letter to William Clement, page four of four, 19 December 1807. 19

Figure 6   "The Cow-Pock-or-the Wonderful Effects of the New Inoculation" by James Gillray, 1802. 24

Figure 7   Portrait of Edward Jenner on the cover of *Health Heroes*, a series commissioned by the Metropolitan Life Insurance Company, 1926. 39

Figure 8   A reference image for Linnaeus's twenty-four classes of plants from the second part, *The Loves of the Plants*, of Erasmus Darwin's *The Botanic Garden*, 1791. 90

Figure 9   The title page of *The Book of Thel* by William Blake, 1789. 93

Figure 10   "The Argument" from "Visions of the Daughters of Albion" by William Blake, 1793. 94

Figure 11   "The Sick Rose" from *The Songs of Experience* by William Blake, 1794. 98

Figure 12   "Comus and His Revellers," commissioned from William Blake by Joseph Thomas, 1801. 116

Figure 13   "Comus and His Revellers," commissioned from William Blake by
             Thomas Butts, 1815. 117
Figure 14   "Map showing how SMALLPOX spread" in *Health Heroes*, a series
             commissioned by the Metropolitan Life Insurance Company,
             1926. 203

Acknowledgments

The work for this book began when Disneyland, the happiest place on earth, got the unhappy news that it was ground zero for a vaccine-preventable outbreak of measles. And it was revised and completed right in the thick of the COVID-19 pandemic. Along the way, I have been fortunate to have generous and brilliant interlocutors to puzzle through this long, interdisciplinary tale of vaccine hesitancy.

As a graduate student at the University of California, Los Angeles, I benefited from the remarkable mentorship of Anne Mellor, Saree Makdisi, Helen Deutsch, and Felicity Nussbaum. There, I discovered from their examples what it meant to develop intellectual curiosity into meaningful research. There, my research agenda was also shaped by my conversations with my fellow graduate students, especially Allison Johnson, Meghan Kemp-Gee, Daniel Williford, Michael Nicholson, and Ian Newman. In my first faculty position at the City College of New York, I lucked into yet another generous cohort that welcomed me to a new city and a new intellectual community. I would like to thank especially Mikhal Dekel, Daniel Gustafson, Robert Higney, András Kiséry, Václav Paris, Harold Veeser, and Joshua Wilner for being so willing to share work, ideas, and conviviality.

The book was finalized as I arrived at the University of California, Riverside (UCR), where I was supported with two years of fellowship at the Huntington Library in San Marino. In the 2016–17 fellowship year, the manuscript was finalized among the learned company of eminent literary scholars like Jon Mee, Laura Forsberg, J.K. Barret, and Tiffany Werth. And in the 2019–20 fellowship year, our fellowship cohort was forced out of our Huntington offices to ponder how humanities scholars can continue to do what they do in a global pandemic. Despite the restrictions on in-person meeting, I managed to keep social and intellectual contact with Dympna Callaghan, Christopher Clark, Stephen Cushman, Jack Hartnell, Dawna Schuld, Ben Davidson, Verónica Castillo Muñoz, Katie Moore, Lauren Cannady, Sarah Rodriguez, and Justina Spencer.

At UCR, I have been able to forge the most wonderful and eye-opening interdisciplinary connections in the medical and health humanities. I have my colleagues here in Riverside to thank for expanding the interdisciplinary scope of my project beyond literary studies. Special thanks go to Juliet McMullin, Carla Mazzio, Padma Rangarajan, Susan Zieger, and George Haggerty for being such attentive and generous partners in this work.

Thanks go also to the amazing editorial team at the University of Toronto Press, especially to my editor Mark Thompson. He shepherded me patiently through the process of anonymous review and revision, making it a truly generative and productive process rather than merely painful. And finally, I want to thank Ronald McGregor, my neuroscientist partner, who gamely listened to fuzzy, humanities opinions about science and medicine without ever telling me to shut up.

Portions of this book have been previously published in the following journals, which I thank for their permission to reprint. Part of the introduction appeared in *Nineteenth-Century Contexts*, 33.5 (2011), and part of chapter 5 appeared in *European Romantic Review*, 22.2 (2011).

PART ONE

Classification

Introduction

This book was partially written and revised during the COVID-19 pandemic, which necessarily sharpened its pragmatic focus. Its medical and health humanities topic, the Romantic-era literary history of smallpox vaccination, might have been much more about the emergence of the benevolent biopolitical state, and the historical and contemporary ways it has built and can continue to foster acceptance of medical science. In short, the story *could have been* about how the biopolitical state can tweak its varyingly successful strategies to encourage, incentivize, or mandate vaccination. However, the pandemic made it even clearer that this was not quite the right story to tell. The absence of state leadership (or even the active harm of bleach, UV lights, and hydroxychloroquine recommendations) characterized the early government responses to COVID-19, and a top-down, biopolitical solution had yet to emerge. Without that much-needed state guidance, we slowly relearned how to listen to and value the largely forgotten genre of the illness narrative. We eagerly shared over Zoom stories of symptomatic and asymptomatic infections, reinfections, breakthrough infections, long haulers, quarantine, restricted travel, and hospitalization, while we listened with rapt attention to the symptomatic progression of infected public figures like Tom Hanks, Chris Cuomo, and Idris Elba. And when the vaccines finally arrived, we related our intimate experiences with the first and second doses of the Pfizer and Moderna vaccines and, from personal experience, my own asymptomatic reaction to the one-shot Johnson & Johnson vaccine, briefly panicking about its temporary FDA suspension due to rare cases of blood clots, and finally settling into some semblance of reasonable calm. From the crucial early days of the pandemic to the weary latter days, these bottom-up illness narratives offered more solace, more hope, and more solutions.

In *AIDS and Its Metaphors* (1989), however, Susan Sontag characterized the pandemic narratives surrounding HIV/AIDS as dangerous, fantastical indulgences in the face of a very real medical catastrophe. We were, as she characterized it, thrown back to the abject conditions of pre-modern medicine. Any quack cure or snake oil mustered enough anecdotal evidence behind it to feed our delusive and dangerous hopes. Metaphors, according to Sontag, could kill, and she wanted "to offer people who were ill and those who care for them to dissolve these metaphors, these inhibitions" (14). According to Sontag, only after taming our wild, imaginative illness narratives would we finally be able to seek proper, evidence-based medical treatment and emerge from the delusions of our pre-modern fog. Even in the wake of Michel Foucault's influential warnings of the coercions of biopower, Sontag nevertheless nudged us towards the benefits of institutional medicine's proven track record of effective health care.[1] And since Sontag's equally influential polemic, the abiding hope has been that a potentially oppressive, Foucauldian biopower could be softened into a benevolent biopolitics, a utopian vision of a gentle caretaker state whose impositions of bodily control are won more through consensus than coercion. At the start of the new millennium, instead of continuing this elusive search for a good and gentle version of biopolitics, Michael Hardt and Antonio Negri, in their influential trilogy of *Empire* (2000), *Multitudes: War and Democracy in the Age of Empire* (2004), and *Commonwealth* (2009), pushed us to find a solution to this prickly problem of life not in the paternalistic biopolitical state but in another elusive utopian vision of "the commons": a diffuse distribution of embodied life without the seemingly objective and necessary controls of state and corporate interests.[2] And most recently, Jeffrey Di Leo and Peter Hitchcock have given a name to this building pushback against the conventional premises of biopolitics in their edited collection of essays, *Biotheory: Life and Death Under Capitalism* (2020). Their new coinage, "biotheory," offers an alternative to biopolitics to envision life as more than just "an extension of the biopolitical in its neoliberal condensation" (16). In this same vein, *The Smallpox Report* leans into this recent theoretical swerve from the conventional premises of biopolitics. Instead of trying to convince a sceptical population to trust a kinder, gentler, and reformed model of biopower, for example, this book privileges what I am calling the Romantic illness narrative and how it shaped the medical, social, and literary history of smallpox vaccination.

This book, in other words, will not *directly* attempt to change the minds of adamant anti-vaxxers from the top down; rather, it approaches the problem at a cultural and systemic level by offering a literary historical example of a time when individual illness narratives were at least as important as the biopolitical calculations of the state. Peering into this Romantic-era literary historical past, I argue, reveals just how much we have devalued or discounted illness narratives. In this way, we have fostered the systemic conditions that produced the anti-vaccination movement in the first place. Instead of continuing the search for a good, alternative biopolitics for our own times, then, *The Smallpox Report* is more interested in a bottom-up rather than a top-down view of Romantic-era medicine, especially in the complex literary history of smallpox vaccination. Instead of asking the biopolitical question about how the state can and should intervene more humanely in tough medical decisions, this book will ask what I believe to be one of the most pressing medical and health humanities questions of our time: how can we learn to value and respect the seemingly unmanageable diversity of illness narratives without conspiratorial indulgence in Sontag's dangerous metaphorical, magical thinking? *The Smallpox Report* will certainly address the top-down view of biopolitics because that remains a crucial component of the evolving conversation. The contemporary voices on eighteenth- and nineteenth-century biopolitics – Robert Mitchell, Richard A. Barney, Warren Montag, et al. – are all richly illuminating how these earlier "systems of life" presage the ways that we structure modern life.[3] In the history of vaccination, however, this story of biopolitical compulsion and systematization is already quite a familiar one. During this pandemic, for example, we have settled into a comforting mantra of "trust the science." *The Smallpox Report* offers a new literary historical account that de-systematizes life by carefully and responsibly inviting the sublime strangeness of illness narratives back into our complex understandings of disease and health.

To do this, I strike a balance between analysing Romantic-era illness narratives and uncovering the era's emergent biopolitical solutions. However, along the theoretical lines of that recent edited collection *Biotheory: Life and Death Under Capitalism*, I consistently privilege the former over the latter, Romantic-era illness narratives over biopolitics. *The Smallpox Report* participates in what the editors of *Biotheory* call "a tradition of moving 'beyond biopolitics' as a condition of governance over life and death" (1). Of course, moving beyond will still require dwelling within these debates, so the book continuously engages with the high philosophical stakes of these biopolitical questions while maintaining its focus on the inoculation narratives of authors like William Wordsworth, Erasmus Darwin, William Blake, John Keats, Mary Shelley, and Arthur Conan Doyle. The COVID-19 pandemic has prepared us to go back to this Romantic era and to take more seriously these seemingly outlandish illness narratives that somehow shaped the development and reception of the smallpox vaccine. It has prepared us also for the strange new close readings that will follow in this book. Moving beyond the story of biopolitics necessarily defamiliarizes these influential authors; it means approaching Dr. Edward Jenner's immunological discovery not just with our neoliberal "trust the science" mantra about vaccines, but also with open ears to Wordsworth's rustic alternatives of human flourishing, Darwin's biological stories of interpenetrating life, Blake's irrational reimagining of health, Keats's poetic turn from his medical training, and Shelley's privileging of local vignettes of sickness and suffering even in the face of a global plague. These Romantic-era illness narratives mattered in a way that we are only just beginning to rediscover as we slowly emerge out of our COVID-19 lockdowns.

Beyond Jenner

In the spirit of restoring the genre of the illness narrative to medical history, I begin with an illustrative anecdote. A peripatetic man rambles through the English countryside to collect rustic stories and shape them into a radical new experiment. After the 1798 publication of the first edition, the critics are ruthless, but national fame closely trails these rural footsteps, and this man's likeness eventually finds a way into the hall of Room 18, "Art, Invention & Thought: The Romantics," on the second floor of London's National Portrait Gallery. This setup's punchline is that this man describes not just the celebrated British poet laureate William Wordsworth, but also Edward Jenner (figure 1), the country physician whose rustic experiments with smallpox vaccination inaugurated an entirely new era of modern preventive medicine. Almost two hundred years after the publication of his *Inquiry into the Causes and Effects of the Variolæ Vaccinæ, Or Cow-Pox* (1798), the World Health Organization would triumphantly declare the scourge of smallpox eradicated. The virulent disease that had decimated entire civilizations in the Americas and had permeated into the political and cultural fabric of eighteenth-century Europe was finally no more.

By featuring Wordsworth's *Lyrical Ballads* (1798) and Jenner's *Inquiry* (1798) together, I argue in this book that smallpox vaccination was as much a triumph of the Romantic literary imagination as it was an achievement of medical science. A larger disciplinary question underlies this perhaps startling claim: Who counts as a producer of medical and scientific knowledge? How could Wordsworth, Erasmus Darwin, William Blake, John Keats, or Mary Shelley contribute anything to the advent of preventive medicine? This study uncovers the surprising literary history of vaccination, which includes poetry and imaginative fiction in the research, discovery, and publicity of Jenner's controversial breakthrough. Most literary critics would exclude Jenner from quintessential Romantic debates about revolutionary politics, the imagination, human perfectibility, utopian schemes, and institutional reform. And most historians of medicine would extract vaccination from its literary historical context to transform it into an exceptional discovery that somehow transcended its Romantic counter-Enlightenment milieu. Vaccination, in this view, was an Enlightenment diamond in the rough, an unlikely success that rose above the era's backwards culture of medical quackery. Instead, *The Smallpox Report* will insist that it was *because* of the pre-disciplinary Romantic culture of medicine that vaccination was even possible to imagine and implement.

Biographies of Jenner tend to take a different, more triumphal tack. Jenner's early tutelage under the most famous surgeon of the day, John Hunter, shapes a convenient origin story of the medical hero as a young man. He was twenty-one years old and already the house pupil of a pre-eminent surgeon, on track to become one of the greatest figureheads in a long line of modern physicians. In John Baron's 1827 biography of Jenner, this tone of hero worship is hard to miss:

If we look at the origin of this discovery from its first dawning in his youthful mind at Sodbury, and trace it through its subsequent stages – his meditations at Berkeley – his suggestions to his great master, John Hunter – his conferences with his professional brethren in the country – his hopes and fears, as his inquiries and experiments

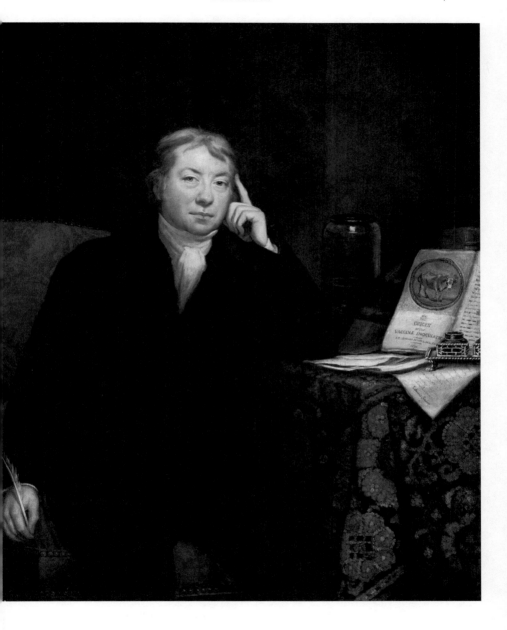

Figure 1. "Edward Jenner" by James Northcote. 1803. © National Portrait Gallery, London.

encouraged or depressed his anticipations – and, at length, the triumphant conclusion of more than thirty years' reflection and study, by the successful vaccination of
his first patient, Phipps; we shall find a train of preparation never exceeded in any scientific enterprise; and in some degree commensurate with the great results by which
it has been followed. (315)

With the benefit of a few decades of hindsight, Baron weaves a tale of inexorable success in which a "youthful mind" carefully marshalled inspiration from a
"great master," intellectual connections to "professional brethren," and unmatched
"preparation" to vanquish the viral foe. Here, Jenner walks in the company of men
of science and men of consequence. At the urging of Hunter, for example, Jenner diligently hones his skills of observation by studying the egg-switching habits
of cuckoos. He debates inoculation procedures with professional clinicians like
Daniel Sutton and Thomas Dimsdale. In a satirical Cruikshank print from 1808
(figure 2), he appears as the "preserver of the Human Race," flanked by the medical authority of Dimsdale on his right and the political authority of George Rose
on his left. With his "professional" coterie in tow, he imperiously turns away the
charlatan inoculators who profit off the dying, pockmarked bodies strewn across
the page. This triumphal story of enlightened science over opportunistic quackery establishes Jenner's vaunted place in modern medical history and cements his
achievement as the work of an inimitable genius.

Such hero worship, however, is barely half the story. First, it is not entirely
accurate. During the 1990s, a bicentennial resurgence of interest in the *Inquiry*
sparked a robust debate about how much credit Jenner actually deserves. That
milkmaids were immune from *human* smallpox because of their handling of
*cow*pox-infected udders was already well-known folklore by the 1770s. And
the older form of inoculation (injecting smallpox instead of cowpox), known
as variolation, had been practised in England at least since Lady Mary Wortley
Montagu brought the idea to England from her Turkish travels in the early
eighteenth century. Thanks to Sutton and Dimsdale, variolation had achieved
an acceptable success rate by the 1790s. Even if the shift from variolation to
vaccination finally erased all risk of unintended infection, it was not the sea
change into something rich and strange that some biographers claim. On the
bicentennial of the successful vaccination of eight-year-old James Phipps, even
Jenner-booster Derrick Baxby admits: "Although probably not the first to try
the experiment, Jenner was the first to *report* it" (770; emphasis mine). *The
Smallpox Report* certainly does not claim to resolve the bicentennial debate
about credit; instead, it documents the complex set of medico-literary conditions for Jenner's smallpox "report." His accomplishment in the *Inquiry*
was less the work of a "professional" scientist or the profound musings of a
solitary genius and more the critically misunderstood success of a Romantic
medico-literary idiom.

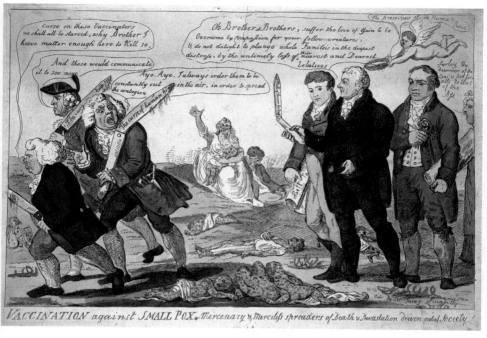

Figure 2. "VACCINATION against SMALL POX or Mercenary & Merciless spreaders of Death & Devastation driven out of society!" by Isaac Cruikshank, 1808. Credit: Wellcome Collection. Public Domain.

Second, the triumphal biographical story is not even a particularly useful fiction. It is typical Enlightenment fare: irrational outrage and hysterical distrust of a new medical procedure are gradually tamed by Reason's patient truth. Vaccination emerges as an inevitable product of the scientific method's teleology of self-correction. Jenner's lionization as the avatar of this Enlightenment science can only end in the unqualified success of biopolitical compulsion and the rational liberal state's benevolent control of immunized bodies. Plot holes, however, emerge immediately. First, smallpox was indeed eradicated in the late twentieth century, but stubborn outbreaks of vaccine-preventable diseases like measles and whooping cough continue to threaten public health. The story fails to explain the continuous history, from smallpox to COVID-19, of what Michael Specter has called "denialism" (*Denialism* 57–102), or the persistent privileging of misinformed patient agency (e.g., vaccine refusal) over established medical authority. Second, the story critically underestimates other Romantic-era medical practices as mere quackery or what Hermione de Almeida refers to as "a hiatus in the history of medicine" (3) even though vaccination emerged from Jenner's participation in that supposedly irrational medical culture. Third, it anachronistically separates Romantic literary production from the history of medicine despite the era's largely pre-disciplinary organization of knowledge. These plot holes have kept the epistemological impasse on the divided Cruikshank page strikingly contemporary. On the one hand are the scarred victims, willing dupes of the old inoculators who peddle their quack cures; on the other hand, are Jenner, Dimsdale, and Rose, wagging their fingers at the unschooled masses. The biographical fiction elects an unaccountable medical elite to arbitrate the common, biopolitical good. No wonder, then, that vaccine refusal has survived into our current age of quarantine and misinformed quackery.

If centring the discovery of vaccination on Jenner is neither entirely true nor particularly useful, what other kinds of stories can be told? Roy Porter's seminal work has pioneered what he calls "doing medical history from below" ("The Patient's View" 175), deliberately recalling what E.P. Thompson did when he reoriented history away from "great men" and towards the continuing struggles of the working class. Fortunately for this study, much of the historical heavy lifting has already been done by bottom-up medical historians like Porter and Mary Fissell. This people's history of health and suffering offers an alternate route for the "the ghost train speeding down the old Whiggish mainline from magic to medicine" ("The Patient's View" 194). No longer must that train make obligatory stops to canonize Jenners along the way. These histories consider instead the social formation of treatment, the shared idioms of medical knowledge, and the significance of lay and folk medicine. Such analysis skews the vaccination archive towards the literary, to the unusual slipperiness of Baxby's heterogeneous smallpox "report." Romantic and Romanticist Paul Youngquist comes closest to capturing that literary texture of knowledge production in his recent engagement with Jamaica's Maroon community:

> Ambient knowledge isn't just *there* like some dusty tome on a bookshelf. It *occurs* as the effect of immersive encounters and exchanges. It *happens* – and it happens to and through you. Errancy names the accidental itinerary comprising your encounters with others, relations – however fleeting – that spark knowledge in the field. ("Accidental Histories" 221)

Speaking of twenty-first-century "encounters and exchanges" in his own humanities fieldwork, Youngquist nevertheless captures the Romantic qualities of Wordsworth and Jenner's "accidental itinerary." The subject of *The Smallpox Report* is the "ambient knowledge" – so pregnant in the Romantic air – that sparked a literary and medical movement.

Argument and method in hand, what is left is just to give a brief disclaimer about what this book is *not*. It is not a corrective attempt at a Jenner biography. Indeed, past part one on "Classification" and the biopolitics of the case study,

Jenner necessarily fades into the background of the medico-literary genres of Romantic "ambient knowledge." It is not about identifying literary metaphors for smallpox. David Shuttleton's book *Smallpox and the Literary Imagination, 1660–1820* ably serves that purpose as a comprehensive reference for that fascinating history of the long eighteenth century as "a crucial era of intensified literary representation" (1). It is also not about cataloguing smallpox or vaccination references in literature. This would demand a kind of distant reading practice to mine the publication data and chart the prevalence of confluent pustules, eyes blinded by scar tissue, congenital infections, and miraculous recoveries. It would privilege, for example, the diligent recovery of obscure Regency novels of fashion such as Elizabeth Meeke's *Conscience* (1814) merely for its first-volume smallpox plot that Meeke largely forgets about in volumes two through four.[4] It is not, in short, a study of how literature imports the independent, larger workings of medical science into its narratives and fictive contrivances; rather, this book documents how Romantic literature *is* medical science. Illness narratives shaped the unique cultural moments that made vaccination possible to imagine, implement, and report. Inoculators like Jenner, Sutton, and Dimsdale were certainly not confined to an Enlightenment bubble. Their work appears in the literary record inscribed in a strange, lost, and pre-disciplinary language. Ultimately, this book is a labour of translation that makes legible the Romantic medico-literary idiom that eventually eradicated smallpox.

The Case of Jenner

Translation means defamiliarizing modern medical genres like the case study. Jenner's *Inquiry*, a late eighteenth-century collection of cowpox cases, is scarcely legible by twenty-first-century medical standards. In the submission guidelines to the contemporary *Journal of Medical Case Reports*, the editorial board emphasizes strict generic parameters, dividing the successful article into two ostensibly complementary sections: the "case presentation" and the "discussion." The former "should include a description of the patient's relevant demographic details, medical history, symptoms and signs, treatment or intervention, outcomes, and any other significant details" and the latter "should discuss the relevant existing literature and should state clearly the main conclusions, including an explanation of their relevance or importance to the field" (Kidd). The case presentation emphasizes the un- or under-reported, the unexpected, the unusual, and indeed the novel. The discussion then absorbs the novel exception into the medical rule.

What does this look like in practice? One of the journal's more popular articles could easily headline a novelty-obsessed tabloid, albeit with a much cruder title than "Pyosalpinx as a sequela of labial fusion in a post-menopausal woman" (Tsianos et al. 1). The article guardedly yet at the same time pruriently speculates on the sexual cause of a post-menopausal woman's labial fusion. The tone immediately turns the medical case legal: "[The 78-year-old Caucasian Greek post-menopausal woman] had been a widow for over 20 years, and *claimed* to have had no sexual relationships since her husband's death" (1; emphasis mine). To her medico-legal prosecutors, the patient is a potentially unreliable witness to her own body. After all, a woman widowed in her fifties and now pushing eighty could not possibly have *claimed* chastity. The remainder of the article reads like a detective story that polices healthful norms, using bodily signifiers as a kind of scientific justification for sexual conformity. The subtext is persistent interrogation: Is it *normal* for a woman to have abstained from sex for over twenty years after her husband died? Is the patient's labial fusion essentially her body's way of saying "use it or lose it"? By the end, the article masks its prurient interest in the case's sexual novelty. Rather than outright sensationalism, it nominally stresses objectivity, consent, and the greater good packaged into a fastidiously managed negotiation between the prying physicians and the compliant patient. The genre of the modern case study, in short, diligently contains its fascination while either ignoring or invalidating the first-person illness narrative. However, its structural tension between the case presentation's irresistible novelty and the discussion's bent towards the objective good never exactly goes away.

Meanwhile, in the early eighteenth century, prurient interest had no use for the cover of medical objectivity. In 1723, Jonathan Bliss, an American physician most likely from Massachusetts, records in a manuscript notebook of case studies his giddy observations about an unusual patient:

> John de Laurier … of Poitou, about threescore years of age, ask'd my advise concerning a gonorrhea, which he had for some months, accompanied with a heavy pain in the loyns. Upon examination of the case, I found by many signs that there was no virulency, but only a mischief contracted by the more violent use of venery, which had wekened the seminary vessels. Wherefore I prescribed him a diet moderately heating & drying, meats of good juice and quick nourishment, to drink unmixed wine moderately and to take some other corroborating and nourishing things. (Bliss)

This "case" of gonorrhea, it turns out, is not even gonorrhea. Bliss nevertheless includes this digression from his subject for mere venereal "mischief." Indeed, other than an entertaining character study of an oversexed, sexagenarian Frenchman, this has little to do with either the presentation or treatment of gonorrhea. The prescription is an extemporaneous afterthought – essentially moderation in all things – because his true interest lies in the case's unburnished novelty. Treatment in Augustan medicine, according to Roy Porter, could not offer much more than that: "in those days before 'scientific medicine' medical know-how was an idiom broadly shared by doctors and patients rather than constituting the kind of esoteric technical monopoly which guarantees professional dominance" (*Bodies Politic* 151). Bliss makes no attempt to discuss the case's "relevance or importance

to the field" or to integrate the story into the "esoteric technical monopoly." Medicine, Porter goes on to argue, was instead a form of mutual storytelling: physicians were self-fashioning themselves into polite gentleman, and patients were
just as involved as their doctors in planning out their own treatment. Rather
than a genre that always veers to the standard, the normal, and the objective,
the eighteenth-century case study made do without the bell curve, demographic
science, and data-driven analysis.

Modern medical professionalism had to wait until at least the beginning of the
nineteenth century. Published in 1803, Thomas Percival's *Medical Ethics* provided
the groundwork not only for the modern case study, but also for the practice of
modern medicine itself. For Percival, the genre of the case study pits an irrational
and unreliable patient against the paternal care of the scholarly physician. In a
startling analogy, a physician, according to Percival, should be to his patient as a
plantation manager is to his slaves:

> Theoretical discussions should be generally avoided: This rule is not only applicable
> to consultations, but to any reasonings on the nature of the case, and of the remedies
> prescribed, either with the patient himself or his friends. It is said by my lamented
> friend Mr. Seward, in his entertaining anecdotes, that the late Lord Mansfield gave
> this advice to a military gentleman, who was appointed governor of one of our islands
> in the West-Indies, and who expressed his apprehensions of not being able to dis-
> charge his duty as chancellor of his province. "When you decide, never give reasons
> for your decision. You will in general decide well; yet may give very bad reasons for
> your judgment." (169)

The patient has no hope to understand the physician's "theoretical discussions";
all that is required is a unilateral "decision." Once a military governor in the West
Indies explains the economics of labour exploitation, for example, there might be
some trouble on the plantation. The advice, then, is to manage and delimit the
patient's participation in every aspect of the case. Here emerges that structural tension in the genre of the modern case study. On the one hand, Percival would still
like to preserve Bliss's unfettered delight in caricaturing French sexual excess, but
on the other hand, that novelty must find its place within a decisive and exclusive
medical archive.

The language of Romantic-era medicine is the exciting historical testing ground
for this still unresolved generic tension between novelty and objectivity. Undoubtedly, one of the most successful results of this transitional moment in the history
of medicine is vaccination. At the peak of smallpox mortality in 1760s London,
the virus was responsible for 6 to 10 per cent of all burials and 35 per cent of
infant mortalities. And perhaps as much as half the adult population bore the disfiguring scars of the disease. Even if by the *late* eighteenth century, variolation had
strengthened herd immunity, vaccination would finally make eradication more

than a pipe dream. By the early 1800s, smallpox mortality rates had plunged, and the disease was on its way to being demoted to a mere "minor cause of death" (Davenport et al. 188). The *Inquiry*, written as a series of crude, unpolished case studies, just could not wait for Percival's ethical rules and generic standards.

Jenner's text details the names, circumstances, and stories of cowpox-infected rustics like the milkmaid Sarah Nelmes (Case XVI). An illustration of her cowpox infection (figure 3) features a large pustule on her hand and two small ones on her wrist that, according to Jenner's leisurely narrative, resulted from an infected "scratch from a thorn" during her daily labours (31). The small pustule on the index finger, however, belongs to no one. Jenner offers that smaller pustule as a point of abstract comparison between early- and late-stage infections. In this single image, the *Inquiry* marks its transitional moment in history. Jenner demonstrates both a willingness to hear the novel stories of milkmaids like Sarah Nelmes as well as a pressing need to catalogue data into a universal medical narrative or Porter's "esoteric technical monopoly" (*Bodies Politic* 151). As we would now put it, "case presentation" is already drifting into conclusive "discussion," but without either Bliss's early resolution to stay with novelty or Percival's later determination of the greater medical good. The *Inquiry* dwells in the ambivalent middle ground, between Nelmes's infected scratches and Jenner's fictitious, exemplary pustule.

Jenner was certainly not the only one working in this awkward idiom of the Romantic case. Wordsworth and Jenner, both publishing their seminal works in the same year, shared a rhetorical style. Wordsworth's lyrical balladeers canvass the countryside for rustic wisdom from curious and novel cases: an idiot boy, an old huntsman, a mad mother, and an aged beggar. Jenner, meanwhile, catalogues cases from dairymaids, servants, and gardeners to track the spread of disease. Both authors present unusual case studies of rural English life while suspending immediate, irritable reaching after fact, reason, and objectivity. Wordsworth's speakers are generously indulgent: they let a little girl persist in her counting error in "We Are Seven," they allow Johnny Foy's non-sequiturs in "The Idiot Boy," and they even hold off on calling the cops on Martha Ray in "The Thorn" even though she may have killed her child in a fit of inconsolable madness. Each novel form of human flourishing is given time and space to make his or her case. Jenner, for example, arrives in the Gloucestershire countryside as an old-fashioned inoculator with the variolation needle in hand. Rather than intruding upon a backwards countryside with Percival's imperialist assurance that "You will in general decide well" (169), Jenner earnestly listens to milkmaids' cowpox stories. Wordsworth's urban speakers do not bluster into rural villages to teach little girls how to count or to offer idiot boys speech therapy. "We Are Seven" ends with the girl's still contradictory "Nay, we are seven!" (line 69). And "The Idiot Boy" ends with the sound of Johnny Foy's onomatopoetic nonsense couplet: "The cocks did crow to-whoo, to-whoo, / And the sun did shine so cold!" (lines 450–1). As with Jenner's composite image, though, Wordsworth embeds eruptive flashpoints of

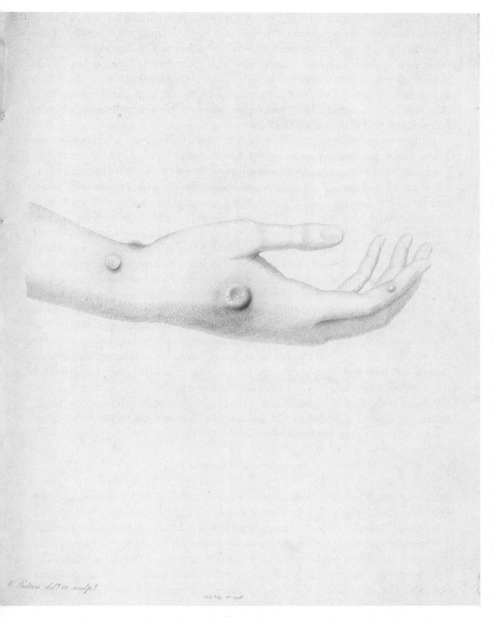

Figure 3. Illustration of the right hand of Sarah Nelmes, Case XVI in Edward Jenner's *Inquiry into the Causes and Effects of the Variolæ Vaccinæ, Or Cow-Pox*, 1798. Call # 335441, The Huntington Library, San Marino, California.

structural tension in the *Lyrical Ballads*. Looming in the background of all these genial conversations is the national project beyond the individual novelty of the case: demographic science or the census in "We Are Seven," social welfare in "The Idiot Boy," child services in "The Thorn," and elder care in "Simon Lee." Even though these marginal voices speak, Wordsworth struggles to translate them into a standard, national vocabulary, a new poetic vernacular of the common folk. Wordsworth's case study, like Jenner's, ultimately prefers to remain structurally inconclusive and ideologically flexible.

As they grew older into the nineteenth century, however, Wordsworth and Jenner began siding more conclusively with Percival's medical modernity as they joined the contested arena of national politics. The rustic Lake poet turned against his youthful radicalism, selling out to become the eleventh British poet laureate. Jenner, meanwhile, abandoned the Gloucestershire countryside for urban, state-sponsored fame. He became fiercely protective of his hard-won reputation, leaving behind the rustic wisdom of the natural world for the heated politics of public health. In an unpublished manuscript letter (figure 4), Jenner privately expresses outrage to his colleague William Clement about upstart vaccinator John Walker, who had refused to follow Jennerian principles and had threatened to start his own vaccination institute. This image is the third page of Jenner's four-page letter dated 19 December 1807. Jenner writes: "With respect to that Vulture Walker, I know not whether he is worth your Powder & Shot" (3). By the end of the same paragraph, he has changed his mind: "on second thought, you must not let Walker escape" (3). So crucial to Jenner are these retributive instructions that he carefully indents the lines on the page to avoid the common paper tear upon breaking the seal. He then folds the letter and reaches for the red wax (figure 5), the official colour of dead-serious business. Such insolence, Jenner concludes, warrants pinpoint punishment. In the end, he decides that proper vaccination procedure is no longer up for debate.

Inoculation as Biopower

From the wandering exploration of novelty to authoritarian retrenchment, the evolving generic form of Jenner's writing career tended towards the consolidation of biopower, or the institutional control and regulation of vulnerable bodies.[5] For inoculation, biopower's most visible consequence has been compulsory vaccination schemes for public servants, university faculty and staff, and students in public schools. Another illustrative and recent example would be the stay-at-home orders of the COVID-19 pandemic. I wrote this introduction in state-ordered lockdown after learning about the efforts to flatten the curve, to protect vulnerable populations, and to keep the virus's R_0 number low via social distancing and mask wearing. Biopower mobilizes these cogent forms of graphed data, demographic statistics, and epidemiological modelling to persuade from above. As my own etymological forty days of quarantine came and went with neither imminent sign of reprieve nor grumbles of protest, this was indeed a cogent strategy that worked on me. To some others, though, biopower inexorably retains the sinister stench of arbitrary authoritarianism. It intrudes upon private notions of the embodied self, and no amount of medical jargon will convince them. Consequently, the recent history of biopower has focused on apologizing to these naysayers for what seem like drastic measures. The pitch is quite simple: the common good tells us that needles are scary, dead or attenuated viruses are gross, and enforced isolation is inconvenient, but all are ultimately necessary.

Even the deeper history of biopower begins with an apology for its unsavory prescriptions. It is perhaps surprising that Jenner's *Inquiry* begins just this way. It inaugurates its vaccination advocacy with a disturbing vignette of bestial cross-contamination:

> The deviation of man from the state in which he was originally placed by nature seems to have proved to him a prolific source of diseases. From the love of splendour, from the indulgences of luxury, and from his fondness for amusement he has familiarised himself with a great number of animals, which may not originally have been intended for his associates. (1)

Civilization's initial deviation from the state of nature long ago, Jenner goes on to hypothesize, had encouraged diseases like horse "grease" (horsepox) to pass among cows and humans. Failing that impossible nostalgia for his prelapsarian Eden, however, Jenner shrewdly makes the best out of a bad situation. After recounting the mess of cross-species traffic, he finds a salubrious exception to the infectious rule:

> Thus the disease makes its progress from the horse to the nipple of the cow, and from the cow to the human subject. Morbid matter of various kinds, when absorbed into the system, may produce effects in some degree similar; but what renders the cow-pox virus so extremely singular is that the person who has been thus affected is forever secure from the infection of the small-pox; neither exposure to the variolous effluvia, nor the insertion of the matter into the skin, producing this distemper. (5–6)

Here, he scarcely masks his disgust; instead, he singles out the cowpox virus from "Morbid matter of various kinds" to an extraordinary outlier that somehow immunizes the human body rather than infecting it. The timidity of Jenner's ostensibly heroic argument feels deeply dissatisfying. Despite the "extremely singular" result, inoculation remains synonymous with filth, infection, and impurity while vaccination is quietly singled out as one of the good ones. In the following case studies, he eagerly links cowpox infection to a reconstructed Eden of unpolluted rustic, English simplicity in Gloucestershire, far away from the cross-species orgy of urban life. He argues for inoculation, in the end, by sheepishly apologizing for it.

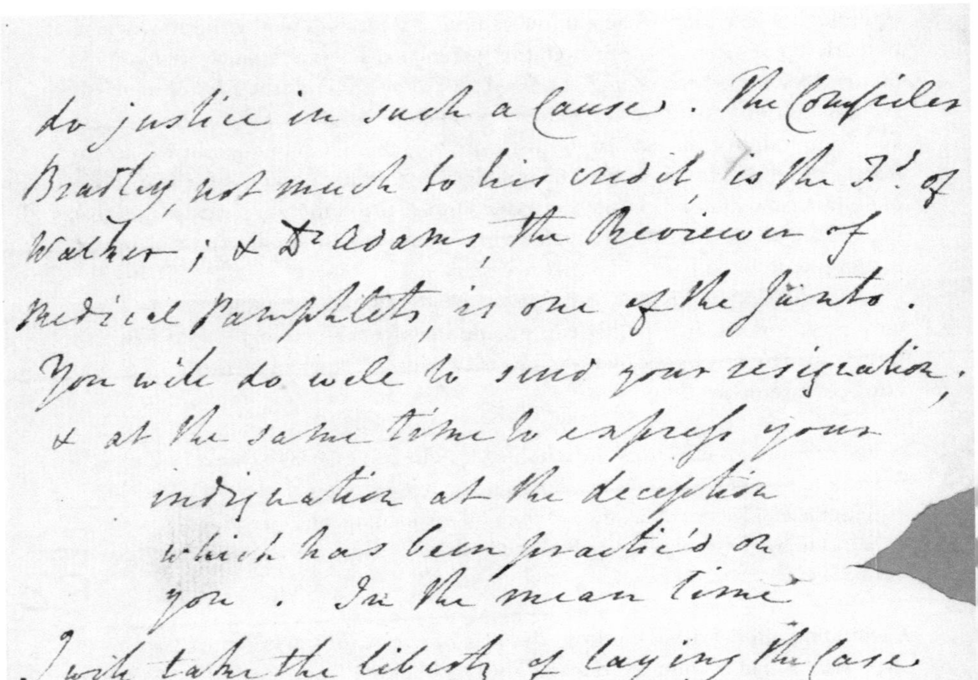

do justice in such a Cause. The Consider
Bratley, not much to his credit, is the Z.? of
Walker; & Dr. Adams, the Reviewer of
medical Pamphlets, is one of the Junto.
You will do well to send your resignation,
& at the same time to express your
indignation at the deception
which has been practic'd on
you. In the mean time
I will take the liberty of laying the Case
before my honest friend John Ring who
like yourself can boast of not having a
single Globule of neuter Blood in his
Body. I will request Ring to write
either to you or myself on the subject.
In justice to the public, on second thoughts
you must not let Walker escape.

Figure 4. Edward Jenner letter to William Clement, page three of four, 19 December 1807. Call # mssHM 74097, The Huntington Library, San Marino, California.

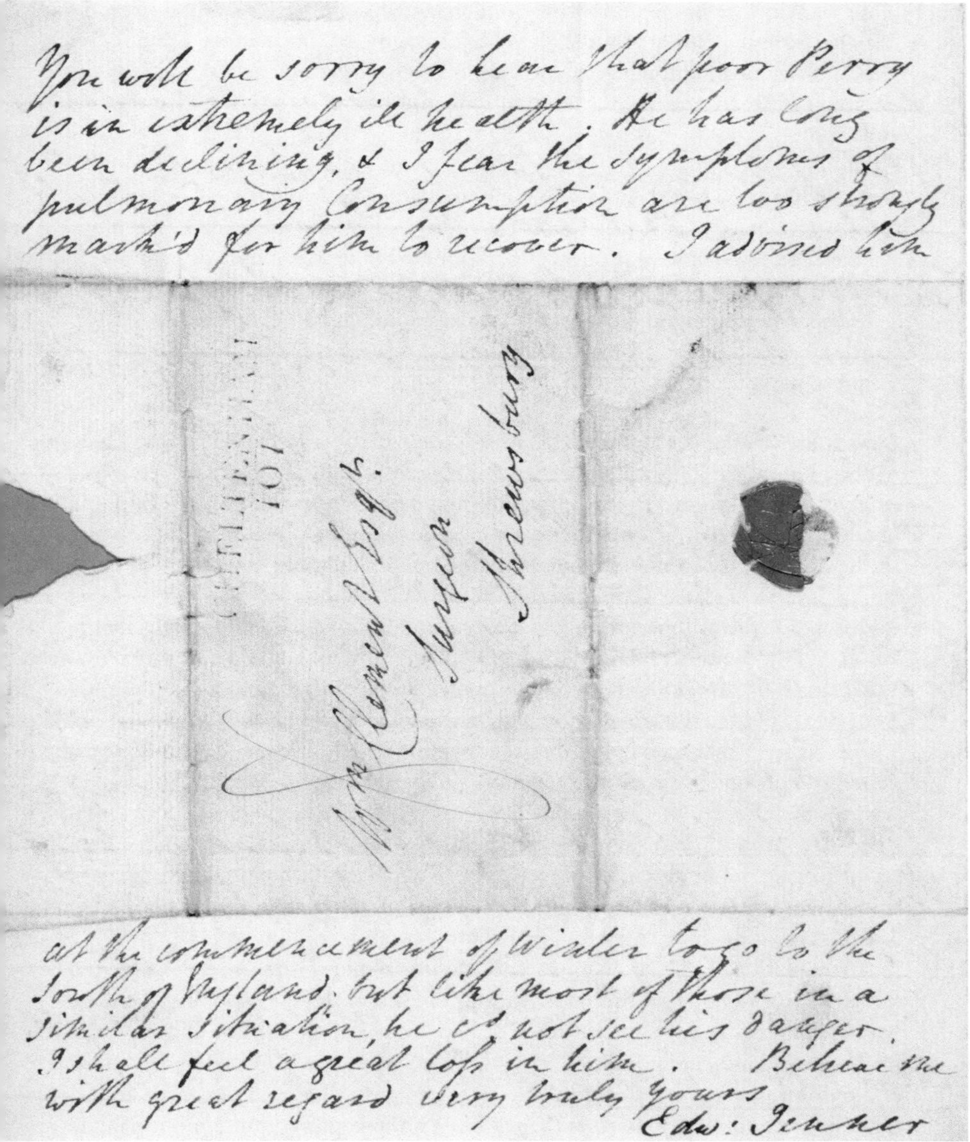

You will be sorry to hear that poor Perry
is in extremely ill health. He has long
been declining, & I fear the symptoms of
pulmonary Consumption are too strongly
mark'd for him to recover. I advised him

CHELTENHAM
107

Wm Clement Esqr.
Surgeon
Shrewsbury

at the commencement of Winter to go to the
South of England. but like most of those in a
similar situation, he cd. not see his danger.
I shall feel a great loss in him. Believe me
with great regard very truly Yours
Edw: Jenner

Figure 5. Edward Jenner letter to William Clement, page four of four, 19 December 1807.
Call # mssHM 74097, The Huntington Library, San Marino, California.

To be fair, this strategy is entirely understandable. Just a few years before the *Inquiry*, Edmund Burke was already using the figure of inoculation to signify his visceral discomfort at unchecked radicalism. In his *Reflections on the Revolution in France* (1790), he equates inoculation with full-blown infection and unnatural violation:

> We wished at the period of the Revolution, and do now wish, to derive all we possess as an *inheritance from our forefathers*. Upon that body and stock of inheritance we have taken care not to inoculate any cyon alien to the nature of the original plant. All the reformations we have hitherto made, have proceeded upon the principle of reference to antiquity; and I hope, nay I am persuaded, that all those which possibly may be made hereafter will be carefully formed upon analogical precedent, authority, and example. (Burke 181)

Burke's use of the word "inoculate" here is a bit tricky and requires some explanation. Before the publication of Jenner's *Inquiry*, "inoculate" largely preserved its etymological origin (*in-* meaning "in" and *oculus* meaning "eye" or "bud") in botanical nomenclature. Our usage, however, does not usually distinguish between Burke's botanical inoculation and Jenner's viral vaccination; the words are now largely interchangeable, both referring to the controlled exposure of a host body to disease for the purpose of immunization. In the Romantic era, though, inoculation and vaccination remained distinct with a profoundly ontological difference. Vaccination (from the Latin *vacca* for cow) is a type of inoculation that develops from cross-species experimentation with cowpox matter whereas inoculation itself is a broad term that merely signifies the "engrafting" (Montagu, *Turkish Embassy Letters* 81) of some form of matter onto a biological substrate. In this telling passage, Burke chooses the word "inoculate" to evoke a rhetoric of contamination that weaponizes a botanical metaphor against the taint of revolution upon a society of magisterial inheritance. Jenner strategically hides in the practised safety of this kind of reactionary rhetoric and tries to construct a postlapsarian Eden free of any impure "cyon alien to the original plant."

If inoculation is just about this trend towards biopower, the questions we can ask about Romantic-era disease remain quite limited. In the biopolitical framework, it is life at all costs or else death. An apologetic biopower can only conceive of disease as an acute condition, a brief way station back to either the comic ending of a normatively healthful life or the tragedy of a final death. Its fearful argument economically narrows the categories of recognized human flourishing. This false dilemma of life and death sometimes binds our topics of study. Medical historians and literary critics of the period, for example, have leaned heavily on this story of biopower. The Romantic body polarizes into biopolitical questions of salvaged life and inevitable death, while sometimes ignoring the untidy middle categories of disease, impairment, and disability; studies of Romantic medicine, in other words, have focused more on topics like vitalism and materialism and less on the lived condition of a disease like smallpox.[6] Though the Romantic theorizers of disease failed to reproduce the enthralling spectacle of the life-and-death vitality debates between William Lawrence and John Abernethy, Hermione de Almeida reminds us that the period still engendered prolific and "unbounded speculation on the character and progress of disease" (139). On the continent, Friedrich Schiller, Friedrich Wilhelm Joseph Schelling, Friedrich Schlegel, and Xavier Bichat all characterized disease as another vital principle – even a precondition for organic life. British theories even started classifying diseases according to Linnaean taxonomies (William Cullen's 1772 work *Nosology; or, A Systematic Arrangement of Diseases by Classes, Orders, Genera, and Species*) and speculating about the body's natural and perpetual state of disease (see John Brown's theory of "excitability").[7]

But biopower's drive towards prescriptive efficiency can hardly afford to think of disease as natural, perpetual, or chronic. It convinces by offering long-term gains in normative health and longevity in exchange for restrictive pain in the short term. Disease is only ever something to be healed rather than managed.[8] The occupation of the medically informed poet, then, has been described consistently as a healer of social ills, of unhealthy colonial environments, and of the diseased body politic. For example, de Almeida assigns Keats the "poetic task as a physician who would heal the sorrows of mankind" (307), Christopher Moylan reads Thomas Lovell Beddoes's drama as "therapeutic theater" (181), Allard describes Thelwall's project to "'heal' the nation at the expense of his own political agenda" (74), Bewell unpacks the logic of Percy Shelley's social "cure [for disease-bearing environments]" (*Colonial Disease* 215) as a recovery of reason and nature, and Gigante focuses her discussion of vitality on "*Naturheilkraft* (natural healing power)" (38). In this ameliorative language of healing, Romantic disease should always reflect Burke's disgust at the inoculated "cyon alien to the nature of the original plant." The stories of these powerful and influential "healer" narratives schedule disease as acute exceptions to normative health. But for many in the eighteenth century, such as Jonathan Bliss's patient John de Laurier, disease was a way of life and prescriptive cures offered little more than empty platitudes.

A Burkean history of inoculation justifies this large body of work on the high-stakes vitality debates and the Romantic poetry of healing, but perhaps more importantly, it has solidified the dominant historical narrative of inoculation as biopower. Michel Foucault's famously imperious proclamation marks this epistemic shift in *The Birth of the Clinic* (1963, trans. 1973): "The age of Bichat has arrived" (*Clinic* 122). In other words, biopower finally triumphs from above. We have digested, internalized, and even axiomatized Foucault's familiar and gripping story of medico-administrative coercion and the socially constructed biopolitical authority of the medical gaze. At the centre of this narrative is Bichat's *Œuvres Chirurgicales de Desault* (1798–9), an anatomical encyclopedia that inaugurates the conception of the modern surgeon and his oppressive gaze. Foucault ominously conflates the history of medicine with this narrowing history of biopolitics. His seminal account of institutionalized biopower leaves little room for patient narratives or literary histories of inoculation. The Foucauldian history must remain untouched by the contributions of medical women, amateur physicians, and the rural poor even if inoculation begins with Montagu's tentative construction of female authority and Jenner's humble origins in rural medicine. The year 1798 *is* a kind of *annus mirabilis* but not just because it trumpets the arrival of Foucault's "age of Bichat"; the year also marks the publications of Jenner's *Inquiry* and Wordsworth and Coleridge's *Lyrical Ballads*. Although it would be glib and inaccurate to substitute "the age of Jenner" or "the age of Wordsworth" for Foucault's proclamation, the literary history of Romantic inoculation, of patient narratives defiantly staring back at the medical gaze, should at least be equally compelling.

The story of inoculation as biopower, however, is enduring for a reason. Jenner's career, for example, faithfully reproduces Foucault's seemingly irresistible biopolitical thesis. Even without reference to Foucault, Tim Fulford and Debbie Lee have tracked this biographical line from his roots as a rural physician, to his sycophantic bid for royal and aristocratic patronage, and finally to his crowning as a national and militaristic hero. They open with quite a Romantic picture of Jenner:

> Jenner's *Inquiry* was beautiful in its simplicity. It was not rooted in visions of national and international conquest of disease, but in the bodies of those who worked in the English countryside. It was not about global politics but about rural health. It was not derived from scientific authorities but from the oral tradition of Gloucestershire villagers. (139)

This rustic "simplicity" must recall the poetic project of Wordsworth and Coleridge, and Fulford and Lee do not disappoint: they track a familiar Romantic path of conservative retrenchment through the rocky reception of the *Lyrical Ballads*, reminding us along the way that both poets eventually abandoned the rural poor for aristocratic patronage and appeal. They claim that, like Wordsworth and Coleridge, "Jenner never won the hearts of Britain's labouring classes – ironically enough since it was with rural laborers that he had begun" (162). That irony proves almost as irresistible as Foucault's account of Bichat. It powers the familiar beats of biopolitical history, from Robert Bloomfield's, Robert Southey's, and Coleridge's poetic propaganda campaigns to publicize Jenner's discovery, to Victorian vaccination protests, and to the state-controlled institutionalization of vaccination in 1908. In tracking these afterlives of Jenner, Fulford and Lee leave behind the "bodies of those who worked in the English countryside" and the "oral tradition of Gloucestershire villagers" (139).

What remains is the ontological "vaccination anxiety" (Fulford and Lee 144–6) that followed Jenner's slippage from mere inoculation to cross-species vaccination.[9] His outrageous proposal that bovine matter was in some way compatible with – and even salutary for – the human body generated a vocal disgust that associated vaccination with bestiality and sexual perversity. Cowpox inoculation threatened both religious and secular notions of the human in its challenge to the Christian metaphor of "an ordered great chain of being" and to Linnaean classificatory systems. Criticism from both the religious orthodoxy and from prominent surgeons and scientists made it necessary for Jenner to embark upon an authoritarian campaign for legitimacy. This dampening of a potentially radical and blasphemous rhetoric is a story that has been told and retold, but *The Smallpox Report* lingers with its literary amplification; the troubled history from inoculation to vaccination extends much further than Jenner's shrewd navigation of dangerous political waters. Michael Specter, for example, reminds us of the enduring "irrational thought and frank denialism" (*Denialism* 6) of contemporary anti-vaccination campaigns. Even though it has saved millions of lives and completely eradicated several pernicious diseases like smallpox and Rinderpest (cattle plague), vaccination still serves as a convenient scapegoat for increased incidences of, to name just a few, diabetes, eczema, asthma, and, most notoriously in Andrew Wakefield's now discredited 1998 *Lancet* study, autism.[10] The COVID-19 vaccines have been falsely linked to magnetism, sterility, and even Bill Gates. The story of Jenner's conservative retrenchment and subsequent elevation to national hero fails to explain the persistent radical kernel in this revolutionary but stubbornly controversial medical breakthrough.

James Gillray, the Regency period's most notorious caricaturist, gives us a striking visual representation of this bifurcated history of Romantic inoculation (figure 6). Jenner, seen cutting into the seated woman's arm, administers his miracle cure while the vaccinated patients on the right deal with some unexpected side effects. Jenner's stiff, supercilious figure provides a visual fulcrum that unevenly divides the image into smallpox victims on the left and patients sprouting bovine appendages on the right. Gillray's satire, at first blush, seems entirely legible. The visual weight of the right half overwhelms the left, and we quickly conclude that the grotesque side effects far outweigh the potential benefits of the vaccine. Fulford and Lee come precisely to that conclusion as they direct their focus to the "wild orgy of transformation": "The cartoon finds a graphic language to articulate widely shared anxieties about the power of new science in the hands of an increasingly assertive medical profession" (144). Gillray surely criticizes the seemingly outlandish idea of vaccination (hence the cartoon's advertised connection to the "Anti-Vaccine Society"), but it also depicts a long queue of desperate smallpox sufferers in the vanishing horizon of the partially out-of-frame doorway, unbalancing the overtly negative critique with a solemn and positive plea for effective treatment. Mike Jay insists that Gillray's "point was not that vaccination was a quack remedy, a folly, or a scam: it was rather that its acceptance into mainstream medical practice did nothing to expunge the underlying grotesqueness of the proposition" (233). Just as Jenner's supercilious air as the "assertive" medical professional begins to

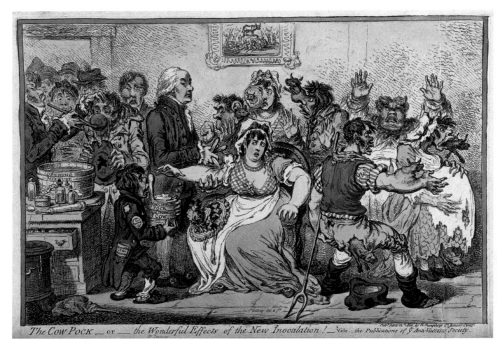

Figure 6. "The Cow-Pock-or-the Wonderful Effects of the New Inoculation" by James Gillray, 1802. Credit: Wellcome Collection. Public Domain.

authorize biopower, a subversive "underlying grotesqueness" persists beyond the biopolitical age of Bichat. The two halves of the image tell two very different stories: on the left is the quiet authority of Jenner and his patient queue of docile bodies, and on the right is the loud, anxious, paranoid, eruptive caricature of inoculation. Any inclusive literary history of inoculation must balance disgust at the cross-species "orgy" on the right with the vast scale of human suffering on the left.

Inoculation as Narrative

Gillray's caricature typified the outraged hysterics of the initial reaction: the country doctor had overreached his station, and his contaminating participation in both the working-class scene of infection on the left and the base, farcical suffering on the right had undercut his portrait's supercilious air of aristocratic professionalism. The grand potential of smallpox eradication did little to assuage patients' prejudicial doubts about a miracle cure gleaned from lowly milkmaid lore. Jenner's medical credentials, impressive as they were, failed to pass muster for a British public that was alternately terrified by the possibility of infection and scandalized by the shameful impropriety of the proposed cross-species cure. Despite his prestigious medical training under John Hunter, Jenner's later decision to return to his native Gloucestershire to practice rural medicine (a move that biographers have attributed to the inherent indolence that shadowed his genius) left him particularly vulnerable to his critics' accusations of amateurish speculation. So, he eventually abandoned his reputation as a competent country doctor as the vaccination controversies swiftly transformed him into a national health advocate. Later, through propaganda campaigns, Jenner became the national hero that we now know, and any erstwhile hint of embarrassment vanished. The triumphal trajectory from zero to hero, as I have already suggested, neglects the explosive and stubborn resistances to vaccination that persist to this day. Compulsory vaccination should have been a reasonable, winning argument for biopower, but it also turned out to be one of its most successful and vocal counterarguments. In this way, vaccination induces the opposite poles of biopolitics: on the one hand, it signals the emergence and legitimization of the state's control over the human body, and on the other hand, it gives rise to a paranoid hermeneutics of health.[11] Romantic medicine, it seems, is much more than a brief eruption of radical experimentalism quickly contained by vaccination's abrupt and unprecedented success in bringing about an enlightened biopolitics.

The familiar story of inoculation as biopower must label Romantic medicine a brief embarrassment in its Whiggish history of Enlightenment science, progress, and rationality. Even de Almeida begins her study of Romantic medicine and John Keats with that sombre disclaimer about Romantic medicine as "a hiatus in the history of science" (3).[12] This, of course, is not the narrative that has survived. Our own contemporary relationship to vaccination remains as vexed as the centuries old Gillray image. Whenever a new vaccine is introduced – most famously with H1N1 and now with the COVID-19 vaccines – the public discourse predictably fixates on the same two concerns: the potential scarcity of the vaccine and the safety of its administration. These concerns recapitulate the two halves of Gillray's portrayal of Jenner: we will clamour desperately for every last drop of vaccine (left) even as we loudly inflate its potential side effects (right). Even though vaccination has been institutionalized and legitimized, we still perceive something radically and ontologically dangerous in the two-hundred-year-old idea. Anti-vaccination campaigns continue to stir up images of grotesque contamination and anecdotal evidence of terrifying side effects to mobilize medical protest and to spread irrational disgust. These issues have only intensified in the globalized twenty-first century, and the biopolitical debates about the large-scale management of disease depend on our historical memory of the first vaccine scares and our attention to the patient narratives of those who lived through the alternatives of disfigurement, disease, and death. In substituting a medical and literary history of Romantic continuity for a history of epistemic shifts towards biopower, a narrative literary history of inoculation can finally start to surface.[13] Romanticism is no zany "hiatus" from either the history of medicine or from literary history; rather, it is an emblem of an embodied politics that has stubbornly survived its legacy of biopolitical revision.

Individual illness narratives, though, have struggled to break through. Even as governors instituted eminently reasonable stay-at-home orders because of the COVID-19 pandemic, thousands of protestors all over the United States mobilized to resist what they saw as the abuses of biopower. The biopolitical state and the individual patient are at an ideological impasse: the former can only flash the graphed abstraction of the CDC's flattened curve, and the latter can only push irrational conspiracy theories. In this polar view, we have thrown away or at least underestimated the potential explanatory power of the illness narrative. Take, for example, the recent media sensation of former CNN anchor Chris Cuomo's infection and slow recovery from COVID-19. His fraternal sparring with former New York governor Andrew Cuomo, his friendly and educational banter with CNN medical correspondent Sanjay Gupta, and his interview with the National Institute of Allergies and Infectious Diseases (NIAID) director Anthony Fauci all put an individual human face on the pandemic. Personal stories like this do as much as epidemiological statistics to explain the greater good. Individual patients need to be a bigger part of the biopolitical prescription, and, as it turns out, Romantic medicine offers a cogent historical model. *The Smallpox Report* moves beyond the biopolitical afterlife of Jenner to develop a deeper literary history that preserves the strange individual narratives of inoculation ever since Mary Montagu's *Turkish Embassy Letters* (1716, published posthumously in 1763). With this in mind, at least two inoculation stories are in sight now: (1) a Jennerian apology for inoculation as biopower, a lamentable but necessary contamination and (2) a more patient-centred history that integrates Romantic-era literary experimentation with larger questions of public health. After briefly documenting the public policy failures of the first, *The Smallpox Report* moves on to detail the mostly untapped explanatory potential of the second.

In this way, *The Smallpox Report* uses literary history to address some of our most pressing contemporary anti-vaxxer concerns. I offer a few possible solutions in the conclusion of the book, but I would just like to flag the issue of audience early on here in the introduction. The anti-vaxxer movement tends to remain unmoved by any top-down, rational arguments. What my argument suggests is that the onus of change should not be on stubborn anti-vaxxers but on *us*, on how we have valued or devalued the illness narrative. In my view, the current dangerous level of medical denialism is a systemic issue that has been produced and nurtured by clinical and institutional medicine's gradual shift away from patient-centred care. Instead of dismissing medical denialism as mere noise against the industrial hum of professional medical progress, I suggest that we listen compassionately to its historical rhythms. I know from personal experience that it is difficult to value narratives that are clearly irrational, misinformed, and paranoid, but the Romantics successfully made the case for vaccination not by touting superior logic against conspiratorial dolts but by valuing the strangeness of how we talk about health. Repairing a systemic issue is not about convincing one person who may already be too entrenched, but instead is about rethinking the biopolitical conditions that fostered the medical denialism in the first place. At the core, anti-vaxxers have historically responded to two basic needs: (1) the need to be heard and (2) the need to be part of a community. Groups, like the recent the QAnon conspiracy, have targeted anti-vaxxers because they feel they are not heard and are cast out from the medical mainstream. The audience of my appeal, then, is not exactly the stubborn anti-vaxxer but those of us who are in positions to effect intellectual and institutional change. My recommendations, in the end, are about systemic, discursive reforms in modern medicine, about changing the ways that we talk about and value the illness narrative.

How, then, can we rediscover these subtle and elusive illness narratives? This new story of vaccination demands some backtracking through the old one, with a keen eye towards what Roy Porter has called the "patient's view" of medical history. But how far back do we need to go to find a medical culture of generative, interdisciplinary, and non-hierarchical exchange? And how do we sort out the good from the bad, the real medico-literary knowledge from conspiratorial nonsense? By the mid to late nineteenth century, the pro- and anti-vaccination battle lines had already been drawn, and patient narratives were already turning bad. The most outrageous and loudest reactions against smallpox vaccination have understandably been the most memorable. The anti-vaccinationist voices included Dr. B. Moseley's warnings about a humanity tainted by beastly diseases, Dr. William Rowley's gruesome image of the ox-faced boy, and Dr. Squirrel's reports about vaccination-related injuries and deaths.[14] In an 1856 issue of his *Household Words*, Charles Dickens cites an unnamed "surgeon" (Moseley) as a leader of the anti-vaccination charge:

> "Can any person," wrote one surgeon, in a book several times reprinted, "Can any person say what may be the consequences of introducing a *bestial* humour in the human frame, after a long lapse of years? Who knows, besides, what ideas may rise in the course of time, from a *brutal* fever having exacted its incongruous impressions on the brain? Who knows, also, but that the human character may undergo strange mutations from quadrupedan sympathy, and that some modern Pasiphaë may rival the fables of old." (Dickens 10, quoting Moseley)

Moral indignation, irrational disgust, and fanciful allusions to mythical bestiality govern Moseley's indignant appeal to medical caution. Dickens capitalizes on this loose logic to poke fun at the anti-vaccinators "who have no right to be remembered with the wise" (10) and to explain the intense controversy that the medical discovery had to endure. Under all the sensationalistic rhetoric, though, is a close interrogation of and reaction against the radically experimental culture of Romantic-era medicine. Moseley argues, as did many medical practitioners of the era, for an increasingly professional medicine that need not resort to strange bestial cures and untested decoctions.

The anti-vaccination movement had, of course, more sober warriors who emphasized the institutional dimension of the complaint. Alfred Russel Wallace, the eminent naturalist whose evolutionary theories eventually pushed Charles Darwin to publish his seminal *Origin of Species* (1859), inserted a long essay titled "Vaccination a Delusion – Its Penal Enforcement a Crime" (213–323) into his retrospective collection *The Wonderful Century: Its Successes and Its Failures* (1898). Beyond his own citation of Moseley, he musters up a much more "scientific" analysis that concludes – with "a statistical, and therefore a mathematical certainty" (vii) – that not only is vaccination not protective against smallpox, but also that its compulsory enforcement will "rank as the greatest and most pernicious failure of the [nineteenth] century" (vi). In Dickens's pro-vaccination satire of Moseley and in Wallace's anti-vaccination editorial, these late nineteenth-century authors based their appeals upon a superior sense of rationality, professionalism, empiricism, and even "mathematical certainty." The undisciplined experimentalism of early scientific trials had finally been honed into a proper method, largely free from error, quackery, and sensationalistic grandstanding. Any kind of patient's history within this nineteenth-century cult of pro- and anti-vaccination "mathematical certainty" would be entirely beside the point. At this point in the nineteenth century, biopower is already all too modern.

Foucault tells a similar tale from a cultural-anthropological standpoint in which the unbalanced ledger of medical signs and symptoms finally organizes itself into ironclad pathological certainty:

> … clinical experience sees a new space opening up before it: the tangible space of the body, which at the same time is that opaque mass in which secrets, invisible lesions, and the very mystery of origins lie hidden. The medicine of symptoms will gradually recede, until it finally disappears before the medicine of organs, sites, causes, before a clinic wholly ordered in accordance with pathological anatomy. (*Clinic* 122)

He traces a sudden retreat from readings of surface symptoms to a continuous medical gaze that penetrates the "very mystery of origins." Pathology takes over with its efficient linkages of cause and effect, of disease and cure. Bichat's anatomical work exemplifies for Foucault an age that had abandoned the subjective diagnoses of bedside medicine for the ostensibly more objective pathology of clinical medicine. The irrational, ambitious, amorphous, and unsuccessful diagnoses of early experimental medicine had been supplanted by the constant vigilance of a discursively constructed rationalism that hinged upon the rigid definitions of a closely policed system of medical signs. Enlightenment medicine, then, arrives at the "age of Bichat" precisely when pathology claims to have purged medical practice of both its erroneous diagnoses and its inefficient prognoses.

From a medical historical perspective, Porter even stakes the very idea of modernity in this epistemic shift when he triumphantly announces that "Modern times dawned with the nineteenth century" (*The Greatest Benefit* 304). Instead of dwelling on the disruptions of medical failures (unlike the extraordinary Enlightenment innovations in physics and chemistry, the medical research of the period yielded significantly fewer success stories), Porter immediately conscripts the discovery of vaccination into a smooth narrative of Enlightenment improvement that ends with the institutional "awakening to the view that health promotion was integral to a well-run state" (*The Greatest Benefit* 277). Porter's failures, though, need not lead us inexorably to the knotty "paradox of Enlightenment medical science – great expectations, disappointing results" (*The Greatest Benefit* 248).[15] Porter pushes swiftly through to later nineteenth-century standards of medical care; by then, he claims that "[Medicine] gained standing for being scientific, and ambitious medical men pressed to learn its procedures and speak its slogans" (*The Greatest Benefit* 305), a Foucauldian end but with a decidedly positive and optimistic historical spin. Moseley's questioning frame, despite its entertaining hysterics, signalled the emergence of a new medical science that valued scrutiny, scepticism, and professional certainty over the novelty of mere experiment. Enlightenment medicine ends with a nineteenth-century discourse of sanitation, proscriptive bioethics, and efficient treatment. These trumpeting pronouncements about the "age of Bichat" or the dawn of "Modern times" portray medicine blazing a singular path towards the birth of biopolitics and the "well-run state."[16] Whether pro- or anti-vaccination (Dickens or Wallace), or pro- or anti-biopolitics (Porter or Foucault), the later nineteenth-century represents medicine's receding into the horizon of the patient's view. What is left is only Foucault's "opaque mass" of medical secrets held behind the veil of state authority and the cloak of superior reason.

Our search continues backwards, then. Instead of Jenner's apologetic and sanitized treatment of inoculation, Mary Shelley's apocalyptic plague novel *The Last Man* (1826) sounds rougher and dirtier; she tarries with disgust and discomfort instead of abruptly fleeing to Edenic safety. Lionel Verney, the eponymous last man in the world, becomes immune to the plague because of his inoculating, diseased embrace of racial alterity:

I lowered my lamp, and saw a negro half clad, writhing under the agony of disease, while he held me with a convulsive grasp. With mixed horror and impatience I strove to disengage myself, and fell on the sufferer; he wound his naked festering arms round me, his face was close to mine, and his breath, death-laden, entered my vitals. For a moment I was overcome, my head was bowed by aching nausea; till, reflection returning, I sprung up, threw the wretch from me, and darting up the staircase, entered the chamber usually inhabited by my family. (*The Last Man* 336–7)

In this fictionalized patient history, there is no safe retreat to either Burke's "analogical precedent, authority, and example" or to Jenner's Edenic Gloucestershire. Verney can only flee in disordered panic from convulsion, horror, and nausea to a family that may already be dead. Whereas Jenner's instinct forces him to slide the "extremely singular" case of vaccination into a neatly generalized discussion of "analogical precedent," Shelley skips directly to speculative fiction with apocalyptic stakes. Set in the twenty-first century, the dire novel nevertheless depicts medical progress in the face of certain annihilation. In a strikingly casual aside, Verney compares the new threat with the old: "That the plague was not what is commonly called contagious, like the scarlet fever, or extinct small-pox, was proved" (*The Last Man* 231; emphasis mine). Shelley predicts, over a century-and-a-half in advance, the World Health Organization's declaration in 1980 of smallpox's official eradication (the last known case being found in Somalia in 1977). Surely, there is none of Jenner's rhetorical timidity here. The incredibly heterogeneous historical developments from variolation to vaccination demand much more than just Jenner and the familiar story of inoculation as biopower. In addition to Shelley's example, inoculation was variously used to model England's engagement with her expansive colonial network, to satirize the troubled domestic absorption of continental notions of reform and revolution, and to shape the changing medical accounts of the human body. In this way, the material and metaphorical deployments of Romantic inoculation traverse several orders of scale: from the physician's locally embodied, anatomical gaze to the politician's global management of empire. Fundamentally, Burke and Jenner feared the wide-ranging idea of inoculation, but there is also a competing Romantic literary history of inoculation entirely unafraid of and unapologetic about the subversive figure.

The Smallpox Report, therefore, lands squarely in the Romantic era for its illness narratives. This study depends not on the later, more familiar voices of the vaccination controversy – Moseley, Dickens, Wallace, Porter, and Foucault – but on earlier Romantic-era patients and storytellers. These earlier authors stare back at Foucault's medical gaze and trouble Porter's selective reading of vaccination's Enlightenment triumph. To understand Romantic medicine's strangeness, William Blake's physician, John Birch, is a good but maybe unlikely place to start. Early on, he advocated for fantastical and experimental electrical cures for menstrual issues, but later recanted with a conciliatory endorsement of experience over experiment. "We live in a capricious age," he laments, "an age that is fond of believing paradoxes, and of grasping at novelty. And this alone might account for the wonderful avidity with which the experiment [vaccination] was adopted" (Birch 34). Here, Dr. Birch associates the Romantic era with capriciousness, paradox, novelty, avidity, and experiment and longs instead for the advent of method, logic, and experience in medical practice. What exactly is this "capricious age" to which Birch alludes? And why do Dickens, Wallace, Foucault, and Porter hasten past this story and towards the more familiar narratives of, for example, Jenner's elevation to the status of national hero, to the consolidation of medical ethics, or to the professionalization of an increasingly pathological medicine? To pin down Birch's "capricious age" is to linger with the complex historical and literary contexts of vaccination. Birch, however, was in a hurry to become modern. He decided that he would rather push through his own degenerate age of Romantic medicine, skipping forward to a staunch anti-vaccination advocacy that depended not on affective disgust, but rather on measured response and rational appeal for medical oversight and experimental caution. Now, our contemporary vaccination debates frequently sound like mad scientists arguing against even madder anti-intellectual reactionaries who balk at real medical progress; but, as Birch's case demonstrates, Romantic medicine is something far less glamorous. It is neither Birch's derogatory assessment of an irresponsibly "capricious age" nor Porter's dramatic dawn of "Modern times" and rational professionalism; instead, it is a deeply conflictual and transitional medical culture that productively pits professional science against patient scepticism, resolved into a careful ecology of experimental theory and ethical practice.[17]

Romantic Disease Discourse

These Romantic illness narratives are sometimes full of Birch's caprice, paradox, and novelty, but I will shorthand these properties more generously as a Romantic disease discourse. I borrow Foucault's sense of the word "discourse" from the *Birth of the Clinic* to capitalize on its currency in the history of medicine. There, he famously defines the birth of the clinic as the ostensible closing off of medicine to the niggling semantics of discourse:

> The clinic – constantly praised for its empiricism, the modesty of its attention, and the care with which it silently lets things surface to the observing gaze without disturbing them with discourse – owes its real importance to the fact that it is a reorganization in depth, not only of medical discourse, but of the very possibility of a discourse about disease. (*Clinic* xix)

Of note here is that Foucault does not entirely foreclose the post-clinical "possibility of a discourse about disease." The clinic, Foucault's metonym for medical pathology, succeeds in foreclosing a "discourse about disease" only insofar as it reorganizes "in depth" the *visibility* of its discursiveness. COVID-19 protests will still happen, in this view, but the modern clinic will (or should) reorganize or reconceptualize any such resistance as hysterical nonsense, rendering it invisible, impotent, and illogical. Here, he carefully reworks the more lucid claim of his mentor, Georges Canguilhem, that the normalization in clinical pathology represents a "really naïve dream of regularity in the absence of rule" (Canguilhem 241). In other words, pathology authors its objective norm by carefully obscuring the very discourse that produced it. In effect, then, the "observing gaze" of modern medicine should only be minimally perturbed by destabilizing questions of subjective discourse.

Romantic medicine, as a "discourse about disease," is an altogether different story. This book explores three defining aspects of Romantic disease discourse. The first pertains to the era's peculiar culture of experiment. Birch called it a "capricious age" for a reason. For example, physician Thomas Beddoes and his oft-lampooned Pneumatic Institute brazenly applied nitrous oxide to various unrelated ailments, sexologist James Graham advertised the amazing health benefits of electromagnetic beds, and Jenner found his unlikely cure for smallpox in the udder of a cow. This experimental culture led to both blatant quackery and medical breakthrough. Yet the history of medicine has been quick to forget about the latter while almost exclusively focusing its attention on the often hilarious consequences of the former.[18] Even though the contemporary medical discourse of immunity and prevention has its roots in this boldly experimental method, Romantic medicine's experimental transgression and its unusually high tolerance for methodological error have rendered it particularly vulnerable to bioethical criticism. Surprisingly, though, this period also managed to produce two of the foundational texts of bioethics: from a literary perspective, Mary Shelley's *Frankenstein* (1818) helped to model an ethic of care to regulate the excesses of an overreaching science, and from a medical perspective, Thomas Percival's *Medical Ethics* pioneered efforts to codify professional conduct in medical practice. Paul Youngquist provides a useful historical account of what happens to the conception of the body given this volatile balancing act between a normative ethics and transgressive experiment: he argues that "monstrosity" (the non-normative body) simultaneously constructs and resists "the social project of proper embodiment in liberal society" (*Monstrosities* xxix). In other words, it constructs the regulatory notion of a "normal" body while, at the same time, offering transformative possibilities in the abnormal and the experimental. The modern medical discourse of eugenic purity and bodily defence had not yet begun to crystallize; instead, Romantic medicine made do with this dual sense of monstrosity and a remarkably porous disease discourse that could admit tweaking, error, correction, invasion, and contamination, all while carefully preventing medical practice from falling into an experimental free-for-all.

Such an agile and experimental medical practice naturally resists strict categorizations, for to name a disease is to mark, with potentially coercive precision, the border between the normal and the pathological. The second important aspect of Romantic disease discourse is its refusal to classify abnormality. In the eighteenth century, nosology (the study of disease classification) had just begun to take up Linnaeus's famous challenge to organize the world. Standardized nomenclature, however, had to wait until the International Classification of Diseases (ICD-1 in 1900). Romantic medicine sits chronologically and ideologically in the middle of this medical history: whereas William Cullen devoted long medical tracts to classify diseases according to increasingly specific categories of genus and species, his apostate protégé, John Brown, was touting a novel theory of "excitability" which provided a serious challenge to nosological classifications. He explained diseases qualitatively as types of irritability and excitation: on the one hand, disease is caused by "too great excitement," but, on the other hand, "*Life is a forced state*; if the exciting powers are withdrawn, death ensues as certainly as when the excitability is gone" (82). Cullen's strict taxonomy of disease and Brown's deliberate blurring of those same categories managed to coexist (albeit uneasily) during the Romantic period. And despite Cullen's drive to pathologize, the body largely remained a loose amalgam of affective drives, psychology, vital force, organs, and pathways rather than a localized network of discrete organic parts. In short, disease was a hotly disputed category, and any attempt at classification faced serious challenges. This medical culture of conflictual nomenclature does not exactly mean that Romantic medicine floundered hopelessly in lexical disarray. Rather, disease existed as more than just a normative exception to health. Health was not just the absence of disease; as Nicholas Jewson puts it, "diagnosis was founded upon extrapolation from the patient's self report of the course of his illness" (228), and health remained a largely amorphous and discursive conceit. Despite (or perhaps because of) this willful suspension of definitional precision, Romantic medicine gave rise to some of the most important landmarks in the history of medicine, from the theoretical innovation of Brown's revolutionary medical paradigm of excitability to the practical research into Jenner's disease-eradicating procedure.

George Grinnell has even gone so far as to dub Romantic medicine "the age of hypochondria" because of these contested notions of health and disease and the heated narrative negotiations between patient and physician.[19] The third and final aspect of Romantic disease discourse that I wish to discuss is this interface between amateur and professional, layperson and expert, and patient and physician. Foucault and Jewson have both provided convincing accounts of the Romantic period's complicated reconfigurations of medical authority. In both histories, the "bedside medicine" of the late eighteenth century gets replaced by the "hospital medicine" (or in Foucault's language the "clinic") of the early nineteenth.[20] They agree on a marked movement away from patients' experiential reports to physicians' professional opinions, but whereas Jewson seems content to adopt a triumphalist stance of Enlightenment progress from the speculation, dispute, and weak disciplinary boundaries of bedside medicine to the definitional precision and clinical observation of hospital medicine (and later, "laboratory medicine"), Foucault remains sceptical about this consolidation of clinical power. This Foucauldian scepticism proves helpful in explaining Romantic literature's easy and productive access to the cutting edge of medical debates. In the Romantic era, strange medico-literary interventions stood comfortably alongside the ostensibly more legitimate accounts of medical practitioners. And Jenner's case certainly shows that Jewson's picture of a medical science in "cosmological" disarray does not necessarily preclude methodical research, innovation, and discovery.

Romantic disease discourse only becomes legible to us if we are willing to unlearn our preconceptions about proper medical writing. In 1985, Karin L. Yanoff and Fredric D. Burg undertook a survey of American medical schools to determine which types of medical writing were considered most important to the modern physician. And in 1988, the authors published their widely cited results: "According to the responding schools, the five most important types were: write-up of the patient history and physical examination, progress note and discharge summary (tied), peer-reviewed published paper (of either clinical or laboratory research), and grant proposal" (30). *The Smallpox Report* takes these five most popular genres of modern medical writing back to the historical drawing board to defamiliarize the genres of medical discourse. The first part of the book about classification schemes rewinds "patient history and physical examination," "progress report," and "discharge summary" back to the Romantic case study, to Jenner's and Wordsworth's delicate balancing acts of spectacular novelty with biopolitical intervention in the cases of their rustic patients. Without an institutional need to classify health as either normal or abnormal, Jenner and Wordsworth worked out the shifting first principles of professional medicine. The second part of the book on Romantic experimentalism locates Romantic antecedents to the "peer-reviewed published paper (of either clinical or laboratory research)" in Erasmus Darwin's medico-botanical theory and William Blake's transgressive experiments with the figure of inoculation. The third part of the book on Romantic interdisciplinarity reads John Keats's and Mary Shelley's speculative fiction with an eye towards the medical genre of the "grant proposal" and Romantic medicine's outrageous promise to eradicate human disease. The future directions of medicine, for both Keats and Shelley, required thinking outside and around entrenched disciplines. Teasing out the medico-literary genres of Romantic disease discourse is not merely the task of finding medical qualities of literary genres or literary qualities of medical genres. Romantic medical writing relies on no such disciplinary divide and ventures far outside "clinical or laboratory" settings. Wordsworth, Darwin, Blake, Keats, and Shelley are not just first responders to the seemingly miraculous advent of immunology in Jenner's smallpox report; they were writing it themselves.

I begin in the first chapter with Wordsworth because his biopolitical argument will seem the most familiar to us. Wordsworth's medico-literary case studies in *Lyrical Ballads* balanced unique illness narratives against a very modern vision of the biopolitical greater good. His vision gradually developed a naive faith in biopower, in a gentle paternalism that can glean universal lessons from individual cases. Wordsworth's early poetic ambivalence about classifying the normal and the pathological eventually aligned quite closely with the utilitarian priorities of modern medicine. He is more familiar to us because he tends towards the modern model of professional medicine's clinical efficiencies. Even though Wordsworth, in the end, sides with this brand of medical modernity, I include him in the story of Romantic disease discourse because of his transitional commitments to both Birch's "capricious age" of Romantic medicine and the newer top-down biopower of professional medicine. The second chapter focuses on another transitional figure, Erasmus Darwin. *The Loves of the Plants*, a poem ostensibly about Linnaean classification schemes, becomes more about the breakdowns of botanical structures and his experiments to reassemble biological life along more expansive horizons. Writing at about the same time as Wordsworth, Darwin would take medical writing someplace stranger and wilder. His utopian, cosmopolitan vision of life imagined the biological world through provocative stories of inoculation. Strict classification became less meaningful as Darwin experimented with this central metaphor to expand his constructed world into the interdependent and interpenetrating inoculated forms of nature.

Once Romantic authors like Darwin started experimenting with inoculation, in all its figurative, botanical, and medical registers, Jenner and Wordsworth's familiar road to biopower gets significantly bumpier. In chapters 2 through 5, the close readings of *The Smallpox Report* become much stranger because they are defamiliarizing these Romantic texts to strip away our modern medical biases about what counts as medical knowledge. These unconventional close reading practices will demonstrate how the Romantics valued the illness narrative as more than just throwaway anecdotal evidence. Only after we unlearn our tendency to separate the medical from the literary can we begin to take these texts seriously as illness narratives. Darwin's anthropomorphic botanical world, for example, is as much fanciful poetry as it is medical narrative. Blake's worm metaphors have been misunderstood because they are both figurative *and* rooted in medical and scientific argument. For Blake, the worm's seeming parasitism (in the purely literary sense) becomes his favourite figure for a kind of inoculating, violative health (in the underappreciated medical sense). While Wordsworth had a naive faith that biopower would eventually eradicate disease and purge infection, Darwin and Blake both imagined a messier biology that lingers with these infected stories of inoculated bodies. Blake's inoculating worm articulates a much darker, but ultimately still positive, illness narrative. Blake exhorts us to listen to Oothoon's illness narrative in "Visions of the Daughters of Albion" even if it is an illness narrative as strange, irrational, distasteful, and paradoxical as an anti-vaxxer's. After being raped by Bromion and rejected by her lover Theotormon, Oothoon tells the outrageously problematic story of how her inoculating violation liberated her from false morality and objective norms. She claims most strikingly (for my close reading in chapter 3), "sweetest the fruit that the worm feeds on" ("Visions" plate 6, line17). Theotormon, however, is too disgusted by her contamination to hear her, and Bromion has already moved on to his next conquest. Blake's point about medicine here is that as soon as it starts to overlook the sublime peculiarity of individual illness narratives, it ossifies into either Theotormon's religious dogma or Bromion's utilitarian scientism. At great cost to her own body, Oothoon had purchased the inoculating, medical knowledge to heal the world, but no one was willing to listen to her uniquely distasteful illness narrative. Oothoon's outrageous story ultimately refuses easy assimilation into any kind of institutional medical archive.

The hallmarks of Romantic disease discourse – reluctance to classify abnormality (Part One on Jenner and Wordsworth), experimentation (Part Two on Darwin and Blake), and interdisciplinarity (Part Three on Keats and Shelley) – allowed Darwin, Blake, Keats, and Shelley to achieve more unfamiliar visions of medical knowledge. Each vision is about doing the hard work of listening to the illness narrative without immediately zooming out to the scale of modern, Jennerian or Wordsworthian biopower. This means getting past Theotormon's religion and Bromion's science to see the value of Oothoon's advocacy of strange new medical knowledge, no matter how disgusting it may sound. Keats would eventually leave a professionalizing medical institution because he sensed the coming loss of this illness narrative. Keats wrote in the era immediately after vaccination, when the new medical procedure inaugurated radical new possibilities of medical treatment and life extension. In "La Belle Dame Sans Merci," Keats shows how the old – the knight, the ballad structure, and the fairy – is potentially left out of this new, modern world of Jennerian and Wordsworthian biopower. He depicts a knight who has outlived his purpose and the quest romance, and his illness narrative is wasted on his interlocutor who can ask only narrow, diagnostic questions. The fourth and fifth chapters on Keats's poetry and Shelley's *The Last Man* document powerful warnings against ignoring the swiftly vanishing illness narrative. Instead, both Keats and Shelley recommend a more generously interdisciplinary medicine that honours the outlier stories of aging knights, ailing Titans, and dying plague victims.

The fourth part of the book on Doyle and medical modernity documents the end of Romantic disease discourse and the arrival of Foucault's modern biopower in my radical detour in the literary history of inoculation.[21] The familiar narrative of inoculation as biopower hardly brooks delay; it passes abruptly from beginning to end, from Jenner's tentative case studies to our modern sense of opaque, clinical authority and compulsory vaccination. *The Smallpox Report* instead reveals history's occluded but crucial middle: Romantic illness narratives' central role in shaping vaccination history. The Romantic era remains important for *The Smallpox Report* because it was one of the last historical moments that truly valued the illness narrative. In the early modern period, for example, there was no question that patient stories should inform treatment and shape medical knowledge. The authors that I consider in this study wrote in an age of institutional transition, the last gasp of the illness narrative. Perhaps because of this, the Romantic anti-vaxxer movement (unlike ours) was remarkably short-lived because patients still felt that their stories were being heard. Biopower would eventually capitalize on this hard-earned consensus, and by the 1840s, compulsory vaccination schemes started to emerge. The anti-vaccination movement came roaring back with a decidedly contemporary spin. With conspiracy theories now amplified by social media, vaccination is still engendering raucous controversy despite its institutional legitimacy. Here, Alan Bewell's reminder that "Disease was both a metaphor and a sad reality" (*Colonial Disease* 4) becomes particularly salient. Wild, irrational "metaphor" and objective, clinical "reality" have not always played our high-stakes, zero-sum game. This book balances Romantic "metaphor" with diseased "reality"; it tracks both the literary and medical uses of inoculation from its botanical prehistory, to its experimental anxieties, to its dilation to global politics, and finally to its Victorian consolidation into biopower. By documenting Romantic disease discourse and its principles of classification, experimentation, and interdisciplinarity, I tell the untold radical story of a medical practice that continues to challenge both our notions of medical authority and our understanding of Romantic literature's long disciplinary reach.

Chapter One

Wordsworth's Romantic Path to Biopower

Wordsworth and Jenner

Part one on "Classification" compares the career trajectories of William Wordsworth and Edward Jenner because their parallel claims to fame – the *Lyrical Ballads* and the *Inquiry*, both published in 1798 – highlight the distorting nature of success. Wordsworth is remembered as the heroic father of vernacular English poetry, and Jenner as the conqueror of smallpox. According to our modern disciplinary script, these two authors are the big Romantic-era success stories of poetry and medicine, respectively. Wordsworth belongs in the vaunted Big Six of Romantic poets, and Jenner has been conscripted into a triumphalist narrative of modern medicine. In 1926, Jenner was even inducted into Metropolitan Life Insurance's educational series and appeared on the cover of *Health Heroes* brochures (figure 7). This level of success, however, tends to obscure their bumpy paths towards an eventually triumphant biopower and towards classification schemes that presage the diagnostic coercions of modern medicine. Like Wordsworth, Jenner was once just a humble wanderer who stopped to hear rambling tales of rustic wisdom. The *Inquiry* was not exactly a *magnum opus* of a singular genius or a health hero, but rather a product of a cultural landscape that made such a report possible. Wordsworth's and Jenner's parallel narratives of success are gripping, but we must also remember the intersections, twists, and turns that got them there. After his *Inquiry*, Jenner spent the rest of his life in the business of polishing the clinical story of uninterrupted rational progress, purging the detours, mistakes, and dead ends along the way. His biopolitical argument for compulsory vaccination evolved into a revisionist, partial view of inoculation as biopower, as an objective, medical truth heroically plucked from the tree of scientific knowledge. Recently, the cracks in this clinical façade have begun to show. The anti-vaccination movement is back with a vengeance, and the two sides hardly speak the same language: medical authorities can only wag their fingers at public ignorance while anti-vaxxers cling to their misguided sense of being in the right. If we could

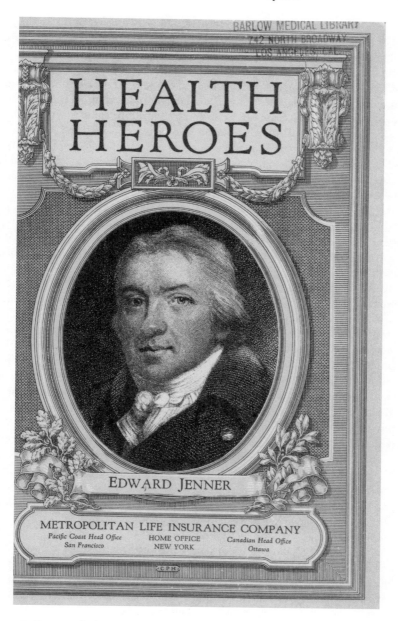

Figure 7. Portrait of Edward Jenner on the cover of *Health Heroes*, a series commissioned by the Metropolitan Life Insurance Company, 1926. Call # R489.J5 H3 1926, The Huntington Library, San Marino, California.

remember the searching dialogues and narratives of Wordsworth among beggars and of Jenner among milkmaids, before their overshadowing successes, we might find some common language after all.

Back in 1798, that searching debate and pre-disciplinary language were alive and well. Like Jenner, Wordsworth remained relatively undecided about the uses and abuses of clinical authority. Their parallel case studies shuttled back and forth between symptom and diagnosis, between novel forms of embodiment and their classification into an indelible medical archive. Together, Jenner and Wordsworth seed my developing tale of Romantic-era medicine, and this chapter reads *Lyrical Ballads* as both illness narratives *and* an unlikely Jennerian urtext of modern biopower. Wordsworth and Jenner may not have tamed entirely the wild whims of Romantic patient agency, but they certainly started to work out the imperatives of the modern case study. Unlike the diagnostic impatience of modern medical writing, though, the Romantic-era case study gently balanced the novelty of the patient's unique presentation of symptoms with its need to absorb abnormality into its generalized medical discussion. As some of the most influential transitional voices of the era, Wordsworth and Jenner have set the agenda for both literary and medical history with their peculiar cases, but the major problem is that those cases remain stubbornly illegible to us. To our post-disciplinary eyes, a poem like Wordsworth's "We Are Seven," for example, reads exclusively as an adorable vignette of a rustic child's triumph against an oddly solicitous and overly rational biostatistician. And Jenner's *Inquiry* makes sense to us only in the familiar paradigm of the modern case's relentless clinical objectivity. To us, poetry is always about our feelings over our rationality while medicine must feature objective rationality triumphing over irrational hysteria. If Wordsworth's poems, however, are read alongside the imperatives of the Jennerian case, Wordsworth's transitioning commitments from the Romantic illness narrative to modern biopower start to surface. And if Jenner is read alongside this burgeoning biopolitical Wordsworth, his argument for vaccination begins to sound much more like a literary project. In the end, the *Inquiry* and *Lyrical Ballads* are not as ideologically or disciplinarily far apart as we might suspect.

The Census and the Clinic

Obstacles to this biopolitical reading of Wordsworth, however, come into view immediately. "We Are Seven" seems to feature a bean-counting avatar of the administrative state who sinisterly forbids a little cottage girl from honouring her deceased siblings in the household count. But even if this *dramatis personae* of the calculating villain and the precocious heroine has remained unwaveringly durable, this chapter insists that Wordsworth strategically avoids casting definitive, polarized roles in this early Romantic case study. Wordsworth's sparse poem tends to be felt before it is understood. Even armed with Jerome McGann's incisive caution against the self-replicating readings of Romantic ideology, readers continue to romanticize.[1] The first reaction is affective and visceral. The speaker is a cruel usurper of idyllic cottage life or an abrasive bully who inexplicably spends an entire poem trying to make a little girl cry. The Romantic ideologue gleans a rustic lesson from the cottage girl's brave intransigence when she insists that John and Jane, her deceased brother and sister, be counted in her eponymous refrain of "we are seven." The second reaction is Fredric Jameson's old saw, "always historicize."[2] For McGann, though, the problem of Romantic ideology is that this second thought ends up as mere wasted energy: no matter how much literary historical context one musters, the affective reading remains as intransient as the little cottage girl. Whatever does not unequivocally brand the speaker villain and the little girl hero is reflexively jettisoned. "Comprehensiveness," McGann concludes, "is achieved by definitional exclusion" (*The Romantic Ideology* 24) as the sly cloak of historicized reason pre-emptively confirms the obdurate bias of passion.

My reading attends to the interpretive impasse but not just by substituting some attempt at a rational reading for an ideological one. That would miss the point of the poem entirely. There *is* the sobering ground of literary historical context – the first British census as well as some post-Revolutionary biopolitical rumblings – but that does nothing to capture the swell of unburdened passion on first looking into Wordsworth's "We are Seven." Just as the belaboured joke is often robbed of its punchline, this sort of contextual explication threatens to snuff out the initial breath of the poem's "pure serene" (Keats, "On First Looking into Chapman's Homer" line 7). This double bind – damned with historical context and damned without – unravels in this chapter in two parts. First, situating the poem within post-Revolutionary demographical debates takes care of the Jamesonian due diligence. Second, John Keats will model for us a contemporaneous readership of "We Are Seven" for whom contextual reason is not out of step with visceral passion, for whom complete readerly intimacy and immediacy is not only possible but necessary. Recovering and recreating this lost moment of reception through Keats finally explains, to continue the simile, Wordsworth's abstruse joke, and, perhaps more importantly, keeps it funny.

While the discussion of Keatsian biopolitics will be suspended until the fourth chapter, I introduce Keats into the conversation now because without Keats, we just cannot see past the unprovoked cruelty of Wordsworth's speaker. Aaron Fogel illustrates the problem by rehearsing some of the standard readings: "Younger readers especially," he claims, "see [the adult speaker] as a destructive teacher reduced to exclamation points and insisting." In perhaps the only oppositional reading, Geoffrey Hartman sympathizes with the adult speaker's hardened pragmatism and echoes Wordsworth's own acknowledgement that the poem reveals deficits in both the child and the adult when he describes "the perplexity and obscurity which in childhood attend our notion of death, or rather our utter inability to admit that notion."[3] Wordsworth's own words do nothing to budge entrenched positions, and the argument becomes, in Fogel's appropriately knotty language, a "moral-imaginative perspectival tangle and unresolvable dialogue" (39–40). But before all the noisy, "unresolvable dialogue" and the circular hermeneutics of Romantic ideology, Keats had it all figured out. He had already obliquely revised the poem himself into his own critical, balladic narrative of forced encounter.

"La Belle Dame Sans Merci" illuminatingly and incisively rewrites the elder poet's "We Are Seven" and exposes a Wordsworth in covert collusion with his bureaucratic speaker. Both poems ostensibly represent the unwelcome encroachment of the modern liberal state on a deliberately constructed romance of the past. As a few critics have now noticed, Wordsworth's emergent figure of looming modernity is the census canvasser who insists that the little cottage girl omit her deceased brother and sister in her sibling count. In a reading that I will develop more fully in the fourth chapter, Keats's speaker similarly accosts a lovelorn knight-at-arms with the polished, diagnostic language of the modern clinic, eager to claim bodies for his dissecting table. Both, as Wordsworth would say, seem to "murder to dissect" ("The Tables Turned" 28). Those siblings buried in the churchyard have no immediately recognized right to be included in the census count, and Keats's knight-at-arms has no legal right to dispute his deathly diagnosis. And yet they do. The girl insists until the end that they are seven, and the knight reads back his dumbfounded diagnostician's initial question – "O what can ail thee, knight-at-arms / Alone and palely loitering?" – with his unhelpfully ironic answer: "And *this* is why I sojourn here / Alone and palely loitering / Though the sedge is withered from the lake / And no birds sing" ("La Belle Dame" 273–4; emphasis mine). Where Keats valorizes dogged resistance and patient agency, Wordsworth struggles to tame the illness narrative; the census canvasser is not cruel but merely doing his job. Wordsworth mobilizes disputations of population against biopower to erect a brave new demographic order in the wake of an anarchic and destructive Revolution.[4] What Keats intuits correctly is that "We Are Seven" is not only a tragedy of lost childhood, but also a calculated satire of childish things.

The affective reading, that of McGann's enervating Romantic ideology, must judge both bureaucratic bodies – Wordsworth's census and Keats's surgical clinic – guilty of violating the rights of their experimental subjects.[5] This reflexive mode of Romantic reading underestimates the great ideological distances between the two poets. Keats's "La Belle Dame" instead looms as the dark dissenting counterpart of his predecessor's "We Are Seven." In Keats's perceptive reading, Wordsworth succumbs to his rude speaker's urgent call to register the rustics of the Lake District into his census ledger. Keats emphasizes instead the vulnerability of marginal populations to schemes of biopolitical engineering. He exposes Wordsworth as an emergent poet of biopower who takes his speaker's persistent question of "How many may you be?" ("We Are Seven" 15) much more seriously than previously imagined. Wordsworth's Jennerian cases in *Lyrical Ballads* blend Romantic feeling with this serious consideration of the biopolitical greater good, but because of the modern disciplinary gulf between literature and medicine, we listen earnestly for the former while doing our best to muffle the latter. When Wordsworth is read within the proper genre of the transitioning Romantic illness narrative, however, his poetic collection's buried biopolitical argument begins to take shape as a Jennerian agenda.

We Are Seven Million

Early census history provides a good foundation for constructing this biopolitical Wordsworth alongside Jenner. A handful of critics now see Wordsworth's counting poem as an answer to the question of population. Both Fogel and Charlotte Sussman have surveyed the ways in which literature, including poems like "We Are Seven," imagines the historical movements and demographics of populations.[6] Hollis Robbins has linked the poem to several specific Parliamentary proposals that led to the first British census of 1801.[7] The census emerged from the centuries-old contest between the daunting grandeur of the ancient world and the progress of modern society.[8] By the 1750s, more and more Britons started to wonder if modern populations had finally outstripped the glory days of ancient Greece and Rome. In 1753, this gathering storm made it to Parliament in "The Act for Taking and Registering an Annual Account of the Total Number of People and the Total Number of Marriages, Births, and Deaths; and also the Total Number of Poor Receiving Alms from every Parish and Extraparochial Place in Great Britain" (*Journals of the House of Commons* 1860). The 1753 act was roundly defeated, and in 1758, yet another proposal was struck down, largely due to fears of governmental intrusion into the private sphere. Only after the French Revolution did this movement pick up steam again, as it became critical to determine England's military strength against an encroaching France. Perhaps revolutionary fears in England had made the measurable health of the body politic a vital talking point. Seven years after revolutionaries stormed the Bastille, a young Oxford man by the name of John Rickman published "Thoughts on the Utility and Facility of a General Enumeration of the People of the British Empire," an essay that brought him to the attention of future speaker of the House of Commons, Charles Abbot (who served from 1802–17). In 1800, Abbot appointed Rickman his Private Secretary, and together, they finally passed the Census Act of 1800. A few months later, the first modern census of Great Britain estimated the 1801 population of England and Wales to be 8.9 million.

Since Rickman ran in the Wordsworth circle, the poet of "We Are Seven" was no doubt familiar with the debates surrounding the emergent science of demography. If "We Are Seven" is Wordsworth's preliminary answer to the population question, is it, as Fogel puts it, an "*anti*-census" poem in the vein of Robert Frost's "The Census-Taker" (1923), an example of "literature against demography" (24)? In the conclusion of her meticulously researched essay, Robbins answers affirmatively and attempts to work through the thematic import of population:

In "We Are Seven," the poetic speaker's task as an official recorder of the population is deliberately opposed to the romantic and visionary work of the maid's poetic sensibilities. While both register some kind of truth, the object of official representation is enrolling material truths and facts, whereas the object of poetry, as Wordsworth argues in his 1802 Preface, is expressing "truth, not individual and local, but general, and operative; not standing upon external testimony, but carried into the heart by passion." The convention of counting a person as "present" stimulates the narrative of ghostly presence. And this, not surprisingly, is what most readers recall about the poem. (210)

However, "what most readers recall" is not always exactly the "ghostly presence" that the "maid's poetic sensibilities" evoke. Nor is it always, as Susan Wolfson suggests, the girl's spiritual, Romantic notion of familial "presence" asserted against the stupidly unimaginative question of "How many may you be?" (*The Questioning Presence* 50). In my experience teaching and discussing the poem, readers often remember the blustering adult before the innocent child and the stupid question before the poignant answer; it is the absurd callousness of the adult speaker that persists in the mind. The child's perspective quickly fades because it is easily understood by us, but the adult speaker's bizarre behaviour demands further explanation. The context of the first British census can bridge that interpretive gap by historicizing the speaker's baffling interrogation, but these "new" readings have hardly deviated from that first, visceral reaction. The census context has merely enlarged the target of scorn to include the speaker's invasive bureaucratic project. With newly hardened hatred for the speaker, the Romantic ideologue continues confidently reading from the gut.

Perhaps what is needed is a deeper history of Wordsworth's surprising sympathy for the emergent census bureaucracy. His collection of *Lyrical Ballads* emerges from a particularly turbulent decade of European history. In the 1790s, a guillotined king and a bloodthirsty Jacobin Reign of Terror had sent panicked, war-weary French émigrés to English sanctuary. Charlotte Smith's dedication to her 1793 blank verse epic *The Emigrants* describes the scene as an occasion to reconsider Anglo-French antipathies. She laments that "the very name of Liberty has not only lost the charm it used to have in British ears, but many, who have written, or spoken, in its defence, have been stigmatized as promoters of Anarchy" (133–4). Despite having penned the more enthusiastically radical novel *Desmond* the year before, Smith writes with new circumspection, not exactly disillusioned with the French Revolution but certainly disappointed by the unchecked rise of demagoguery in France. The "undistinguishing multitude" and the "promoters of Anarchy" (Smith 133) threaten to derail the vaunted promise of *liberté, égalité, fraternité*. Now, rather than cheering on the fall of the Bastille, Smith yearns for the healing of old wounds by proposing more amicable relations with an embattled France. England becomes the potential distinguishing principle of the "undistinguishing multitude," now able to absorb French exiles into an ordered, cosmopolitan citizenry. Meanwhile in a chaotic and lawless France, the "infuriate crowd" presides over "the ruin'd mass, / Flush'd with hot blood" and brandishes "The headless corse of one, whose only crime / Was being born a Monarch." She decides rather bleakly that the rational (English)man is left only to "Blush for his species" (bk. 2, lines 50–68).

Five years later, Wordsworth would identify in "We Are Seven" the missing technology in Smith's jeremiad as the sort of biopower manifested in Rickman's national census. For Foucault, the late eighteenth century was an era of volatile social reform that led to the "discipline" of the nineteenth century and the "bio-power" of the twentieth.[9] In Smith's "species" discourse is what Foucault would call the nascent "massifying" ideology of "biopolitics": "Unlike discipline, which is addressed to bodies, the new non-disciplinary power is applied not to man-as-body but to the living man, to the man-as-living-being; ultimately, if you like, to man-as-species" (*Society Must Be Defended* 242). Smith imagines both French-man and Englishman ordered into an idealistic cosmopolitan "species," but lacks a pragmatic method of institutional governance, a proper technology of unifying power. Foucault explains that such a technology would have to mould population into "a global mass that is affected by overall processes characteristic of birth, death, production, illness, and so on" (243). Biopower as the subtle privileging of species health over individual life is a foregone conclusion for Foucault, but Smith and Wordsworth live it as an anguished formational process. Smith's "massifying" imagination absorbs French refugees into a cosmopolitan body politic but stops short of linking concept to implementation; instead, she is left only with a kind of species shame – that anguished "Blush" – about the inability to achieve true international cooperation. The poem's proleptic ideal is precisely this partnership between feuding nations, a kind of Kantian "perpetual peace" governed by an airy sense of internationalism (*Perpetual Peace* 93–130). Smith's revolutionary ambivalence here would prove terribly suggestive to someone like Wordsworth. On the one hand, humanity has expanded beyond the tyrannical oppression of the *ancien régime* to form individual subjects, free from sovereign power. On the other hand, Smith's "massifying" population remains dangerously unshapen, moldering as a "ruin'd mass" and a "headless corse."

After Smith died in 1806, Wordsworth famously remembered her as a poet "to whom English verse is under greater obligations than are likely to be either acknowledged or remembered."[10] If "We Are Seven," published just five years af-ter *The Emigrants,* is about population, it makes sense that Wordsworth's poem inherits his poetic predecessor's biopolitical concerns. Instead of an increasingly cosmopolitan England learning to take in emigrants from her historical foe, Wordsworth reduces the question from Smith's grand geopolitical scale and the high style of blank verse to the Jennerian Romantic illness narrative. He presents a modest scene of rustic conversation between the "undistinguishing multitude" of uncounted cottagers and the distinguishing task of the census canvasser. Wordsworth, unlike Smith, brashly articulates the missing technology of power in the concrete form of a national census that realizes Foucault's "global mass." The census, for Wordsworth, becomes his national project for the good of the "massifying" conception of man-as-species. Both Smith and Wordsworth understood that, as the sway of absolute sovereignty waned, government of the people and by the people was up for grabs. Whereas Smith foresaw only anarchy and mob rule, however, Wordsworth shrewdly found opportunity. When the adult speaker interrogates the little cottage girl, he is not merely crunching numbers, twirling his thumbs, and stroking his moustache menacingly; rather, he is part of a tentative biopolitical experiment to amass enough data to sweep up the decapitated heads of monarchs and the anarchic remains of revolution for both the greater good and the continued flourishing of the new species of liberated man.

The aggression of the speaker's assault reflects the poem's high ambition. The ballad unsettles decorum with its insistence on uncomfortable conversation and forcing a little cottage girl to explain herself. Wordsworth's ballad begins and ends in this mode. The first stanza of the poem expresses what Wordsworth anoints in the "Preface" (1802) as "truth, not individual and local, but general, and operative" (605). The speaker immediately forgoes the former for the latter: his first stanza reads, "A simple Child, / That lightly draws *its* breath, / And feels *its* life in every limb, / What should *it* know of death?" ("We Are Seven" 1–4; emphasis mine). It matters little that the child is female (hence the gender-neutral pronouns) and even less that she dares to present an alternative perspective on death. The speaker pre-emptively brands the child "simple" before she is even allowed to mount her defence. Only after this biased testimony does he deign to recount the conversation: "I met a little cottage Girl: / She was eight years old, she said; / Her hair was thick with many a curl / That clustered round her head" ("We Are Seven" 5–8). She insists that even though her sister and brother "in the church-yard lie," they are still seven siblings in total. Instead of allowing this nice sentiment, the speaker presses on until the end, when he concludes in the final stanza that his words are wasted on this simpleton:

> But they are dead; those two are dead!
> Their spirits are in heaven!
> 'Twas throwing words away; for still
> The little Maid would have her will,
> And said, "Nay, we are seven!"   ("We Are Seven" 65–9)

Even though the final words nominally belong to the "little Maid," the desperate "Nay" transforms her joyous "we are seven" into a petulant error. Interestingly, this ending also abandons the four-line ballad stanza in favour of a five-line, prosodic echo of the speaker's "you are five" that drowns out the girl's concluding "Nay, we are seven" (also five syllables). Thus, the poem is not so much about the triumph of Robbins's "ghostly presence" of brother John and sister Jane; rather, it ends with the speaker's accounting and recording of cottage experience into his poetic census. The speaker's callous persistence is, of course, shocking, but there is also an urgent need to admit the little cottage girl's family into a kind of common-sense understanding. The debate does not end with happy acknowledgment of the girl's difference; instead a poetic, imaginative, and active comprehension finally incorporates the statistical outlier neatly into a "general, and operative" truth that continually reasserts the speaker's positivistic "five" ("We Are Seven" 36).

The "egotistical sublime" of this poetic bluster depends on the continual forcing of encounter to regulate the "ruin'd mass" of the world through conversation, friction, and debate.[11] When Wordsworth ruminates on the new bureaucratic form of the census, he reacts not with suspicion but with a cautious optimism about its world-building potential. The poem delights in enumeration and data collection: it uses a four-line ballad stanza with a four-syllable title, there are two siblings in Conway, two at sea, two in the church-yard, five living siblings, seven total, the little girl is eight years old, and the church-yard is twelve steps away from the mother's door. The speaker sneaks in an extra line to the ballad stanza and a "Nay" to the girl's refrain to end confidently with the chiming sounds of five lines and five syllables. What, then, is the fate of the girl's "seven"? Why does that "seven" deserve its titular pride of place? According to recent scholarly extrapolation from the first official British census of 1801, the population of England numbered between seven and eight million. When Wordsworth was composing "We Are Seven" in Alfoxden about a decade earlier, that rough, unofficial number would have been quite close to seven million, an estimate that Wordsworth would probably have been familiar with given his association with the emerging class of demographic scientists.[12] The girl's "seven" powerfully evokes England's bustling millions; with this number, Wordsworth imagines a "massifying" life at two disparate scales: the girl's local "we are seven" meets the national declaration of "we are seven million." The chiming numbers of the poem insist on the ideological convergence of the local with the national, of the individual with the state. Both the census-taker and the little girl are right and wrong in different ways, but in their disputation lies the tantalizing hope of a fair, biopolitical schematization of the English population. In this way, Wordsworth becomes quite dissimilar from the usual Romantic picture of the freethinking, counter-cultural nature poet; his gentle endorsement of a form of Foucauldian governmentality makes him not only an apologist for census bureaucracy, but also a poetic forefather of modern biopower.

Well before his state-sponsored tenure as Poet Laureate from 1843 to his death in 1850, this early Wordsworth is, in a sense, already a statesman. His benevolent biopolitical state is hardly authoritarian, but he welcomes its gentle guidance in the aftermath of revolutionary anarchy. Whereas Smith throws her hands up in outrage and exasperation, Wordsworth takes up the challenge of his poetic predecessor to imagine and implement in verse the nascent technology of democratic power. The telling impasse between the census canvasser and the little cottage girl dramatizes the still imperfect nature of this biopower. At the heart of Smith and Wordsworth's conception of "man-as-species" and their search for its organizing, political principle is a set of unanswered post-Revolutionary questions. Without kings and queens, who should govern? How can government hope to function? Smith poses these as provocatively open questions, but Wordsworth claims a partial solution, not exactly in the speaker's census per se, but in the tortuous and torturing process of census taking. Wordsworth is, of course, not exactly the cruel speaker of the poem. Indeed, the speaker's bizarre insistence on finishing off his poem with a flourish of five household members, five lines, and five syllables is a clear crime against balladic prosody. Wordsworth merely suggests that the census taker is onto something. In that impasse – among the speaker's positivistic fives, the girl's ghostly sevens, and the cosmopolitan millions of England – lies Wordsworth's case study of a liberal state governed by the new institutional technology of benevolent biopower that can reconfigure the new species of free men and women into political life.

Keats's Awkward Affair

Since modern readings must encounter a Wordsworth filtered through the brutal history of twentieth-century biopolitics, his naive faith in the benevolent neoliberal state seems dangerously unhinged. Consequently, we tend to reduce "We Are Seven" to a safe, cute, and straightforward exercise in rustic satire that targets the speaker's dictatorial arrogance. Nazi-era eugenics and concentration camps, though, remained largely inconceivable to someone like Wordsworth, and he persists throughout the collection of *Lyrical Ballads* in his belief of a positive, unifying power over human life. It is not only "Romantic ideology," then, but also the history of totalitarianism that occludes our view of Wordsworth's utopian biopolitical future. Keats could be quite a bit more ideologically agile in his rewrite of "We Are Seven." Even with the watershed history separating "We Are Seven" from "La Belle Dame," Keats could still make sense of Wordsworth's burgeoning commitments to biopower. In 2011, the world population reached seven *billion*, three entire orders of magnitude beyond Wordsworth's paltry seven million. In an intervening history of genocide and mass incarceration, there is hardly any historical evidence to convince the modern reader of biopower's salutary ends. Only by deferring to Keats's revision of his predecessor's poetic census can a more historically situated Wordsworth emerge. Jamesonian historicizing can only go so far, and Wordsworth eventually demands a better reader.

For Keats, the census is only half the story. Just as Wordsworth's lyrical ballad anticipates the first modern British census of 1801, Keats's oblique revision participates in the debates leading up to the Anatomy Act of 1832. By the time Keats was in medical school (1815–16), the demand for fresh corpses had exceeded the supply, and there was a great push to free up more bodies for medical use. Prior to the Anatomy Act, only recently executed criminals were to be used for experimental purposes. The gist of the legislation was to remove these strict regulations regarding the acquisition of surgical cadavers. The debates were incredibly heated since the new law required a serious overhaul of cultural perspectives on the embodiment of death. Ruth Richardson explains that a "fundamental shift" in funerary practices allowed for "the invasion of commerce into the rite of passage" (4). She argues that the Anatomy Act allowed medical schools to snatch up droves of new corpses from economically blighted neighborhoods; in effect criminalizing poverty by treating the body of the pauper like the mutilated corpse of an executed murderer. Along with this utilitarian advocacy of "commerce" and economic expedience, proponents of the Anatomy Act piggybacked on the rhetoric of a secularizing world that insisted on displacing superstitious rituals of death with positivistic science.[13] Whereas Wordsworth learned second-hand about the national census from his friend Rickman's proposal, it was Keats's own medical career that granted him access to this latest incarnation of biopower. Both the Census and Anatomy Acts explain why these characters are talking to each other in the first place: while Wordsworth's speaker roams far into the margins of the countryside to gather demographic information, Keats's speaker conveniently times his arrival to coincide with the farm's seasonal downturn (winter) to collect the starved bodies of the poor for the dissecting table and for the secular good of an increasingly industrial and commercial nation.[14]

Like the census canvasser, the inquisitive speaker of "La Belle Dame" blusters into the bucolic space of romance with his diagnostic question, but rather than revealing the human species to itself, he gets everything wrong; his diagnoses are mere wild guesses.[15] The poem functions as Keats's strategic wet blanket to Wordsworth's biopolitical optimism. Indeed, the echoes are not only ideological, but also formal. Keats preserves Wordsworth's ballad stanza without resorting to a rambling five-liner. Like Wordsworth, Keats begins the encounter with an arrogant interlocutor who asks, "O what can ail thee, knight-at-arms?" only to answer the question himself ("La Belle Dame" 1). Keats even directly borrows his predecessor's language: he rewrites Wordsworth's "I met a little cottage girl" ("We Are Seven" 5) into "I met a lady in the meads" ("La Belle Dame" 13). The descriptions of hair and eyes proceed in almost perfect parallel: "Her hair was thick with many a curl / That clustered round her head" ("We Are Seven" 7–8) and "Her hair was long" ("La Belle Dame" 15); "Her eyes were fair, and very fair" ("We Are Seven" 11) and "her eyes were wild" ("La Belle Dame" 16). Wordsworth's child is "wildly clad" and Keats's belle dame has "wild wild eyes." And most interestingly, Keats refines Wordsworth's twos, fives, sevens, eights, and twelves into a single enumerated image: "And there I shut her wild wild eyes / With kisses four" ("La Belle Dame"

31–2). In his well-known, tongue-in-cheek explanation of these bizarre lines to George and Georgiana Keats, he explains:

> Why four kisses – you will say – why four because I wish to restrain the headlong impetuosity of my Muse – she would have fain said "score" without hurting the rhyme – but we must temper the Imagination as the Critics say with Judgment. I was obliged to choose an even number that both eyes might have fair play: and to speak truly I think two a piece quite sufficient – Suppose I had said *seven*; there would have been three and a half a piece – a very awkward affair – and well got out of on my side. (*Letters* 227; emphasis mine)

This indirect jab snidely judges the most famous poetic "seven" of the time as a "very awkward affair" that demands some straightening up.

For Keats, Wordsworth's mashups of lyric and ballad, and census bureaucrat and little cottage girl are productive, procreative encounters that are nevertheless empty. Children, dead and alive, densely populate the thin 1798 volume of *Lyrical Ballads*, yet the actual procreative act, what Blake more explicitly and more joyfully dubs "happy copulation," is noticeably absent.[16] Keats, doubtful of the quick productive potential of the forced encounter, prefers aimless recreation to procreation. In Keats's rewriting, Wordsworth's little cottage girl grows up a decade later as the vengefully domineering belle dame, and the narrative action of the ballad lingers on the embodied language of the "moist" forehead, the "sweet moan," and the "kisses four." Unlike Wordsworth's perfected case study and its concluding equation of five, seven, and seven million, Keats's end is much less determinate. His speakers are frequently left in stunned silence or in aching doubt. "Ode to a Nightingale" complicates the speaker's sensual, ecstatic moment with a bodily jolt: "Do I wake or sleep?" (80). "Ode on a Grecian Urn" ends the speaker's rhapsodizing with an ambiguous talking urn and no one left to interpret it: "Beauty is truth, truth beauty, – that is all / Ye know on earth, and all ye need to know" (49–50). Similarly, "La Belle Dame" abruptly concludes just before the bureaucratic voice of the clinic can respond to the knight's frenzied tale. Keats dwells with all the sensual confusion and meandering of the sexual act, while Wordsworth forgoes sexual process for pragmatic product. And while Keats dwells with the feverish poetics of the morning after, Wordsworth jumps straight ahead to the sober, compromising poetics of nine months later, to the "simple child" who says the darndest things.

When Keats's speaker asks the diagnostic question, he is not Wordsworth's rustic canvasser. He is the predatory anatomist who scouts out fresh, viable corpses for his dissecting table, and his probing questions seek only to establish a legal claim on the knight's body. The speaker's goal in the first three stanzas is to persuade the knight that his life is as good as over and that he should begin getting his affairs in order. Rather than shelter or nourishment, the speaker offers long odds, and given the environmental vulnerability of the rural poor, he warns against foolish persistence. He upsells the modern lie of the common good, urging the knight to sacrifice his supposedly ailing body for a homogenizing conception of the human species. Just as the census canvasser's ledger demands an accurate count, the surgeon requires the knight's willing concession to authorize this new biopolitical vision of the world. But instead of finding a starving labourer who has finally failed to make ends meet, the speaker encounters a digressive knight-at-arms who tells an antique tale of ghostly kings and a cruel fairy's child. While Wordsworth's case study soberly mediates between seven and seven million, citizen and nation, and liberty and biopower, Keats's speaker clams up three stanzas into the poem, and the patient's bizarre illness narrative dominates entirely. Keats short-circuits the biopolitical pitch: he imagines an alternative biopolitics in which the knight's digression is not just the adorably wrong "seven" of Wordsworth's little cottage girl. The knight understands the speaker's dire prognostication, but he finally decides that he is not buying what the eager biopolitician is selling. In the end, the speaker finds himself unable to stake any claim on the knight's body. Biopower ultimately fails to convince.

But for us, biopower is what we remember and celebrate in popular culture. For example, Spock's now famous paraphrase of Romantic-era utilitarianism in *Star Trek II: The Wrath of Khan* – "the needs of the many outweigh those of the few" (Meyer) – makes both Wordsworth's census and Keats's clinic sound innocent enough. Keats's powerful ending, however, sours the honeyed allure of species safety. Foucault's "man-as-species" demands both Wordsworth's brand of compromise and Smith's massifying imagination to stamp out the ostensibly selfish desires of "the few." Mary Shelley, perhaps the most cogent critic of the Romantic imagination's impossible ambition, succinctly dramatizes Keats's scepticism about this biopolitical calculation. After initially agreeing to construct the creature's female companion, Victor Frankenstein reveals his seemingly magnanimous reason for refusing the creature's request: "I shuddered to think that future ages might curse me as their pest, whose selfishness had not hesitated to buy its own peace at the price perhaps of the existence of the whole human race" (*Frankenstein* 119). Here, Frankenstein styles himself the selfless martyr, sacrificing his "own peace" for the benefit of the "whole human race." For Shelley, this utilitarian magnanimity turns out to be the mere self-delusion of an entirely unreliable narrator. Whereas Wordsworth's expansive concept of species goes out of its way to bring all walks of marginal life into the biopolitical fold, Shelley's mad doctor and Keats's morbid anatomist sinisterly choose who deserves to inhabit the human world and who is worthy of political life.

Wordsworth, Shelley, and Keats are the first interpreters of what Rosemarie Garland-Thomson calls a kind of "liberal eugenics" that thrives even in the absence of totalitarian control:

Proponents of eliminating disability and disabled people under various rationales and practices such as selective abortion, euthanasia, the right to die, and genetic engineering contend that reproductive technology and euthanasia are not eugenic because they are voluntary and noncoercive, a blend of pragmatism, liberalism, and consumerism. (Garland-Thomson 77)

In their consideration of the "normal" family, Faye Ginsburg and Rayna Rapp continue to challenge these ostensibly "voluntary and noncoercive" processes: "the 'choice' regarding who is admitted to the human community has shifted from the state to the family, assisted by emergent professions such as genetic counseling" (83). The medical profession, for example, boxes families into the "choice" to terminate pregnancies because of genetic abnormalities such as Down's syndrome.[17] Frankenstein and Keats's speaker, early models of such genetic counsellors, mark out the strictly policed parameters of human flourishing. Wordsworth, however, sees no sceptical scare quotes around the "choice" for the good of family, community, and species. Whereas Shelley and Keats caution against mad scientists as genetic tyrants, Wordsworth holds onto the post-Revolutionary possibilities of individual choice to shape a utopian and cosmopolitan brotherhood of free and equal men.

At this point, it is important to point out that history has proven Wordsworth's biopolitical optimism wrong and Shelley and Keats's scepticism right. As Giorgio Agamben explains, the neoliberal belief in man-as-species has led not to the realized dream of Wordsworth's case study but to the concentration camp and to the lawful justification of genocide. Unlike Foucault, who marks biopower as a recent technology rife with creative possibility, Agamben diligently uncovers variously masked versions of this power over life from antiquity to the present. Foucault's history is one punctuated with epistemic breaks that demands situational vigilance because of the constant reconfigurations of the structures of power. Agamben's more-or-less continuous history of power renders Wordsworth's mad dream of political agency in the wake of a watershed, revolutionary moment entirely nonsensical. There is no rich, new Foucauldian era of post-Revolutionary potential from which to craft a kinder and gentler biopower.[18] For Agamben, the eternal recurrence of the ancient Roman figure of *homo sacer* confirms that biopower demands a eugenic principle. Whether a Roman exile, a political prisoner in Guantanamo Bay, a Jewish person stripped of citizenship in Nazi Germany, a comatose patient in a persistent vegetative state, or a child who refuses to count down to five, these *homines sacri* exist within a blurry "zone of indistinction" in which biopolitics – positive power over these massified bodies – almost imperceptibly slips into thanatopolitics, a lawful power over death. Agamben would argue, against Wordsworth's rosy biopolitical future, that this line of thinking always inheres an exclusionary thanatopolitics in which genocide and concentration camps are lawful, justifiable, and even moral. This is no mere slippery slope for Agamben but is precisely the lived history of sovereignty. Wordsworth, defiant against this history, maintains steadfast faith in biopower and has his solicitous bureaucrat glean enlightening lessons from his rural rambles to seek fair compromises.

Keats rewrites the case of "We Are Seven" to expose the dangerous thanatopolitical within Wordsworth's conception of benevolent biopower. The speaker presumptively maps out the knight's end-of-life journey to claim a kind of rational, juridical power over death. He deliberately underestimates the chances for survival in the wintry conditions given the knight's deathly symptoms of pallor, fever, and perspiration.[19] This speaker is no mere peripatetic gentleman taking a stroll through cottage towns; rather, he blusters into the blighted countryside and imperiously demands his pound of moribund flesh. Like Agamben, Keats unmasks the eugenic drive within biopolitics and warns of a genocidal impulse towards the "loitering" poor that seeks to repurpose worthless life into practical medical use. Whereas Wordsworth's demographic ideology appears generously inclusive, Keats's critique exposes the exclusionary principle of biopower that necessarily relies on the exile of *homo sacer* whose body is forfeited to preserve the fiction of species. By the time he wrote the poem, Keats had seen more of the calamitous fallout from the idealism of the French Revolution: Robespierre's Reign of Terror, the rise and fall of Napoleonic tyranny and empire, and the real possibility of perpetual war. With these warning signs in mind, he breaks with Wordsworth's optimistic reconfiguration of biopolitical sovereignty. While stopping just short of Agamben's central image of the concentration camp, Keats nevertheless imagines a thwarted dystopian moment of malicious gentrification in which the wasting bodies of the loitering homeless become mere fodder for biopolitical legislation to assemble its gleaming, post-Napoleonic cosmopolis.

Paternalism without Patriarchy

Wordsworth shrugs off these critiques and continues to shape the gentle hand of paternal biopower. There is no shortage of solicitous, bureaucratic speakers elsewhere in the case studies of *Lyrical Ballads*, and similar questions persist throughout the collection. Wordsworth mobilizes literal-minded provocateurs to stumble into the margins of the human species to narrate their subjects into biopolitical life. In his explanation of the pleasures of "metrical language," Wordsworth observes that the mind derives pleasure from these encounters of "similitude in dissimilitude" ("1802 Preface" 610). Familiarity from unfamiliarity serves as both the collection's aesthetic principle as well as its moral imperative. So rather than knee-jerk deference to the wisdom of the little cottage girl's contrarian spirituality, Wordsworth's speakers surely deserve some more analytical patience. Reading the poetic collection as a series of confrontations between rustic folk heroes and doltish villains greatly misjudges Wordsworth's calculated poetics and politics of compromise. Far from mere straw men to be blown away, these obtuse canvassers are the "awkward" spokesmen of biopower who gently mould difference into unity, dissimilitude into similitude. The collection's cases do not merely celebrate the rural margins of England; rather, it documents how rustic folk are to be conceived, philosophically digested, and integrated into the modern, vernacular world. The poems journey across all walks of life – the mad, the idiotic, the poor, the disabled – to bring the marginalized into a newly imagined human species. Each chime of dissimilitude needs harmonizing. Any "spontaneous overflow of powerful feelings" requires ruminative "tranquility" (Wordsworth, "1802 Preface" 611) from which to structure new social hierarchies and political configurations of power.

The speakers' paternal care represents for Wordsworth the latest scions of kingly power. Even as little girls and boys create powerfully moving teachable moments, father still, in a sense, knows best. Like the census canvasser of "We Are Seven," these speakers exhibit stunning failures of compassion and comprehension, but in that gap lies not exactly bald satire but biopolitical prescription. The bungled narrations manufacture a kind of urgency to intervene in rustic tragedies and to shape dangerously unshapen dissimilitude into governable life. In a cluster of poems about absent fathers, for example, Wordsworth insists on domestic hierarchy writ large: the speaking fatherly presence manages the mad, nurturing passion of the mother and the fanciful flights of the abnormal child.[20] About a hundred years earlier, after civil war and the restoration of monarchy, Robert Filmer healed a wounded nation by crafting the same family-as-state argument in *Patriarcha* (1680) to justify the divine right of kings:

> for as Adam was lord of his children, so his children under him had a command and power over their own children, but still with subordination to the first parent, who is lord-paramount over his children's children to all generations, as being the grandfather of his people. (6–7)

After revisiting the trauma of his own experience of violent republican revolution, Wordsworth retreats to the familiar solace of paternal order.

He stops short, however, of endorsing Thomas Hobbes's *Leviathan* (1651), an unambiguously monarchical vision of the social contract between subject and absolute sovereign. Since the French Revolution ends in the déjà vu of regicidal violence, Wordsworth tweaks the idea of sovereignty itself. Instead of staunch, filial loyalty to a protective king, Wordsworth's social contract subjects man to the normalizing rule of species. The mad, the idiotic, and the arithmetically challenged outliers fall under the paternalistic care of his fumbling but well-intentioned spokesmen of biopower. Perhaps anticipating the objections later voiced by Shelley, Keats, and Agamben, Wordsworth makes clear that he is no patriarchal authority himself. The first volume of the second edition of *Lyrical Ballads* (1800) is shrewdly bookended with poems that turn the potentially menacing biopolitical gaze against himself, against the fever-dreaming poet "William" in "Expostulation and Reply," and against the nostalgic lyricist of "Tintern Abbey." From beginning to end, Wordsworth struggles to mount a convincing case for a unifying human power beyond archaically patriarchal conceptions of authority: liberal paternalism without monarchical patriarchy. Wordsworth's lyrical ballads never rise to the level of Keats's and Agamben's worst case scenarios of an exclusionary thanatopolitics; instead, he constructs a healing account that reconstructs both the individual and the state from the ruins of Revolutionary violence.

One of our favourite stories to tell is that of Wordsworth's political apostasy: the young poet as a peripatetic revolutionary and the older poet laureate as a reflective, reactionary, and idle statesman. He begins as a French Revolutionary, ready to abandon it all and set up a Pantisocratic utopia in America, and ends up a conservative old man. Gripping as it is, the story is an oversimplification. As Keats astutely points out, the Wordsworth of the 1798 *Lyrical Ballads* is already a conservative plotter. He plots the embodied vulnerabilities of the rural margins and enters their names into his inclusive, biopolitical ledger; an act that Keats would later strategically distort into a despicable scene of morbid intrusion. This, in the end, is not to charge Wordsworth with doe-eyed optimism or political naivety; rather, it is to credit the impossible ambition of this "experiment" to discover the "real language of men" ("1802 Preface" 595). At the end of the "Preface," he even invites us to read as sceptically as Keats:

> From what has been said, and from a perusal of the Poems, the Reader will be able clearly to perceive the object which I had in view: he will determine how far it has been attained; and, what is a much more important question, whether it be worth attaining: and upon the decision of these two questions will rest my claim to the approbation of the Public. ("1802 Preface" 615)

Although Keats and modern history have finally answered no to the "important question," it was still worth asking.

Indeed, Wordsworth's biopolitical question survives in altered form. The uneven afterlife of the Romantic-era case study suggests that the question has matured into a dangerous false dilemma. The contemporary answer pits biopower against patient agency: either we can have nice things like vaccination and the eradication of smallpox, or we can value patient narratives in our discussions of medical care. Fortunately, decentring vaccination from Jenner as "health hero" makes ample room for both. Smallpox vaccination was not solely about the elevation of Jenner's clinical authority over the silenced voices of suffering patients. Jenner was no singular conqueror of smallpox and has no monopoly on the Romantic medico-literary idiom of the case study. Wordsworth asked the same productive questions. And Romantic medicine asked even more. Vaccination is not just a story about Jenner, and Romantic medicine is not just a story about Wordsworth's and Jenner's case studies. The following chapters highlight just how generically diverse Romantic medical writing was, and how far from Jenner the story of smallpox eradication eventually veers.

PART TWO

Experimentation

Chapter Two

Darwin's Evolutionary Metaphor

The Grandfather of Evolution

After part one on the classification schemes of Jenner and Wordsworth, the story of compulsion, of inoculation as biopower, seems ready for takeoff. Even if the Romantic case began in ambivalence, both Jenner and Wordsworth eventually succumbed to the biopolitical allure of the greater good. Jenner took up the mantle of imperial vaccinator who culled the frauds, the charlatans, and "that Vulture Walker" from his vision of national public health.[1] Wordsworth's encounters with his rustic patients balanced the scales of public good and private indulgence to register marginal life into his bioethical ledger. The Romantic case always wants it both ways: it listens to Sarah Nelmes's novel tale of daily labour even as its attention drifts towards big data and its massifying catalogue of cowpox pustules. The little cottage girl's seven was cute but of increasingly limited use to Wordsworth's national census. It is tempting to draw a straight historical line from this transitional Romantic ambivalence all the way to modern medical authority. For Michel Foucault, the line is impatient: "an entirely free field of medical experiment had to be constituted, so that the natural needs of the species might emerge unblurred and without a trace" (*Clinic* 38). For Roy Porter, the line is laser-focused: "the emergence of this high-tech scientific medicine may be a prime example of … the kind of myopia which (literally and metaphorically) comes from doggedly looking down at a microscope" (*The Greatest Benefit* 8). For Nicholas Jewson, the line is ruthless: "the triumph of blind physio-chemical law over the idiosyncratic individual experience of the sick-man within the worldview of the medical investigator did not occur until the latter had achieved a degree of detachment from the demands of the sick" (240). It seems the triumph of biopower has indeed arrived at this point.

Mary Fissell's historical through line, however, instead traces the stubborn persistence of patient agency and what she calls "vernacular medicine" all the way back to eighteenth-century Bristol. Her medical history forestalls what Foucault calls the clinical "age of Bichat": "What had been a set of shared assumptions, a belief system held by high and low alike in the seventeenth century, became the purview of the poor by the early nineteenth century" (2). The "waning of vernacular medicine," Fissell strategically understates, "was a complex process" (2). According to her account of this process, patient agency does not disappear so much as it is redistributed along class lines. And on the forty-year anniversary of Jewson's medical-cosmological thesis, Stephen Gillam finds that patient agency, or what Jewson called the "idiosyncratic individual experience of the sick-man," has returned in "e-scaped medicine" (661), the newly unbalanced social contract between patient and physician in the information age. Gillam explains,

> Modern-day "healthism" – so familiar to GPs – has been described as in part a response to the disappearance of Jewson's sick man. This "postmodern" phenomenon is characterised by high health awareness and expectations, information-seeking, self-reflection, and a partiality towards alternative, folk models of illness. All too often it is associated with mutually distrustful patient-professional relationships. (617)

Either the sick man's "healthism" has returned suddenly, or it never left at all. Since Wordsworth and Jenner had already made the Romantic case for biopower as early as 1798, the emergence of "information-seeking" patients on WebMD and "distrustful" naturopaths may seem a retrograde and unwelcome surprise. Patient agency, though, has a long, continuous history that only recently has been taken up by bottom-up medical historians like Fissell. My own patient's view of inoculation emphasizes the deep continuity of this medical distrust. Instead of drawing that straight line towards homogenous biopower – Foucault's birth of the clinic, Porter's "high-tech scientific medicine," or Jewson's "triumph of blind physio-chemical law" – this second part on experimentation shows how Romantic illness narratives tinkered with the metaphor of inoculation, even before Wordsworth and Jenner, and offered telling precursors to what we now call e-scaped medicine, healthism, or medical denialism.

This kind of persistent patient agency does not emerge out of the blue from the Romantic case study. Jenner and Wordsworth represent only a fraction of Romantic medical writing's generic diversity. Lady Mary Wortley Montagu, for example, had advocated controversially for variolation, a primitive and more dangerous form of smallpox inoculation, after her early eighteenth-century Turkish tour. Later in the same century, Erasmus Darwin had challenged the orthodoxy of Linnaean classifications with the strange inoculated botanical forms of his *The Loves of the Plants* (1789). Inoculation generated more than enough controversial medical writing even before Jenner's *Inquiry* and Wordsworth's *Lyrical Ballads*. Darwin, a respected Lichfield physician, had published his medico-botanical experiment nine years earlier. Its fanciful analogies and heroic couplets might make it hard for us to take seriously as true medical or scientific research, but Darwin's arguments about Linnaeus's twenty-four classes of *species plantarum* are as earnest as any peer-reviewed research article from prestigious contemporary periodicals like *The New England Journal of Medicine*. Darwin's research just had stranger priorities and wilder experimental methods. In contrast, *NEJM* is succinctly transparent about its editorial goals. The journal boasts of its authority and exclusivity: "At least five experts review and edit each Original Article or Special Article manuscript published by *NEJM*. Of thousands of research reports submitted each year, about 5 per cent are eventually published by *NEJM*." It also touts its preference for calculated understatement: "The peer review process works to improve research reports while preventing overstated results from reaching physicians and the public." The modern pace of scientific research ensures that new medical knowledge immediately affects lives, so any sensitive information is strictly policed by the profession's expert gatekeepers. According to this publication model, the continuous and ravenous demand for new medical knowledge must not dictate the carefully regulated supply of peer-reviewed research; instead, readers of the journal are reassured that the 5 per cent of research that eventually makes it to print is as far as possible from sensational hucksterism. The published research, in the end, is the understated, refined, and distilled product of a trusted process.

Next to the impressive editorial rigour of *NEJM*, Montagu's epistolary correspondence and Darwin's *The Loves of the Plants* might have the ring of barbaric nonsense. Instead of carefully peer-reviewed understatement, Darwin luxuriates in expansive metaphor and impossible experimental trajectories. Instead of refining Linnaeus's twenty-four classes of plant life, Darwin gleefully and arbitrarily enlarges the botanical world into literary, anthropomorphic, and cosmopolitan networks. However, rather than relegating Darwin to the realm of pure fantasy in the old garb of heroic couplets, what would it mean to read him seriously as a medico-botanical experimenter? After all, Erasmus Darwin *is* the grandfather of Charles Darwin's evolutionary theory, and he deserves some patience if not credit. Darwin's unique experimental mode is what Nobel Prize winner biologist François Jacob has said of evolution itself. In his seminal 1977 essay in *Science,* "Evolution and Tinkering," Jacob crafted an enduring metaphor of evolution as tinkering as opposed to engineering; it makes do with bricolage without the need for a complete toolset.[2] Darwin's inoculation metaphor functions not as Wordsworth's and Jenner's biopolitical engineering but as evolutionary tinkering, experimentally assembling bits and pieces to suit the evolving needs and desires of a contingent life. Instead of inoculation as a constricting biopower, Darwin's inoculation metaphor experiments, unfolds, tinkers, and expands the stories of the natural world. Instead of biopower's relentless endgame of strict classification, Darwin charts increasingly expansive and amorphous ontologies. In challenging the botanical categories of his eminent botanical peers – Linnaeus in the early eighteenth century and Michel Adanson in the mid-eighteenth century – Darwin discovers strange metaphorical, political, philosophical, and scientific uses of the medico-botanical figure of inoculation. That radical metaphor, in the end, helped Darwin reimagine nature as an experimental tinkerer in the large-scale project that we now refer to more agnostically as the principle of natural selection.

Since the word "inoculation" has botanical origins, Darwin winds back the clock and revisits Edmund Burke's sense of inoculation as the engrafting of a scion (a bud) onto a stock plant.[3] Unlike Burke's disgust at the engrafting of an alien scion onto the original plant, Darwin takes advantage of this metaphor's radical possibilities in his hybrid verse forms. In the preface to *The Loves of the Plants*, eventually published as the second part of his long poem *The Botanic Garden* (1791), Darwin frames his poetic undertaking with Linnaean taxonomy on the one hand, and inoculated varieties on the other. He faithfully lists Linnaeus's twenty-four classes of plants, but also offers a subtle caveat that reveals the extent of his own poetic intervention into botanical science:

> The Species are distinguished by the foliage of the plant; and the Varieties by any accidental circumstance of colour, taste, or odour; the seeds of these do not always produce plants similar to the parent; as in our numerous fruit trees and garden flowers; which are propagated by grafts or layers. ("The Botanic Garden" 284)

Many critics have focused on his gendered revision of Linnaeus and his description of the sex lives of plants through botanical representations of stereotyped women – the blushing virgin and the *femme fatale*, for example. Rather than the "Species" of the sexed parents, my approach to Darwin fixes on the "Varieties" of the "grafts or layers" that frequently differ from the parents in radical ways. Here is the locus of Darwin's radical research, his attention to "the possibilities of a new age dawning" (Teute 319) in the French-revolutionary fervour of the 1790s. In this way, inoculation becomes one of Darwin's favourite metaphors to explore radical new ideas in both botany and medicine. These kinds of inoculation stories, Darwin argues, are essential to the unfolding and expanding distribution of these stories in the natural world. Instead of disciplining these narratives into Linnaean classification, he luxuriates in the slow and sometimes perverse stories of interpenetrating and inoculating life.

Inoculation's medical, philosophical, political, and literary registers, however, all hinge on the figure's etymological origins in the botanical controversies of the eighteenth century. The word itself emerges from a rich debate concerning plant grafts and their proper classification within various taxonomic schemes.[4] Since Darwin's inoculation metaphor freely transgresses across the categories of plant, animal, and human, it will not do to just leave it as a historical accident that both botany and immunology should converge upon this single, convenient term. In the early eighteenth century, Linnaeus's seminal work on biological classification led to a comprehensive organizational scheme that purported to account for the entire world of plants with just twenty-four categories. Perhaps inevitably, such a rigidly finite structure raised doubts in the circles of natural philosophy, generating numerous exceptions to the botanical rule in the form of baffling mutations, varieties, and grafts. It is this botanical origin of inoculation – as a vexing figure that troubles grand efforts to categorize and schematize – that becomes particularly salient when Darwin adapts the botanical trope to the discussion of one of the most controversial and successful discoveries in the history of medicine.

Darwin's epic poem, *The Loves of the Plants*, makes just this kind of disruptive literary intervention into the Linnaean debate. His project purports to delight and instruct through personified representations of Linnaeus's twenty-four botanical classes. In transposing botanical science to heroic couplet, Darwin pokes holes in the veil of Linnaean order, perhaps quite an unlikely feat for someone like Darwin. As a physician who dabbled in natural philosophy, botany, and poetry, he may appear the very image of a dilettante. The more generous account, however, paints him as a poet-physician, a jack of all trades whose intelligence and genial nature gained him admission into some of the most impressive intellectual circles of his day. But a jack of all trades is frequently a master of none. He tends to subsist as a minor figure in the history of medicine, in the history of science, and even in literary history. His eccentric genius is overshadowed by the more canonical figures that follow him. Even Desmond King-Hele, Darwin's biographer and most ardent contemporary advocate, casts him as a sort of father figure to British Romantic poets, as if his only possible appeal is as a precursor to worthier poets like Wordsworth and Coleridge. Darwin's eclectic body of work explored the evolutionary ideas that paved the way for the theory of natural selection, but again he is overshadowed, this time by his more famous grandson Charles. His interdisciplinary approach, his strange formal experimentation, and his seemingly haphazard methodology have marked Darwin's literary and scientific legacy with an off-putting whiff of empty erudition and aimless dilettantism.

Yet recent scholarship is eager to recuperate his reputation. We have learned about his close participation in the Lunar Society's often madcap adventures in scientific and technological invention, his cautiously radical and cosmopolitan politics, his honing of the scientific analogy, and his proto-feminist appropriation of botanical science.[5] His poetry's effortless meandering perhaps increasingly speaks to our concerns over the boundaries of knowledge and the dangers of insular notions of discipline. And Darwin nicely exemplifies Romanticism's constructive encounter between scientific discovery and literary representation. This chapter marshals this increasing interest in the recuperated Darwin to show that he is not a mere popularizer of the Linnaean system; instead, Darwin boldly reimagines botany, as I will detail later, via three increasingly grand architectural metaphors: the prison, the mansion, and the temple. The architectural trajectory moves from carceral confinement towards expansion, exploration, and humanization while eschewing the Linnaean strictures of botanical nomenclature. Throughout *The Loves of the Plants* and later in *The Temple of Nature* (1803), Darwin mediates this expansion with the trope of inoculation in both its botanical and medical senses. He lingers in botanical strangeness, in mutations and grafts, to draw connections with the two major medical developments of the 1790s that he lived long enough to see: variolation (smallpox inoculation) and vaccination (cowpox inoculation). The controversies surrounding both forms of inoculation allowed Darwin to articulate his imaginative, political vision of a cross-pollinating community of nature and a mutually beneficial ecology of belonging. His botanical personifications expand scientific vocabulary to a more inclusive notion of the human body and its place in the natural world. Where does humanity call home: the prison, the mansion, or the temple? In finding his answer to this provocative research question, Darwin liberates botany from the silence of imprisoned flowers, manages the fragile economy of the vegetable mansion, and finally locates his cosmopolitan utopia in the temple of nature. Inoculation, for Darwin, is always about this constant renovation and evolution.

This second part on Romantic disease discourse's experimentation begins with Darwin because he trailblazes a divergent Romantic path away from Wordsworthian biopower. Even before Jenner and Wordsworth, Darwin tinkered with the idea of inoculation beyond strict classificatory schemes. While Darwin saw inoculation as an *evolutionary* metaphor, William Blake, as I will explain in the following chapter, experimented with it as *revolutionary* metaphor. In François Jacob's formulation, Wordsworth and Jenner were instead engineers; even as they dallied with the stories of rustics and milkmaids, they were already gravitating to the idea of reforming society from scratch. They eventually started to engineer this new world from the top down, from an enlightened sense of being in the biopolitical right to enforce their utilitarian vision of the greatest benefit for mankind. Darwin and Blake had more modest, but no less influential, experimental methods. They dallied with strange and provocative individual narratives in a slow, contingent experiment rather than a grand feat of biopolitical engineering. For Darwin and Blake, the Romantic illness narrative was less an occasion to enumerate, sort, and classify, and more an invitation to tinker continuously. Whereas Jenner apologized in his *Inquiry* for the distasteful cross-species traffic of modern life, Darwin mostly delights in the inoculated world. Instead of settling on strict classification, Darwin broke from eighteenth-century botanical science with his mutable botanic garden that abounded with unique inoculated forms, each with an amazing story to tell.

The Prison House of Botany

The eighteenth-century botany that Darwin inherited was largely about categorical confinement. Before Darwin, Linnaeus had formulated a provocative nomenclature to understand the natural world through an increasingly secularized science.[6] From his modest, eleven-page first edition of *Systema Naturae* (1735) to the sprawling three-thousand-page thirteenth edition (1767), Linnaeus worked tirelessly to contain animals, plants, and minerals within manageable categories. This meticulous organizational impulse hardly seems compatible with the stereotyped caricature of the Romantic poet, mired in gothic excess, unbounded variability, and intractable vision. Nevertheless, Darwin, now more or less (probably less) a canonical representative of what we have come to call first-generation Romanticism, productively mined Linnaeus's scientific legacy of botanical classification for poetic inspiration. During the same tumultuous year that marked the beginning of the French Revolution, Darwin seemed oddly content to merely reproduce Linnaeus's botanical system in his epic poem *The Loves of the Plants*. Darwin's seemingly tame subject, however, belies the botanical metaphor's long and complex medical history. As David E. Shuttleton has noted in his study of smallpox poetry, seventeenth- and eighteenth-century poets were already invoking the "floral analogy" (200) to check stark reality with ameliorative metaphors that could, for example, transform pockmarks into roses. By the late eighteenth century, Darwin was armed with an already robust medico-botanical lexicon to align his shifting figure of inoculation – as both botanical grafting and medical procedure – with the period's radical and revolutionary politics.

Such an alignment might seem odd at first since Shuttleton's prehistory of the metaphor often reads like a staunchly conservative tale of loyalty, nationalism, and patronage. One of the earliest texts to connect smallpox and botany was Dryden's first published poem, "Upon the Death of Lord Hastings" (1649), an elegy for a schoolmate who had died of smallpox at the age of nineteen. Rather than shying away from the diseased body, Dryden's poem relies on a startling strategy of bodily exposure and metaphorical containment:

> Was there no milder way but the small-pox,
> The very filthiness of Pandora's box?
> So many spots, like naeves on Venus' soil,
> One jewel set off with so many a foil;
> Blisters with pride swell'd, which through's flesh did sprout
> *Like rose-buds, stuck i' th' lily-skin about.*
> Each little pimple had a tear in it,
> To wail the fault its rising did commit:
> Which, rebel-like, with its own lord at strife,
> Thus made an insurrection 'gainst his life.
> Or were these gems sent to adorn his skin,
> The cabinet of a richer soul within?
> No comet need foretell his change drew on,
> Whose corpse might seem a constellation.   (lines 53–66; emphasis mine)

The figural density of the passage does not escape Samuel Johnson's sharply critical eye. He extends his well-known discussion of Cowley's overwrought "metaphysics" to include what he refers to dismissively as Dryden's puerile "school performance": "Lord Hastings died of the smallpox; and his poet has made of the pustules first rosebuds, and then gems; at last exalts them into stars" (Samuel Johnson 121). Dryden's sustained metaphorical sequence rewrites Hastings's untimely death and bodily disfiguration as a euphemistically idealized narrative of natural beauty ("rose-buds" and "lily-skin"), human artifice ("jewel" and "gems"), and finally heavenly reward ("comet" and "constellation"). Meanwhile, the poetic strategy smuggles in some political subtext: the "little pimple" learns to regret the "insurrection" that causes both lord and subject to perish – no doubt an allusion to the beheaded Charles I and Oliver Cromwell's dream of a fledgling republican Commonwealth. It is no surprise then that Dryden's royalist poem was published in *Lachrymae Musarum*, a collection of aristocratic, occasional poems about Hastings's death. As Dryden's ill-advised pustular rebellion exemplifies, the collection was almost certainly a conspicuously political lamentation for the death of the king.[7] The poem achieves its political end by imagining the site of fatal infection as a hybrid body of "rose-buds" and "lily-skin" (the doubling of the floral metaphor as well as the mirrored hyphenation both underscore this line's invocation of botanical hybridization), which firmly links the inoculated body to a project of conservative, royalist amelioration.[8]

More than a century later, Burke's botanical warning against contaminating English purity with the infection of French Revolutionary ideology –"inoculat[ing] any cyon alien to the nature of the original plant" (181) – reverses Dryden's ameliorative figure of botanical inoculation while preserving its politically conservative tenor. Montagu's earlier popularization of variolation (in the 1720s) had medicalized, humanized, and embodied the figure of botanical inoculation, so Burke's hierarchical argument in *Reflections* could not possibly condone the free circulation of biological matter. For Burke, Dryden's bodily idealization becomes sociopolitical contamination. Despite Burke's negative appropriation of the metaphor, as Shuttleton points out, "botanical analogies" still remained a "plank in the Jennerian counter-attack against charges that vaccination is unnatural" (200). For example, Robert Bloomfield's *Good Tidings* (1804), a long poem dedicated to the legitimization and popularization of Jenner's vaccine, recycles the same floral images that Dryden used more than 150 years before:

> In ev'ry land, on beauty's lily arm,
> On infant softness, like a magic charm,
> Appear'd the gift that conquers as it goes;
> The dairy's boast, the simple, saving Rose!   (123–6)

Here, the body is even more explicitly hybridized: the "lily arm" is injected with the "saving *Rose*" of the cowpox vaccine, a striking materialization of Dryden's "rose-buds, stuck i' th' lily-skin about" (58). Dryden's euphemistic rose becomes

Bloomfield's "saving *Rose*"; instead of merely dressing up the disease in a floral metaphor, the "Vaccine Rose" has become much more than ornament. In pursuing his vision of public health, Bloomfield revives Dryden's botanical metaphor from Burke's injunction. But instead of a radical relocation of medical expertise from the bustling city to the "simple" country, Bloomfield settles for an instrumentalized pastoral, nationalistic, and triumphal vision "conquer[ing] as it goes" and extracting propaganda out of syrupy images of country life.[9] Bloomfield offers figural repetition with a significant medical difference: rather than figuratively healing a mourning nation that has just decapitated its monarch, Bloomfield's metaphor promises to erase the bodily traumas of the smallpox victim and to finally reclaim an idyllic vision of a pastoral Eden.

Each of these three authors – Dryden, Burke, Bloomfield – argues for the persistence of a pastoralized status quo: Dryden's royalist regret urges England to bring back her King, Burke's idealized society of continued inheritance mobilizes the sublimity of hierarchical vision to quell enthusiastic stirrings of revolutionary levelling, and Bloomfield's return to Edenic health peddles idyllic rustication to aristocratic appetites for the picturesque. Yet, as Johnson perceptively notes, Dryden's politics were anything but stable: he later elegized Cromwell in his "Heroic Stanzas" (1658) only to turn around yet again to celebrate the restoration of Charles II in "Astraea Redux" (1660). Johnson accounts for these shifting politics by historicizing a nation of changing allegiances: "The reproach of inconstancy was, on this occasion, shared with such numbers, that it produced neither hatred nor disgrace; if he changed, he changed with the nation" (Samuel Johnson 122). In Dryden's case, as well as Burke's and Bloomfield's, the botanical metaphor strives to temper large-scale unrest and anxiety with a conservative disavowal of change. It purports to offer a metaphorical distraction that draws attention away from radical stirrings, whether they be experiments in popular governance, agitated discussions about the rights of man, or controversial new medical procedures. But if the figure of botanical inoculation so easily flips between the negativity of Burke's "alien" contamination and the triumphalism of Bloomfield's "saving" gift while preserving its solidly conservative politics, then the metaphor threatens to become flatly instrumental: a blank figure that merely absorbs the political. If it just "changed with the nation," then inoculation essentially means nothing at all.

As the *material* histories of inoculation push against a purely *figurative* and instrumental botanical discourse, however, the metaphor begins to refuse its conservative script. Dryden, for example, unaware of the later, mid-eighteenth-century practice of variolation, can happily use the figure of a hybridized plant to euphemize the bodily excess of the smallpox victim. Burke invokes the botanical metaphor only to reject it because of its potentially radical association with variolation; a medical practice packaged with a dangerously egalitarian corollary: a suggestion that biological matter – *diseased* biological matter, no less – was essentially interchangeable across his sacrosanct and inherited boundaries of gender and class. By the time Bloomfield writes *Good Tidings*, the accumulation of medical history begins to exceed political containment. Bloomfield, with the blessing of Jenner himself, wanted to capitalize on the historical success of the botanical metaphor by naming the poem "The Vaccine Rose," but he eventually changed the title to "Good Tidings; or, News from the Farm." Critics have cited publisher issues to explain the name change, but I would add a more literary rationale. In this medical and literary history from Dryden to Bloomfield, the *metaphoric* distance between medical tenor (variolation and vaccination) and botanical vehicle (hybridization through inoculation or grafting) began to collapse into an uneasy *metonymic* identity; the finalized title "News from the Farm" wisely substitutes a much safer pastoral *metaphor* ("the Farm") for the increasingly freighted botanical *metonym* ("The Vaccine Rose"). At this point, the figure of inoculation becomes inseparable from grotesque species abomination, and the poetics of botanical euphemism falters. Indeed, John Birch, physician to William and Catherine Blake, purges vaccination from his conservative vocabulary altogether: "we shall soon see what yet remains of popular opinion favourable to the cause of Vaccination, *vanish into thin air* ... the speculatists in physic, like the speculatists in politics, will be brought back to the old standard of sober reason, and experience" (2). He links experimental medicine ("speculatists in physic") with radical politics ("speculatists in politics") and finally makes impossible Bloomfield's initial attempt to tame the figure of inoculation with a conservative botanical poetics.

A conservative history of the botanical metaphor, then, is not enough, and many critics have already begun to uncover Romantic botany's radicalism, especially in relation to Darwin. For example, Alan Bewell has read the Romantic period's surging interest in botany as a product of new cosmopolitan and globalized ideologies, and Richard Sha has suggested that botany provided Romantic authors the means to imagine perverse and emancipatory sexualities.[10] Romantic botany expresses a diverse range of radical utopian impulses: cosmopolitan purpose, sexual liberation, gender equality, and class levelling. In my readings of Darwin (this chapter) and Blake (the next chapter), I integrate the conservative prehistory of the botanical metaphor of inoculation (Dryden, Burke, Bloomfield, and Birch) into this emerging picture of botanical radicalism. My synthetic account of conservative and radical literary histories envisions a Romantic botany that includes the related material history of inoculation and vaccination. Radicalism, mediated through this botanical metaphor, reflects the political volatility of the 1790s. The shifting figure of inoculation alternately imagines a utopia of sexual freedom under an egalitarian government and a circumscribed vision of hierarchical order. Darwin (and especially Blake, as I discuss in the following chapter) works to unveil the radical kernel hidden beneath inoculation's conservative trappings: the latent sense of unnaturalness that Johnson's identification of unnaturalness in Dryden, Burke's frantic political tweaking of the metaphor in *Reflections*, Bloomfield's strategic name change, and Birch's ultimate abandonment of vaccination metaphors.

Whereas Darwin's cautious radicalism is still deferential to the metaphor's history of conservative concealment, Blake's plants plot to overwhelm their botanical categories and prisons. Despite Darwin's radical pedigree, his deployments of the botanical metaphor retain some of Burke's disgust. He prefers a dual calculation that radicalizes botany while concealing the dangerous excess of botanical life; the surplus that always threatens to overwhelm sense, category, and understanding. Blake would ultimately reject such "mind-forged manacles" ("London" 8). His botanical poems unhinge desire, joy, and revolution from any kind of ethical hedging or Urizenic, botanical containment.

This is not to say that Darwin is aesthetically timid or entirely naive about his radical politics. In an era of popular revolution and reactionary terror, Darwin's political circumspection represents an orchestrated response to a set of political debates about radical reform and social responsibility. Burke's *Reflections* set the tone of this debate as well as its figural parameters. To invoke the botanical metaphor is also to invoke its conservative history, to legitimate Burke's voice in the Revolution Controversy, and to participate in a culture of polite conversation – as opposed to combative controversy – that selectively constrains the free generation of revolutionary ideas for the sake of harmonious discussion and exchange.[11] Botany's Linnaean origins encouraged slow and careful organization, lexical categorization, and the narrow production of scientific authority. Botany functions as containment, as an expression of an Enlightenment ideal of rational discussion and the easy purchase of authority and truth through regulated conversational friction. Within this figural framework, Darwin still managed to find a radical – albeit circumscribed – voice. Blake, as I show in the next chapter, suspects that Enlightenment reason and conversation are just as likely to produce oppressive authority as scientific truth. Together, Darwin and Blake map out two paths: Darwin produces a contained Linnaean radicalism whereas Blake originates new, revolutionary discourses, detached from botany's literary history. Darwin's radical metaphor of inoculation remains mostly confined to the prison house of botany, restrained by its literary prehistory, the figural parameters of Burkean politics, and the empirical categories of Linnaean taxonomy.[12]

Darwin *does* occasionally pry himself loose. In a paratextual note, he takes a shot at Burke's rhetorical style while keeping quiet about his politics: "Some parts of Mr. Burke's eloquent orations become intricate and enervated by superfluity of poetic ornament; which quantity of ornament would have been agreeable in a poem, where much ornament is expected" ("The Botanic Garden" 327).[13] Instead of directly attacking Burke's adherence to inherited hierarchies, ideological inconsistencies, or logical faults, Darwin's complaint (the only explicit reference to Burke in the poem) takes exception only to the incongruity of the rhetorician's formal extravagance. And even that complaint feels warmly sympathetic since Darwin finds himself struggling to match medium to message in *The Loves of the Plants*. After all, a text on botanical classification is hardly a place "where much ornament is expected" ("The Botanic Garden" 327). A 1798 issue of *The Anti-Jacobin* transformed Darwin's muddled ornament into "The Loves of the Triangles," a parody that poked fun at the botanical poem's formal strangeness, the overuse of personification, and the dangerous yet oblique references to Revolutionary politics.[14] If Burke deserved censure for the "superfluity of poetic ornament," then Darwin was certainly guilty of his own formal trespasses.

The important difference, however, is that Darwin was right and Burke was comically wrong. In the *Reflections*, Burke's metaphor of the inoculating "cyon" that contaminates the original plant awkwardly relies on botanical hybridization to represent the debilitating effects of foreign (French) influences on a genetically pure state of inherited health (England). In his "eloquent" rhetorical performance, Burke depends on an ultimately unconvincing metaphorical correspondence. Since plant grafting – the hybridization of different plants to propagate desirable traits – was a common practice with an ancient track record of success, Burke's botanical contamination makes little to no scientific sense, and the rhetoric quickly degenerates into pure "ornament" with only a minimal connection to the material world. Darwin's own handling of the botanical metaphor carefully measures the ratio of imaginative ornament and scientific explanation. In his oft-cited advertisement to *The Botanic Garden*, Darwin balances imaginative metaphor and scientific reality:

> The general design of the following sheets is to inlist Imagination under the banner of Science; and to lead her votaries from the looser analogies, which dress out the imagery of poetry, to the stricter ones which form the ratiocination of philosophy. While their particular design is to induce the ingenious to cultivate the knowledge of Botany, by introducing them to the vestibule of that delightful science, and recommending to their attention the immortal works of the celebrated Swedish Naturalist, LINNEUS. ("The Botanic Garden" 12)

Burke's "looser analogies" fall short of achieving the "ratiocination of philosophy," a charge that amplifies Darwin's light formal critique into an ideological confrontation. His insistence on the meeting of "poetic ornament" with botanical science challenges and revises both the rhetorical form and the political content of Burke's *Reflections*. In this way, Darwin confidently claims to demonstrate how botany can *properly* manage Revolutionary politics.[15] Instead of weaponizing botany as an empty figure that relentlessly pushes towards an independent political articulation, Darwin connects botanical material with political metaphor in a more convincing correspondence that takes Linnaean classification just as seriously as any program of radical politics or Revolutionary ideology. Burke was content to remain a politician of the status quo, while Darwin always found more to tinker with.

Mansion of Twenty-Four Apartments

The Loves of the Plants is Darwin's earliest attempt to achieve such a system of correspondence between the conservative prison house of botany and radical politics. The poem is based on Linnaeus's ordering of all plants into twenty-four classes, differentiated by "the number, situation, adhesion, or reciprocal proportion of the males [stamens] in each flower" ("The Botanic Garden" 284). Those twenty-four classes are further divided according to species and variety. Darwin even replicates Linnaeus's tendency to personify and sexualize the intimate lives of plants. In the preface, for example, he tasks himself with the lofty goal of transforming vegetable into animal and plant into person:

> Whereas P. OVIDIUS NASO, a great Necromancer in the famous Court of AUGUSTUS CAESAR, did, by art poetic, transmute Men, Women, and even Gods and Goddesses, into Trees and Flowers; I have undertaken, by similar art, to restore some of them to their original animality, after having remained *prisoners* so long in their respective *vegetable mansions.* ("The Botanic Garden" 289; emphasis mine)

Despite these scientific origins and faithful Linnaean echoes in Darwin's expansive project, the poem is no mere regurgitation of decades-old botanical knowledge. For those musty "vegetable mansions," he refers the reader elsewhere: first to Linnaeus's original works, "exactly and literally translated into English, by a Society at Lichfield, in four Volumes Octavo" and then to a translation "of Dr. ELMSGREEN, with the plates and references from the Philosophia Botanica of LINNAEUS" ("The Botanic Garden" 288). The poem is, in other words, no substitute for the primary sources of scientific knowledge. Instead of mere scientific recapitulation or poetic ornamentation, Darwin's goal is to liberate those botanical "prisoners" from scientific orthodoxy, to attract the reader to botany with delightful verse, to direct that interest to more serious studies, and to advocate a more speculative science that effortlessly integrates imaginative conjecture with the rationalist and empirical observations of Enlightenment science. This convoluted plan, however, leaves him vulnerable to critique. In the simultaneous pursuit of science and poetry, he runs the risk of being bad at both. Linnaeus's modern biographer, Wilfrid Blunt, complained that Darwin "reduced Linnaeus's concept to charming absurdity" (248) while a cantankerous Coleridge put it much more bluntly: "I absolutely nauseate Darwin's poem" (164).[16] Darwin's strange brand of speculative science and his eccentric verse have drawn criticism from scientists, poets, literary critics, and historians alike. Nevertheless, a growing group of scholars seeks to absolve Darwin of these scientific and literary sins and to recover him from undeserved obscurity. Darwin's floral metaphors, the literary construction of his radical politics, and his deliberate departures from Linnaeus's botanical script are far from the incoherent ramblings of a bored rural physician.

Rather, in this recuperative view, his botanical project productively pushes the limits of Enlightenment science (liberating "prisoners") even as it insists on a bounded, empiricist, and rationalist discourse (Linnaeus's "vegetable mansions").

Such calculated madness requires formal method, and since poetic form for Darwin is tantamount to a kind of political commitment, the heroic couplet is, at first blush, a strange choice. If one were asked to identify radicalism's poetic form, the fast answers might include the subversive prosodic experiments of Milton's blank-verse epic, Wordsworth's lyrical ballad, or Whitman's free-verse autobiography. By the 1790s, the epic was almost certainly out of fashion, and the heroic couplet was hardly revolutionary. What possible ideological work could Darwin squeeze out of such a stodgy form? The couplet belongs to polite Enlightenment discussion, a rational discourse mediated by mnemonic opposition, metrical balance, and didactic clarity. The chiming end-rhymes convey a precarious yet perfect sense of balance and precision – the universe reduced to finite and discrete "prisons" of metrical feet. Indeed, most critics have over-emphasized Darwin's Enlightenment credentials perhaps out of some suppressed embarrassment at the strangeness of his awkward couplets. Stuart Harris has dubbed *The Botanic Garden* an "Enlightenment epic," Donald Hassler has enumerated Darwin's many scientific accomplishments, and Jenny Uglow has documented his close ties with the Scottish Enlightenment.[17] And Darwin's reference to "vegetable mansions" recalls John Locke's earlier use of the phrase "our mansion" to describe the fixed embodiment of the self – the archetypal model of Enlightenment subjectivity.[18] Darwin's poem certainly inherits the Lockean impulse to compartmentalize, contain, and classify according to finite, phenomenological categories. The preface of *The Loves of the Plants* faithfully echoes Locke's *Essay Concerning Human Understanding* (1690) with its neat divisions of all botanical life according to "number, situation, adhesion, and reciprocal proportion of the males in each flower" ("The Botanic Garden" 284). Unlike Locke, though, Darwin troubles the architectural metaphor as he liberates his botanical "prisoners" from "their respective vegetable mansions." For Darwin, Linnaean categories are simultaneously mansions and prisons, the central paradox that motivates his unique brand of botanical science and his ambitious goal to recover nature's "original animality" from the threat of scientific complacency. Even as he clings to the gilded cages of Enlightenment mansions, Darwin leaves ample room for a prison break.

The paradox of "prisoners" in "vegetable mansions" suggests that Darwin's couplet belies a formal complexity beyond the musical endings of his pentameter lines. As J. Paul Hunter reminds us, the couplet's neatly oppositional binarism is an over simplification, and he urges us to look past the *local* binarism to the "binaries in the total text" (116). Indeed, Darwin's poem is not even merely couplets; most of it is an extensive critical apparatus of footnotes, illustrations, dialogues, digressions, and essays. The generic diversity swiftly moves the poem past even the ostensibly easy management of local binary form to a sprawling and chaotic global paratextuality. Between cantos I and II of *The Loves of the Plants*, for example, Darwin inserts a strange dialogue (Interlude I) between the Bookseller and the Poet on the differences between poetry and prose ("The Botanic Garden" 326–31). The Bookseller worries out loud to the Poet about the profitability of a botanical poem and complains, "Your verses, Mr. Botanist, consist of *pure description*; I hope there is *sense* in the notes" ("The Botanic Garden" 326). This is a playfully meta-fictional moment in which the Bookseller talks about the notes within the notes while the Poet muses about genre within a curious, generic blend of botanical verse and prosaic exposition. In drawing attention to questions of genre, Darwin recalls the historical relationship between the heroic couplet and the eighteenth-century dialogue, which Hunter ably summarizes:

> Perhaps it is something they [poets of the long eighteenth century] learned from the disastrous binary choices that public institutions and political structures tended to enforce, but the antithetical discourse of the period – in poetry and prose – repeatedly and systematically breaks down and redefines easy oppositions, which is one reason that the dialogue was so popular a form. That process of redefinition and refinement is almost a description of what philosophical discourse was in the post-Hobbesian moment, and it is virtually the program assumed by the Anglophone pentameter couplet. (116)

Not only does Darwin prefer dialogic forms, but he also amplifies the irony of such a form – the manufacturing of "easy oppositions" only to subject them to a simultaneous "process of redefinition and refinement" – by proliferating his increasingly complicated paratextual apparatus. The poem's hybrid form, then, stretches the parameters of eighteenth-century Enlightenment discourse to its limit and prevents those Lockean "vegetable mansions" from contracting into vegetable prisons.

This hybrid dialogic form turns out to be an appropriate match for the hybrid botanical content. Darwin privileges varieties, grafts, and layers over more fixed Linnaean categories of order, genus, family, and species. In the preface, his botanical system is described as a series of nuptial pairings:

> The illustrious author of the Sexual System of Botany, in his preface to his account of the Natural Orders, ingeniously imagines, that one plant of each Natural Order was created in the beginning; and that the intermarriages of these produced one plant of every Genus, or Family; and that the intermarriages of these Generic, or Family plants, produced all the Species: and, lastly, that the intermarriages of the *individuals* of the Species produced the *Varieties*. ("The Botanic Garden" 288; emphasis mine)

In typical Darwinian fashion, he personifies the propagation of plants as the "intermarriages of the individuals." His plants are endowed with *individual* Lockean

subjectivities beyond Linnaeus's flowery prisons. Plants instead have an anthropomorphic free will that explains the long and mysterious process of botanical variegation, cultivation, selective breeding, and grafting. In this sense, Darwin works
within the Enlightenment tradition's deistic worldview, "*Deus creavit, Linnaeus
disposuit*"; or, in Darwin's variation, God created the "Natural Order" while "individuals" continue to produce the future "Varieties" of that order through their
increasingly mixed assemblages. "Varieties," rather than "Natural Orders," are the
end point of Darwin's botanical lineage; he gives them pride of place in both preface and poem. Unlike Linnaeus, who suppresses his uncertainty about the nature
of varieties (genetic mutation was not yet part of botanical science's vocabulary)
in favour of fixed, unchanging categories, Darwin prefers to dwell on the unex-
plained (and unexplainable, at the time) complexities of botanical variegation. Yet
this is not just a simple case – like Burke's inoculated plant – of excessive poetic
licence carelessly overrunning scientific precision. Darwin's departure from Linnaeus intervenes in a very real eighteenth-century scientific debate about the fixity
of species. Remarkably, his discussions of botanical variegation (codified later by
Gregor Mendel and his law of segregation) anticipate evolutionary theory without
any recourse to genetic evidence. These metaphorical leaps would culminate in
Charles Darwin's later empirical verification of his grandfather's conjectures.

The eighteenth-century debate about species variation in which Darwin's poem
intervenes is perhaps most ably summarized by Bentley Glass, one of the twentieth century's most distinguished geneticists. According to his account, Linnaeus,
in the *Systema Naturae* of 1735, originally "accepted the foregoing conception of
the nature of species without troubling himself greatly about the problem of variation – a mere vexatious complication in the way of the great task of classification"
(228). Later, when he could no longer sustain his plausible deniability about the
problem of botanical variation, Linnaeus devised a new strategy of disavowal:

> In the *Philosophia Botanica* of 1751 Linnaeus makes clear the basis of the distinction.
> Species were not only those entities created in the beginning, but individuals of a
> species "multiply and produce, according to the laws of generation, forms always
> like themselves. This is why there are just so many species as there exist today diverse
> forms of structures." Varieties, on the other hand, were simply "plants of the same
> species modified by whatsoever occasional cause," such as "the climate, sun, warmth,
> the winds, etc." They relate only to "stature, color, taste, odor," and upon the return
> of the plant to its original environment, they revert to type. (Glass 228)

In this later work, Linnaeus takes tentative steps to account for the "diverse forms
of structures" in botanical life. Even as he begrudgingly acknowledges the incredible, observable variations within species, he still tries to explain them as just
"occasional" traits incurred through some ill-defined environmental stimuli: "the
climate, sun, warmth, the winds." The human hand, he argues, has a negligible

role in the proliferation of botanical varieties, and the diversity we observe in the botanical world is just a result of temporary and passive variation. Even though Darwin cites the *Philosophia Botanica* in his preface as the primary Linnaean reference of *The Loves of the Plants*, he acknowledges that Linnaeus's scientific hand-waving is not much of an explanation, and he sets out to translate Linnaeus's equivocation into a more figurative and speculative language.

Darwin was not the first to take Linnaeus to task for his unsatisfactory answer to the botanical problem of variation. Michel Adanson, a French naturalist who contributed to some significant and enduring revisions to Linnaeus's botanical nomenclature, had similar qualms in his paper, "Examen de la question, si les espèces changent parmi les plantes; Nouvelles Expériences tentées à ce subjet" (1769). In this paper, he systematically refutes Linnaeus's stubborn exclusion of varieties in his botanical system and puts forth a proto-evolutionary view of plant life. After experimenting with different forms of plant propagation for almost a decade, Adanson concluded that many of the varieties that Linnaeus lumped into different species designations were in fact mutant varieties. In successive generations, these mutants, which Adanson dubbed *monstres* (monsters), would begin to produce "normal" progeny, proving that they belonged to the same parent species.[19] Adanson expressed these results in a more colourful language: "these monstrosities and variations have a certain latitude, necessary without doubt for the equilibrium of things, after which they return into the harmonious order preestablished by the wisdom of the Creator" (qtd. in Glass 231). Whereas Linnaeus refused to reconcile the "monstrosities" of the botanical world with God's "harmonious order" in favour of a more comfortable notion of species fixity, Adanson brazenly suggested that such divine "equilibrium" admits – and most likely even requires – variants, mutants, and even *monstres*. That provocative word *monstres* must have caught Darwin's ear during his botanical studies. Adanson's *monstres* enjoy "a certain latitude" to transform the "harmonious order" of species without entirely dismantling it. The Linnaeus-Adanson controversy, fixity against flux, authorized Darwin to expand the terms of that "certain latitude" to explain the organization of botanical life without a slavish adherence to Enlightenment orthodoxy, and to amplify Adanson's metaphorical *monstres* into fully fleshed-out botanical characters, teeming with vibrant life, sexual desire, and unpredictable psychologies. Adanson's throwaway metaphor would find full expression in the indeterminate realm of Darwin's imaginative fiction.[20]

Darwin's treatment of the wild fig tree, for example, begins with indulgently poetic trappings – "Closed in an azure fig by fairy spells / Bosom'd in down, fair CAPRI-FICA dwells" ("The Botanic Garden" II.iv.429–30) – but is packaged with a dense gloss about the variation, cultivation, and development of the plant. The verse itself is much more impatient. After the introductory couplet about "CAPRI-FICA," the poem immediately turns to a rapid-fire series of four analogies: "So sleeps in silence the Curculio" ("The Botanic Garden" II.iv.431); "So the pleased Linnet, in the moss-wove nest, / Waked into life beneath its parent's breast" ("The Botanic Garden" II.iv.435–6); "So with quick impulse through all Nature's frame / Shoots the electric air its subtle flame" ("The Botanic Garden" II.iv.447–8); and "So turns the impatient needle to the pole, Tho' mountains rise between, and oceans roll" ("The Botanic Garden" II.iv.449–50). This descriptive chain of fig, weevil, bird, lightning, and compass attempts to explain caprification – "A process resorted to for ripening figs by means of the puncture of insects produced on the wild fig (*Caprificus*), or by puncturing them artificially"[21] – through imaginative analogies in the verse and the more literally descriptive essay in the footnote. In both cases, Darwin describes caprification as a type of beneficial inoculation, an enervating penetration that can nonetheless prove salubrious. The "curculio," or weevil, is a parasite that feeds – with a long needle-like proboscis – on the kernels of immature nuts, preventing the tree from propagating its seed. The second analogy recasts penetrative inoculation as a type of birth, while the third and fourth analogies expand the figure towards the awful sublimity of atmospheric and geological phenomena. Caprification as inoculation wavers between the thematic registers of death (the curculio's parasitism on the nut tree) and birth (the linnet's piercing birth through the egg), of destruction (the lightning's noisy disturbance through "Nature's frame") and structure (the earth's fixed magnetic poles). The schizoid verse posits questions that it ultimately does not answer by itself. Do the benefits of these forms of inoculation outweigh the risks? Is inoculation an unnatural act, an abomination, or a sublime blasphemy? Shall we choose the curculio's deathly and parasitic proboscis or the linnet's liberating beak as the poem's representative take on the inoculating needle? Or perhaps the forking destruction of the lightning bolt or the invisible line of magnetic north that runs through mountain and ocean?

These eleven couplets about the wild fig are accompanied by a long botanical essay that begins to answer these questions. At this point, Darwin's essay on the wild fig is worth reproducing in full:

> *Capri-ficus.* l. 430. Wild fig. The fruit of the fig is not a seed-vessel, but a receptacle inclosing the flower within it. As these trees bear some male and others female flowers, immured on all sides by the fruit, the manner of their fecundation was very unintelligible, till Tournefort and Pontedera discovered, that a kind of gnat, produced in the male figs, carried the fecundating dust on its wings, (Cynips Psenes Syst. Nat. 919) and, penetrating the female fig, thus impregnated the flowers. For the evidence of this wonderful fact, see the word Caprification, in Milne's Botanical Dictionary. The figs of this country are all female, and their seeds not prolific; and, therefore, they can only be propagated by layers and suckers. Monsieur de la Hire has shewn, in the Memoir. de l'Academ. de Science, that the summer figs of Paris, in Provence, Italy, and Malta, have all perfect stamina, and ripen not only their fruits, but their seed; from which seed other fig-trees are raised; but that the stamina of the autumnal figs

are abortive, perhaps owing to the want of due warmth. Mr. Milne, in his Botanical Dictionary (art. Caprification), says, that the cultivated fig-trees have a few male flowers placed above the female within the same covering or receptacle; which, in warmer climates, perform their proper office, but in colder ones become abortive. And Linnaeus observes, that some figs have the navel of the receptacle open; which was one reason that induced him to remove this plant from the class Clandestine Marriage to the class Polygamy. Lin. Spec. Plant. ("The Botanic Garden" 407)

In the first paragraph, he restates the problem of variation in the context of the fig's unusual mode of fecundation: "a kind of gnat, produced in the male figs, carried the fecundating dust on its wings, and, penetrating the female fig, thus impregnated the flowers" ("The Botanic Garden" 407). The English fig tree, which has only female flowers, must then be a species variation that "can only be propagated by layers and suckers"; that is, only through human and insect caprification. The second paragraph documents different varieties created through human intervention in France, Italy, and Malta, ending with Darwin's dissatisfaction at his botanical mentor's explanation of this botanical diversity: "Linnaeus observes, that some figs have the navel of the receptacle open; which was one reason that induced him to remove this plant from the class Clandestine Marriage to the class Polygamy" ("The Botanic Garden" 407). Just as Adanson had done before, Darwin objects to Linnaeus's stubborn adherence to notions of species fixity and offers his own "conjecture." His concluding paragraph even borrows from Adanson's monstrous language:

From all these circumstances I should conjecture that those female fig-flowers, which closed on all sides in the fruit or receptacle without any male ones, are *monsters*, which have been propagated for their fruit, like barberries, and grapes without seeds in them; and that the Caprification is either an ancient process of imaginary use, and blindly followed in some countries, or that it may contribute to ripen the fig by decreasing its vigour, like cutting off a circle of the bark from the branch of a pear-tree. ("The Botanic Garden" 408; emphasis mine)

Adding to his already unwieldy list of analogues, Darwin proceeds to make comparisons with barberries, seedless grapes, and pears. Each analogy brings caprification closer to the language of smallpox inoculation; the "cutting," "prick[ing]," "punctur[ing]," and "wounding" of plants to ripen or sweeten fruit, along with the botanical etymology of the word inoculation, are deliberate evocations of the medical procedure. Consequently, Darwin's description of spinster fig flowers – "closed on all sides in the fruit or receptacle without any male ones" – as "monsters" incurs a triple meaning: (1) an uncharitable (and misogynistic) valence that invokes sensationalistic visual representations of smallpox victims as grotesque "monsters," (2) a scientific classification derived from Adanson's botanical mutants

(*monstres*), and (3) a synthesis that reclaims smallpox victims as "monsters" inoculated against the diseases of the "normal." Monstrosity – in both figurative and
scientific senses of the word – produces sweeter fruit, stronger trees, easier propagation, and healthier bodies. The wavering verse begins to make more sense with
the footnote's diligent regulation of inoculation that the volatile medico-botanical
figure that confounds and unsettles even as it preserves and enhances the fragile
economy of botanical and human health. Darwin, in this sense, is an advocate for
inoculation, but with none of Jenner's apologetic disgust with the cross-species
traffic of modern life.

This "economy of vegetation" is the poem's central theme (and the title of the
first volume). Animals, plants, and humans interact with each other in an intricate
network of what Darwin calls "depredations" (what we would call the food chain).
These intermixed ecologies are natural and salubrious unlike Jenner's introductory
description of "The deviation of Man from the state in which he was originally
placed by Nature." However, when Darwin describes a family of poisonous plants –
Dictamnus, Mancinella, Urtica, and Lobelia – he encounters a dangerous and
exceptional world apparently full of what Coleridge would call "motiveless ma-
lignity," of venomous and nefarious plants that continuously pollute our air with
toxin, gas, and disease:

> Round the vex'd isles where fierce tornadoes roar,
> Or tropic breezes sooth the sultry shore;
> What time the eve her gauze pellucid spreads
> O'er the dim flowers, and veils the misty meads;
> Slow o'er the twilight sands or leafy walks,
> With gloomy dignity DICTAMNA stalks;
> In sulphurous eddies round the weird dame
> Plays the light gas, or kindles into flame.
> If rests the traveler his weary head,
> Grim MANCINELLA haunts the mossy bed,
> Brews her black hebenon, and, stealing near,
> Pours the curst venom in his tortured ear. –
> Wide o'er the mad'ning throng URTICA flings
> Her barbed shafts, and darts her poison'd stings.
> And fell LOBELIA's suffocating breath
> Loads the dank pinion of the gale with death.
> – With fear and hate they blast the affrighted groves,
> Yet own with tender care their *kindred Loves*! – ("The Botanic Garden" II.iii.179–96)

The villainous "DICTAMNA" invades the mostly idyllic tropical climate of the
first four lines with its "sulphurous eddies" of flammable gas, the ghostly "MANC-
INELLA" stealthily murders the unwary passerby with her Shakespearean venom,

the bellicose "URTICA" fires her poisoned arrows upon "the mad'ning throng," and the insidious "LOBELIA" resorts to merciless germ warfare. These "gloomy," "grim," and "fell" assassins seem to be the botanical world's unrepentant criminals, plants curiously excepted from nature's otherwise strictly regulated and caprified economy. Yet significantly, Darwin chooses to make no reference to Coleridge's motiveless and malignant Iago, preferring instead to cast Mancinella as Claudius, the repentant avuncular villain of *Hamlet*, and Urtica as Falstaff, the genial fool of the Henry plays. Early on in *Hamlet*, the ghost of Hamlet's father narrates Claudius's plan to pour "the curst venom in his tortured ear": "Upon my secure hour thy uncle stole, / With juice of cursed hebenon in a vial" (*Hamlet* I.v.61–2). This, of course, is echoed in the "black hebenon" of Darwin's Mancinella. The subsequent reference to *Henry V* is less explicit. Falstaff's mostly beneficial influence on Prince Hal is described in botanical terms: "The strawberry grows underneath the nettle [Urtica] / And wholesome berries thrive and ripen best / Neighboured by fruit of baser quality" (*Henry V* I.i.62–4). With both Shakespearean references, the violent depredations of these poisonous plants move towards an uneasy symbiosis. Mancinella as Claudius recalls the redemptive potential in "the conscience of the King" (*Hamlet* II.ii.605) and Urtica as Falstaff reminds us of Prince Hal's debt to his formative debauchery. And the final couplet's portrayal of Lobelia as a fierce protector of her family succeeds in humanizing her "suffocating breath." Still, the quickness of the chiming couplet mostly obscures these quieter moments and leaves us with a lasting impression of these poisonous plants as brutal, mercenary, violent, and treacherous.

As in the case of the wild fig, Darwin relies on the explanatory footnotes to slow down the rapid-fire verse. His discussion of Dictamnus – the burning bush of the Old Testament – provides him an occasion for a lesson in the uses of essential oils as narcotics, analgesics, and restoratives. Of particular interest is his extended anecdote about turpentine, a resin from the pine tree now used mostly as an industrial solvent: a "M. de Thosse" noted that "a small quantity of oil of turpentine" could destroy insect infestations and prevent future parasites from feeding on his trees, but when applied to a nectarine tree, the turpentine mixture "killed both the insect and the branches" ("The Botanic Garden" 363). The poisonous Mancinella fruit and the deadly Lobelia flower have similarly beneficial uses as emetics and perfumes. These "vegetable secretions" ("The Botanic Garden" 363) walk the fine line between debilitating poison and medical palliative, a point that Darwin makes by placing Urtica (the nettle) in the same figurative company as smallpox inoculation. In an analogy to inoculation procedures, Darwin pays close attention to both the quantity of poison and the method of exposure when he explains human interactions with the nettle:

> *Urtica.* l. 191. Nettle. The sting has a bag at its base, and a perforation near its point, exactly like the stings of wasps and the teeth of adders. Hook, Microgr. p. 142. Is the fluid contained in this bag, and pressed through the perforation into the wound made

by the point, a caustic essential oil, or a concentrated vegetable acid? The vegetable poisons, like the animal ones, produce more sudden and dangerous effects, when instilled into a wound, than when taken into the stomach; whence the families of Marfi and Psilli, in ancient Rome, sucked the poison, without injury, out of wounds made by vipers, and were supposed to be indued with supernatural powers for this purpose. By the experiments related by Beccaria, it appears, that four or five times the quantity, taken by the mouth, had about equal effects with that infused into a wound. ("The Botanic Garden" 363–4)

Just as M. de Thosse had discovered that turpentine can effectively destroy aphids without killing the tree, Darwin finds unconventional and potentially dangerous ways to cure disease – through vomiting, purging, or intoxicating – without killing the patient. The wounding penetration of the stinging nettle, the wasp, and the adder can easily pass "without injury," depending on the control of "quantity" and the circumstances of exposure. Those ostensibly "supernatural" healers of ancient Rome, for example, could orally extract poison "instilled into a wound" without succumbing to the fatal venom themselves. Here, Darwin follows through on his ambitious mission statement – "to inlist Imagination under the banner of Science" ("The Botanic Garden" 12) – with his Enlightenment-inspired drive to purge superstition and "supernatural powers" from science. The empirical demystification of Roman fantasy draws much of its force from the material example of smallpox inoculation, a proven example of infectious matter *safely* "instilled into a wound." Immunity no longer had to subsist on "supernatural" explanation.

The figure of inoculation, in both its botanical and medical registers, regulates the poem's balancing act between verse and footnote, imagination and science, and metaphor and material. With the case of caprification, Darwin confines the penetrative metaphor to plants and insects, but with the poisonous plants, he starts to explore more adventurous inoculations of the *human* body. The association of Urtica with Falstaff, for example, introduces the idea that controlled exposure to the filth, disease, and poison of the tavern eventually leads Hal to be an effective king, immunizing his mortal body against the infection of the "fruit of baser quality" (*Henry V* I.i.64). In his notes, Darwin literalizes his reading of *Henry V* with the medical adaptation of poisons into balms: "These pungent or nauseous juices of vegetables have supplied the science of medicine with its principal materials" ("The Botanic Garden" 363). Just as Falstaff preaches excess to teach kingly moderation, poisonous plants like Mancinella serve as "purge, vomit, intoxicate, &c" ("The Botanic Garden" 112) to re-establish a healthful bodily economy. The economy of vegetation overgrows its vegetable prisons and mansions because of these incredibly unpredictable, messy, and even perverse interactions of the botanical world. Adanson's *monstres*, Darwin's "grafts and layers," and the hybrids of botanical science branch out into tangled relationships – poisonous, salutary, parasitic, symbiotic – among plants, animals, and even human beings.

Even though Darwin's poem constantly threatens to break out of his carceral metaphor, it falls short of dramatizing Burke's catastrophic vision of botanical pollution from a "cyon alien to the nature of the original plant." Darwin's mansion remains standing long enough to match Burke's own botanical terms, never contracting into the "prison" of Burke's "body and stock of inheritance" (181). Darwin's exposure of Burke's mistake about inoculation wins a political point by tightening the "looser analogies" of Burke's confused imagination into the "stricter ones which form the ratiocination of philosophy" ("The Botanic Garden" 12). Darwin's post-Enlightenment refutation of Burke clarifies what at first seems like a paradoxical politics. On the one hand, his radicalism insists on cultural contamination, cosmopolitan cross-pollination, and fluid dialogue while rejecting a stodgy Burkean society based on chivalric inheritance. On the other hand, he wants to prove that "alien" inoculation is not the terrible cultural pollution that Burke imagines in *Reflections*, forcing Darwin to contain all that potentially eruptive excess – monstrosity, bodily violation, and penetrative contamination – into a neat quasi-Linnaean system of botanical nomenclature that collects the supposedly dangerous residues of revolution into manageable categories and Lockean mansions. Darwin's radical politics have been notoriously hard to gauge because of this hedging. Critics have speculated that Darwin's proto-evolutionary thought might indicate a radical belief in a kind of Godwinian perfectibility. Others vaguely link his promiscuous plants to a Kantian history of cosmopolitanism.[22] The botanical metaphor provides further insight into Darwin's speculative politics. His radical evolutionary theory is a path of organic progress that nonetheless requires diligent mapping. Enlightenment "ratiocination" closely polices the cosmopolitan perversity of his medico-botanical world. Despite Burke's botanical error and the challenge to conventional medical and botanical taxonomies, the Burkean and Linnaean prisons remain standing as both an organizing principle and a limiting factor of Darwin's radical poem.

The Temple of Nature

Darwin eventually moves on up from his vegetable prisons and mansions into a temple. His last long poem, *The Temple of Nature* (1803), loosens the preoccupation with Linnaean containment by expanding his subject well beyond botanical science. Most critics agree that it is the better poem, but perhaps it is less well-known because of its thematic unevenness. The encyclopedic poem catalogues all forms of life in the natural world in an expansive vision that challenges, and even unsettles, botanical economy:

> So erst the Sage with scientific truth
> In Grecian temples taught the attentive youth;
> With ceaseless change, how restless atoms pass,
> From life to life, a transmigrating mass;

> How the same organs, which to day compose
> The poisonous henbane, or the fragrant rose,
> May, with to morrow's sun, new forms compile,
> Frown in the Hero, in the Beauty smile.
> Whence drew the enlighten'd Sage, the moral plan,
> [That] man should ever be the friend of man;
> Should eye with tenderness all living forms,
> His brother-emmets, and his sister-worms.   (*The Temple of Nature* IV.417–28)

The corresponding footnote acknowledges the poem's debt to Pythagoras's theory of the transmigration of souls from which Darwin imagines a "transmigrating mass," a natural world that teems with interpenetrative relations and interchangeable bodies. Here, his architectural paradox opens into a new spatial metaphor that relocates "scientific truth" from prisons and mansions to "Grecian temples," an awkward juxtaposition of the ever-expanding field of scientific knowledge with the ever-contracting dogma of religious orthodoxy.[23] His eponymous temple, though, is far from a dogmatic prison. Whereas *The Botanic Garden* softens the restrictive binary of imagination and science, *The Temple of Nature* undoes it entirely. Darwin is finally able to write a poem in which science and poetry, fact and faith, blend together effortlessly. This passage, for example, replaces Darwin's defensive posture with a positive vision of natural multiplicity; hybrid forms no longer depend on caprification or the inoculating penetration of one body into another, because he imagines instead just an embodied unity of "all living forms" slowly evolving in a majestic "transmigrating mass." Now, when he speaks of poisonous plants ("henbane," or in the earlier Shakespearean version, "hebenon") and botanical perfumes ("the fragrant rose"), he forgoes the Shakespearean hedging and loudly celebrates how these plants "May, with to morrow's sun, new forms compile." All grafts, layers, hybrids, mutants, and *monstres* amalgamate into one inclusive and evolving community of "brother-emmets" and "sister-worms." This concluding cosmopolitan vision of radical intermixing is much more than Linnaean systems, Lockean mansions, and Burkean hierarchies. His renovated temple readily admits faith, speculation, and uncertainty.[24]

Even though *The Temple of Nature* finally frees Darwin's nascent evolutionary theory from the Enlightenment urge to catalogue, classify, and contain, his treatment of smallpox retains a lingering scepticism. By the time Darwin finished the poem, Jenner had already published his *Inquiry* and the cowpox vaccine had already begun making its preliminary rounds. In his first explicit mention of smallpox, Darwin discusses immunity in a lengthy analogy to what he calls the "Approach of Age":

> On the contrary, many animal motions by perpetual repetition are performed with
> less energy; as those who live near a waterfall, or a smith's forge, after a time, cease

to hear them. And in those infectious diseases which are attended with fever, as the small-pox and measles, violent motions of the system are excited, which at length cease, and cannot again be produced by application of the same stimulating material; as when those are inoculated for the small-pox, who have before undergone that malady. Hence the repetition, which occasions animal actions for a time to be performed with greater energy, occasions them at length to become feeble, or to cease entirely. (*The Temple of Nature* II, n. VII, sec. III)

Here, he rehearses the old-fashioned notion of life and human volition as a temporary irritation of dead matter. Just as the inoculated smallpox sufferer becomes immune to subsequent infection, the "perpetual repetition" of "animal motions" causes a kind of accommodative attrition which eventually leads to old age and death. He deftly eschews Jenner's word "vaccine," explaining that those who have already contracted the disease do not undergo stimulating "animal motions" when "inoculated *for* the small-pox" (emphasis mine). That "for" (a simple substitution of "with" would quickly clarify his point as a reference to variolation) strategically obscures his position on the heated debates about vaccine safety. In a poem ostensibly about how all organisms of the natural world exist together in a "transmigrating mass," this evasiveness, perhaps even squeamishness, about cross-species inoculation is quite jarring.

The second mention of smallpox more clearly expresses the explosive force of Darwin's new speculative methodology. The eighth note goes on at length about human reproduction, employing, in typical Darwinian fashion, an explanatory analogy to convey his point:

There is one curious circumstance of animal life analogous in some degree to this wonderful power of reproduction; which is seen in the propagation of some contagious diseases. Thus one grain of variolous matter; inserted by inoculation, shall in about seven days stimulate the system into unnatural action; which in about seven days more produces ten thousand times the quantity of a similar material thrown out on the skin in pustules! (*The Temple of Nature* II, n. VIII, sec. IV)

This striking connection between human reproduction and viral propagation further unsettles Darwin's earlier classificatory project, for if human and animal lives are indeed "analogous in some degree" to the lives of "contagious diseases," then Linnaeus's vision of an ordered universe sounds more and more like a pipe dream. In this passage, Darwin replaces his erstwhile evasiveness and squeamishness about such natural disorder with utter excitement. He marvels at the "unnatural action" of the smallpox virus ("variolous matter"), even punctuating his gleeful observation with an exclamation about the speedy appearance of "pustules" on the skin. Here, Darwin's indulgence in imaginative speculation is on full display.[25] The temple affords Darwin the space to explore the myriad implications of the inoculation metaphor without the pressures of Linnaean fidelity. Now, Darwin not only deviates from Burke's fearmongering about inoculation as cultural contamination, but also from his own handling of inoculation in *The Loves of the Plants*; rather than the incredibly evasive dance around caprification, he bluntly literalizes the connection between plants and bodies with "one grain of variolous matter; inserted by inoculation." In this poem, Darwin decides that inoculation is neither corruptive contamination (Burke) nor monstrous hybridity (*The Loves of the Plants*). Instead, it settles into a gentler metaphor of cosmopolitan unity, of new forms continuously compiling, of a transmigrating mass of natural evolution.

Even in the expanded temple, Darwin's radical metaphor of inoculation remains largely noncommittal. His lingering faithfulness to Enlightenment closure contains the more eruptive corollaries of inoculation – contamination, violation, abomination, and revolution – into the safe, post-Linnaean system of the "transmigrating mass." Darwin's rehearsal of the long, carceral history of botanical inoculation gets him to the cosmopolitan conclusion of *The Temple of Nature*, but along the way he accumulates the Burkean terms of conservative circumspection and hierarchical deference. The utopia of "brother-emmets" and "sister-worms" models a cosmopolitan end in which life has suddenly cast off its need for nomenclature, prisons, and mansions. Frantz Fanon would later accuse this strain of Darwinian cosmopolitanism of under-theorized utopianism:

> The characteristic, virtually endemic weakness of the underdeveloped countries' national consciousness is not only the consequence of the colonized subject's mutilation by the colonial regime. It can also be attributed to the apathy of the national bourgeoisie, its mediocrity, and its deeply cosmopolitan mentality. (98)

The decolonized subject, according to Fanon, merely reproduces the colonizer's regime as a naive and "cosmopolitan" universalism that obscures the real work of revolution. Darwin's handling of the inoculation metaphor – the dizzyingly circuitous figures of *The Loves of the Plants* and the quiet yet exciting taboo of *The Temple of Nature* – marks out his weak political commitment to the cosmopolitan conclusion. By relying on the terms of Linnaean classification, idealistic universalism, and a squeamish neutrality on the vaccination question, Darwin muffles the eruptive metaphor with Enlightenment guilt, a strategy that dreams of a beautiful cosmopolitan end without the messy revolutionary means. In a telling letter to Jenner, for example, Darwin jumps forward to an idyllic future of smallpox eradication:

> Your discovery of preventing the dreadful havoc made among mankind by the small-pox, by introducing into the system so mild a disease as the vaccine inoculation produces, may in time eradicate the small-pox from all civilized countries, and this especially: as by the testimony of innumerable instances the vaccine disease is so

favourable to young children, that in a little time it may occur that the christening and vaccination of children may always be performed on the same day. (qtd. in Baron 541)

In the place of the ox-faced boys and bovine pregnancies of vaccination caricature, Darwin substitutes a calmer image of innocent babes at the baptismal font. His work takes the sting out of the inoculating needle and sacrifices material precision for a more comfortable and ordered medical cosmology. Even without the stomach for the convulsive, lived experience of revolution, however, Darwin's experiments still managed to rescue the radical *potential* of the inoculation metaphor from the Linnaean prison house of botany.

Chapter Three

Blake's Revolutionary Metaphor

Darwin and Blake

Unlike Darwin, William Blake is a poet and visual artist that famously has no patience for Enlightenment hedging. His distaste for our "mind-forg'd manacles" ("London" 88) amplifies Darwin's disruptive poetics of botanical inoculation and shapes a transitional moment of medical history mired in deep, ontological anxieties about vaccination. Blake juggles the same terms – botany, inoculation, and radicalism – while introducing a volatile new one into the conversation: infection. Blake's poems have little of the raucous visual satire of Gillray's human-bovine hybrids (figure 6), but he delights in its outrageous provocation of bodies transformed by cross-species infection. As a commercial engraver for Darwin's *Botanic Garden*, Blake learned from the same medico-botanical sources, but instead of his client's dreamy cosmopolitan utopia, he constructs a mythopoetic world in the violent grip of both evolutionary *and* revolutionary becoming. In the end, Blake's experiment takes him far beyond Darwin's neat architectural bounds.

The young Blake, however, began in the shadow of Darwin's short-lived celebrity. After the publication of the wildly successful *The Loves of the Plants* in 1789, Darwin impatiently sought a suitable engraver for *The Economy of Vegetation* (which became the first volume of *The Botanic Garden* even though it was written later in 1791). Part of that project was a long and idiosyncratic digression about the Portland Vase, a notoriously indecipherable Roman artefact from the first century.[1] In a letter from the radical publisher Joseph Johnson, Darwin learned of some prickly copyright issues: "It is not the expense of *purchasing* Bartolozzi's plates that is any object; they *cannot be copied* without Hamilton's consent, being protected by act of parliament" (*Collected Letters* 386). After Sir William Hamilton purchased the vase in 1778, he commissioned the artist G.B. Cipriani to draw it for the engraver Francesco Bartolozzi. Since Hamilton ran into some financial troubles with the vase, obtaining consent would undoubtedly have proven a costly enterprise. Instead, Johnson proposed another solution: "Blake is certainly capable of making an exact copy of the vase,

I believe more so than Mr. B[artolozzi], if the vase were lent him for that purpose" (*Collected Letters* 386). Since Blake had already begun work on some engravings for *The Economy of Vegetation* with his colleague Henry Fuseli, Johnson thought him an appropriate (and relatively cheap) choice to work on the engraving of the Portland Vase. This is the much recounted story of when Blake met Darwin and of how Blake gained his peculiar employment as a copier (engraver) of a copy (painting) of a copy (Wedgwood replica of the Portland Vase).[2]

Johnson's assignment, to create "an exact copy of the vase," nicely captures Darwin's Enlightenment desideratum in *The Botanic Garden*. Blake's relationship to Enlightenment science, though, was significantly more hostile than Darwin's. Canonical Enlightenment figures such as Francis Bacon, John Locke, and Isaac Newton were frequent targets in Blake's critiques of hegemonic systems. And in one of his most famous statements on the subject, Blake's anti-Enlightenment rancour erupts into an angry analogy: "SCIENCE is the tree of DEATH / ART is the tree of LIFE" ("Laocoön" 403). So, it is not surprising that Blake scholars are eager to locate a falling out between Blake, the great poet-prophet against the relentless industrialization of Enlightenment science, and Darwin, the great proselytizer of scientific progress and invention.[3] The fire at the Albion Flour Mill in 1791, for example, could be a promising start. The factory's ruthlessly efficient machinery was designed by Darwin's fellow Lunar Society members Matthew Boulton and James Watt.[4] Whereas Darwin lamented the destruction of the latest industrial marvel, Blake celebrated the damage done to the Industrial Revolution's "dark Satanic Mills" ("Milton" 295). Here, Blakean protest sounds entirely incompatible with Darwinian scientism.

In "Jerusalem" (1804–20), he invokes the incident at the Albion Mill in the language of the Laocoön annotation:

> Then left the Sons of Urizen the plow & harrow, the loom
> The hammer & the chisel, & the rule & compasses; from London fleeing
> They forgd the sword on Cheviot, the chariot of war & the battle-ax,
> The trumpet fitted to mortal battle, & the flute of summer in Annandale
> *And all the Arts of Life they changd into the Arts of Death in Albion.*
>
> ("Jerusalem" 362; emphasis mine)

In both the "Laocoön" image and "Jerusalem," life and death correspond respectively to art and science, perhaps suggesting a straightforward opposition between Blake's revolutionary poetics and Darwin's Enlightenment propaganda. The "Jerusalem" passage, however, features something stranger than ideological polarity. The instruments of science, industry, progress, and the factory – the plow, the loom, the hammer, the chisel, the rule, and the compass – are not immediately bound up with "death"; instead of the easy equation of science and death in the "Laocoön" image, Blake insists in "Jerusalem" that these instruments "*changd* into the Arts of

Death" (emphasis mine). Just as the trumpet and the flute are not accountable for Scottish warmongering in Annandale, Boulton and Watt's inventions need not signify the unequivocal evils of industrial society. They are but motiveless instruments, the *potential* for industrial capitalism's unredeemable corruption.

There is, to make a long story short, still no explicit evidence of Blake's disenchantment with Darwin or vice versa. Matthew Green has gone even further to lean on the natural affinities between Blake and Darwin's Midlands Enlightenment:

> This approach, which risks reducing comparative reading to the search for Darwinian imagery in a Blakean corpus that is fundamentally hostile to Darwin and to the Midlands Enlightenment more generally, depends upon the representation of Darwin as the purveyor of a dehumanising and totalising scientific logic and of Blake as a straightforward opponent of empiricism and technological progress. In opposition to such representations, however, it is possible to identify in both Blake and Darwin a valorisation of intellectual heterogeneity that welcomes strife and dissension as indispensable to both the increase of knowledge and the progress of democracy. (205)

Part of this chapter's argument about Blake handles the unresolved debate about the Blake-Darwin relationship by tracking their various metaphorical uses of medical and botanical inoculation. Whereas Darwin abruptly imagines a cosmopolitan *end* through a quiet tabling of the vaccination controversy, Blake dwells on the medico-botanical metaphor to represent the chaotic *means* of revolutionary possibilities. Both use inoculation to deal with messy "intellectual heterogeneity" as well as "strife and dissension," but Darwin's instinct is to experiment within Linnaean boundaries while Blake allows the figure to proliferate freely across classifications. Neither is Darwin "dehumanizing and totalizing" nor is Blake a "straightforward opponent" of Enlightenment science; instead, both capitalize on a medical and scientific metaphor to model unique visions of healthful life. Darwin's tinkering trajectory from botanical grafting, to metaphorical inoculations, and finally to his cosmopolitan "transmigrating mass" of biological life excludes the middle terms of inoculation, infection, and revolution. Blake, however, builds unapologetically strange botanical hybrids and cross-species monsters to emphasize the various interpenetrations and violations of his mythologized human history. The figure of inoculation is a striking commonplace of both Darwin's and Blake's radicalisms, but where Darwin is tentative, Blake is borderline reckless. For him, the figure is at once botanical, animal, and human, the material trace of a world in the throes of revolutionary transformation.

Blakean Botany and Miltonic Trial

Blake's associations with two physicians – Darwin and John Birch – ensured that he kept well informed about both botanical and medical matters. William and

Catherine Blake were acquainted with Birch as early as 1801 (*Letters* 65). The most widely discussed contact between the Blakes and their physician – Birch's miraculous electrical cure of Catherine's chronic rheumatism – would have to wait until October 23, 1804 when Blake, in a letter to William Hayley, rejoiced at his wife's convalescence: "Electricity is the wonderful cause; the swelling of her legs and knees is entirely reduced" (*Letters* 136). This well-documented story about Birch's "Electrical Magic" (*Letters* 140) has already begun to inform some promising readings of Blake's poems and shed light on his relationship to Romantic medicine (Sha 216–17; Schott 2114–16). However, what remains untouched is Birch's medical pamphlet *Serious Reasons for Uniformly Objecting to the Practice of Vaccination*, which he wrote in the same month (October 1804, published in 1806) that Blake wrote of Catherine's recovery from her rheumatic pain. In this modest, but forcefully argued, seventy-four-page condemnation of the practice of vaccination, Birch adamantly refuses to "give up Experience for Experiment," and concludes quite definitively "THAT WHAT HAS BEEN CALLED THE COW POX IS NOT A PRESERVATIVE AGAINST THE NATURAL SMALL POX" ("Serious Reasons" 73–4). In this particularly hypocritical moment, he wags his finger at faddish pneumatic (nitrous oxide) cures of venereal diseases to prove his point about the ridiculousness of vaccination without even a word about his own endorsement (just a few years before) of equally faddish electroshock therapies to remove "Female Obstructions" ("Considerations" ii), his uniquely awkward term for irregular menstrual cycles. Birch's inconsistent turn from experimental medicine would prove a disappointment to Blake's increasing interest in radical science. Despite his early endorsement of Birch's "Electrical Magic," Blake resisted Birch's trajectory from transgressive "Experiment" to conservative "Experience," from radical medical trials to a slavish adherence to rational precedents and scientific method. From Birch's sceptical pamphlet, Blake emerged a stubborn advocate of both variolation and vaccination. His poetic work diverges from both medical mentors, Darwin and Birch, in its consistent refusal to equivocate about the pressing issue of vaccination. Neither Darwin's Enlightenment strategy of containment nor Birch's sudden medical apostasy fully captures the unique texture of Blake's revolutionary botanical, medical, and literary experiment.

With Birch out of the way, Blake also sought some ideological distance from Darwin, his erstwhile collaborator. In one of the iconic botanical images of Darwin's *The Loves of the Plants* (figure 8), each of Linnaeus's twenty-four categories of flowers is illustrated with detailed examples, neatly cordoned off from each other with rectilinear frames and displayed with the scientific precision of perfect containment. One can imagine how Blake's aesthetic motto – "Art can never exist without Naked Beauty displayed / No Secresy in Art" ("Laocoön" 403) – encountered this claustrophobic image. As the uncompromising artist of "Naked Beauty" prepared his work on *The Economy of Vegetation*, the "Secresy" of Darwin's Linnaean art must have made a stifling impression. Blake's "Secresy" derives etymologically

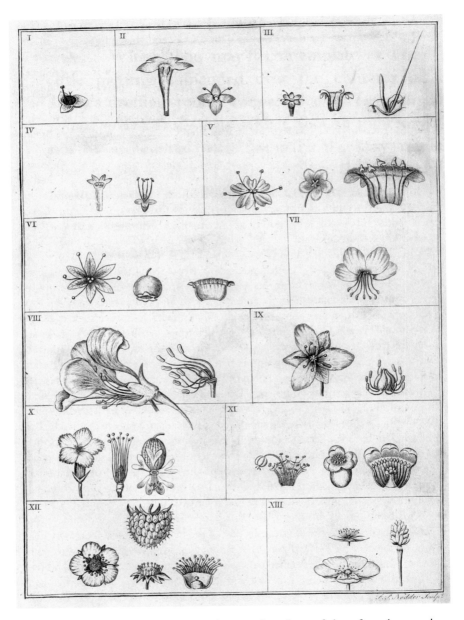

Figure 8. A reference image for Linnaeus's twenty-four classes of plants from the second part, *The Loves of the Plants*, of Erasmus Darwin's *The Botanic Garden*, 1791. Credit: Wellcome Collection. Public Domain.

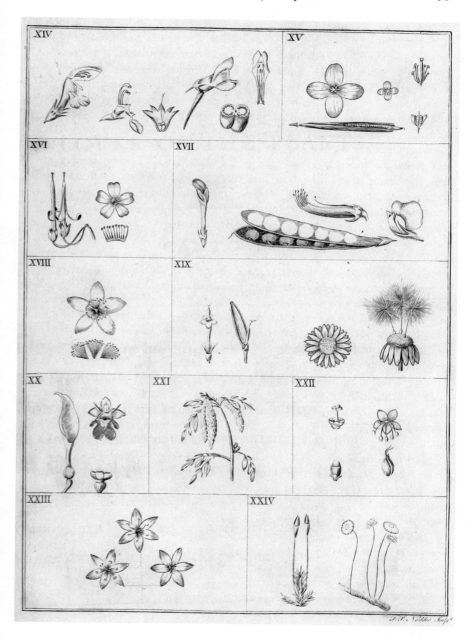

Figure 8. (*Continued*)

from the Latin *secernere*, meaning to separate or divide off, so his proclamation of "No Secresy in Art" surely renders these visual separations and divisions of Darwin's poem utterly unthinkable in Blake's own botanical work.[5] The poems that I consider in this chapter – "The Book of Thel" (1789), "Visions of the Daughters of Albion" (1793), and "The Sick Rose" (1794) – typify Blake's reaction to botany's coercive visual culture. In the botanical images of these three poems (figures 9–11), the flowers have broken out of their frames, forming sprawling, organic borders of tendrils, leaves, and thorns. Strange human images emerge from the flowers in seemingly random proportions. There is "No Secresy" in this "Art," no Linnaean containers labelled with Roman numerals; instead, through the dynamically interpenetrative textual and visual botanical representations of these three poems, Blake begins to shape a protean political allegory that radically rewrites a moral tale of virtuous, feminine chastity – Milton's "Comus" (1634) – into a long, narrative sequence that depends on the proliferating, sexualized image of botanical (and later, medical) inoculation.

That "Thel" references and even rewrites Milton's early masque is already a well-established critical commonplace. S. Foster Damon has even presented this influential interpretation as unerring fact in his *Blake Dictionary*: "*The Book of Thel* is best understood as a rewriting of Milton's "Comus" ... Blake tells the same story, but in biological terms, not moral ones" (52). Critics have followed up on this thread, but they tend to underestimate the extent of Blake's radical rethinking of "Comus."[6] In 1801, under the commission of Reverend Joseph Thomas, Blake began work on a set of eight illustrations from Milton's play. Fourteen years later, under the patronage of his friend Thomas Butts, Blake revised those same eight scenes with significant visual and thematic variations. In this misleadingly punctuated history, Blake references "Comus" only three times in twenty-six years (the publication of "Thel" in 1789, his "Comus" illustrations in 1801, and the revised illustrations in 1815), an unusually discontinuous history for an artist who consistently regarded Milton as his visionary muse. Already responsible for one of the most famous (mis)readings of Milton – his adulatory proclamation that the poet of *Paradise Lost* (1667) was "of the Devils party without knowing it" ("Marriage" plate 6) – Blake also continuously thought about similarly misshaping "Comus" and "Areopagitica" into his ideological mould.[7]

Thel's (and later Oothoon's and the sick Rose's) insistence on purity depends not only upon Milton's puritanical discourse of chastity, virginity, and virtue, but also on the temperamental botanical figure of inoculation. With this embedded discourse in Blake's revisionist arsenal, he grounds Miltonic typology in the material world of botanical science instead of obediently relying on Providence or "right Reason" (*Paradise Lost* 456). More specifically, Blake brazenly reinvents the Lady's constantly assailed virtue as a type of beneficial inoculation. Milton himself recapitulates this theme of virtuous trial throughout his career: (1) in "Comus," the Lady's elder brother insists, "this I hold firm; / Virtue may be assail'd but

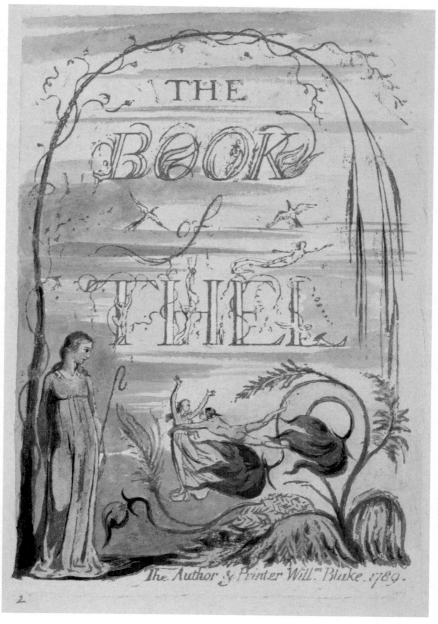

Figure 9. The title page of *The Book of Thel* by William Blake, 1789. Call # 57434, The Huntington Library, San Marino, California.

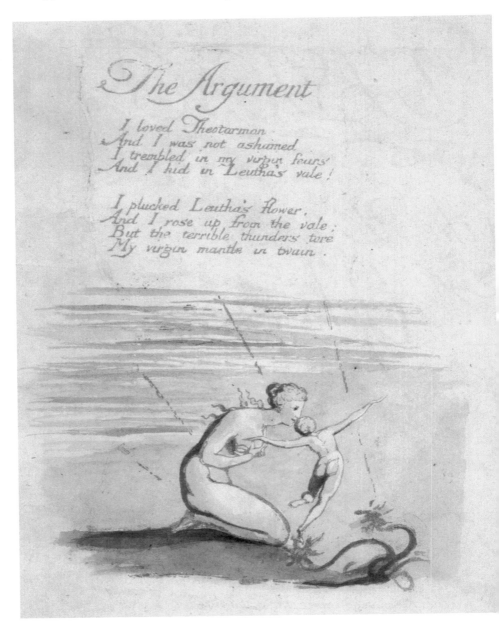

Figure 10. "The Argument" from "Visions of the Daughters of Albion" by William Blake, 1793. Call # 42625, The Huntington Library, San Marino, California.

never hurt, / Surpris'd by unjust force but not enthrall'd" (103), (2) in "Areopagitica," Milton's prose defence of free speech argues, "I cannot praise a fugitive and cloistered virtue, unexercised and unbreathed, that never sallies out and sees her adversary, but slinks out of the race where that immortal garland is to be run for, not without dust and heat" (728), and (3) in *Paradise Lost*, Eve uses a similar argument to convince Adam to divide their Edenic labours: "And what is Faith, Love, Virtue unassay'd / Alone, without exterior help sustain'd?" (386). Virtue unexercised, unbreathed, and unassayed is anathema to both Milton and Blake, but whereas the former holds to an unyielding faith in the organizing power of Godly rectitude, the latter argues from the medico-botanical example of immunity to tell a much more subversive story.

The character of Thel could be seen as a virgin of mindless, retreating purity – of Milton's "fugitive and cloistered virtue" – who finally refuses the poem's Darwinian aphorism, "Everything that lives / Lives not alone, nor for itself" ("Thel" plate 3, 26–7).[8] At the end of the poem, the persistent and inquisitive youngest daughter of Mne Seraphim ultimately rejects the world of horrible experience and returns to her angelic family of divine innocence: "The Virgin started from her seat, & with a shriek / Fled back unhinderd till she came into the vales of Har" ("Thel" plate 6, 19–20). The ambiguity of these last two lines – Thel's fearful "shriek" could just as well be a "shriek" of judicious defiance – leaves the complicated world of experience outside the vales of Har; its dark influence, while menacingly visible across the "eternal gates" ("Thel" plate 6, 1), does not irrevocably contaminate Thel's divine virtue.[9] In this case, Thel is far from a victim of Milton's cautionary tale about "cloistered virtue"; she has braved the considerable trial of "dust and heat," and, like the virtuous Lady of "Comus," has returned to her family stronger and wiser. The quasi-Darwinian title plate (figure 9) illustrates this endorsement of Thel's return to her life in the perfect "economy of vegetation" through an exuberant visualization of botanical life. The brittle arch of the weeping willow, gently constricted by coiling tendrils, suggests both beginning and end in its simultaneous evocation of frontispiece and gravestone. From the blossoms of the pasqueflower (*Anemone pulsatilla*), emerge two joyous human figures, no doubt an allusion to Darwin's observation about the same flower in *The Loves of the Plants*:

> There is a wonderful conformity between the vegetation of some plants, and the arrival of certain birds of passage. Linnaeus observes, that the wood anemone [the pasqueflower] blows in Sweden on the arrival of the swallow; and the marsh mary-gold, Caltha, when the cuckoo sings." ("The Botanic Garden" 316–17)

The entwined willow, the blooming pasqueflowers, the erupting human figures, and the circling swallows that populate the plate all exist in this "wonderful conformity," ostensibly the divine reward of Thel's virtuous choice. An unopened flower bud even leans seductively towards her to invite her to participate in this magnificent spectacle of idyllic nature, completing the robust Darwinian person-ification of Thel's botanical world.

But there is already a creeping sickness in the vales of Har. This early poem introduces the "worm of the silent valley" ("Thel" plate 3, 29), a central figure in Blake's extended visual-poetic meditation on the inoculation metaphor that reap-pears in crucial moments of both "Visions of the Daughters of Albion" and "The Sick Rose."[10] Still apprehensive of her fading life, Thel complains to the Cloud that she will "only live to be at death the food of worms" ("Thel" plate 3, 23). Thel's subsequent encounter with the infant worm quickly corrects her mistaken, morbid image of the ostensibly nefarious parasite:

> Then Thel astonish'd view'd the Worm upon its dewy bed:
> "Art thou a Worm? image of weakness, art thou but a Worm?
> I see thee like an infant wrapped in the Lilly's leaf.
> Ah weep not, little voice, thou canst not speak, but thou can weep.
> Is this a worm? I see thee lay helpless & naked, weeping,
> And none to answer, none to cherish thee with mother's smiles."
>
> ("Thel" plate 4, 1–6)

Like the paradoxical title page, the worm evokes both beginning and end in its "helpless" infancy and its morbid predation on decaying flesh. In Thel's persis-tently interrogative mode, she asks in her disbelieving prejudice, "Is this a worm?," to which the motherly Clod of Clay responds with a gentle version of Darwin's cosmopolitan vision: that even the "meanest thing" ("Thel" plate 4, 11) – Blake's worm and Clod of Clay or Darwin's "brother-emmets" and "sister-worms" – par-ticipates in nature's complex cycles of life and death. In this sense, the worm signi-fies the precise materialization of Milton's morality tale; it provides Thel a glimpse of death, decay, and corruption without compromising her innocent virtue. It is the perfect potion of life and death, of fortified virtue and heroic trial.

Violence and Forgiveness

What changes, though, when "experience" leaves the comfortable realm of medi-ated metaphor and arrives at an embodied site of literal assault? The viscerally embodied violence of "Visions of the Daughters of Albion," for example, weighs blanket forgiveness against the visual sublimity of physical violation. When Blake claims, "The lamb misused breeds public strife / And yet forgives the butcher's knife" ("Auguries" object 14), does he intend to forgive all violence uncondition-ally? This couplet from "Auguries of Innocence" (1803) reveals an "attractive, popular Blake" who mixes "unsparing social insight" with the promise of "hope and healing" through a transformative imagination that resolves Heaven-raging and Hell-shuddering paradoxes with aphoristic consolation (Eaves et al.).[11] But is this sacral forgiveness also an implicit forgetting? In "Visions," Blake tackles the problem of violence not with the ringing aphorisms of "Auguries" or the unsullied virtue of "Thel," but with the fleshly immediacy of diseased human bodies.

Oothoon, the poem's protagonist and ardent advocate of free love, relies on Darwin's botanical metaphor to make her sexual point: "Sweetest the fruit that the worm feeds on" ("Visions" plate 6, 17). She argues against her lover Theotormon that her rape by his rival Bromion does not necessarily mark her with base impurity or fallen desire; rather, she argues that the experience of the sexual act makes her *more* desirable. Notably, Blake arrives at similar images at least two other times: in "The Marriage of Heaven and Hell," he likens the priest's curse on "fairest joys" to "the catterpiller [*sic*] choos[ing] the fairest leaves to lay her eggs on" ("Marriage" plate 9, 16), and in the design of "The Sick Rose" (1794), a parasitic vermicular form attaches itself to one of the largest leaves of the eponymous rose (figure 11). In other words, the "catterpiller" identifies the fairest leaf to feed on, the worm the sweetest fruit. This straightforward interpretation has informed most readings of Oothoon: just as the parasite's voracious interest attests to the botanical value of the host, so too does Bromion's rape of Oothoon confirm her sexual desirability.[12]

The material contexts of Oothoon's argument, however, distinguish it from both the parasitic images of "Marriage" and "The Sick Rose," and the hopeful paradoxes of "Auguries." As several studies of Blake have shown, Blake's intuitive grasp of Romantic-era science shaped his poetic production, so his nod to botanical science deserves greater attention than it has received.[13] When Mark Lussier speaks of Blake and science, he sees double: a poet who famously thundered against Newtonian mechanics and Lockean epistemology but also an amateur scientist who eagerly anticipated the advent of quantum physics.[14] Oothoon's argument about violence and forgiveness depends on our understanding of this doubled Blake who can appropriate, for example, the language of Newtonian calculus – "limit" and "fluxions" – to his own visionary ends. With these scientific contexts in mind, Oothoon's argument starts to sound quite different. Whereas the "catterpiller" actively consumes both the "fairest leaves" and the largest leaf of the sick rose, Oothoon deftly flips the image's negativity in her grammatical inversion of subject and predicate by imbuing the sweetest fruit with the provocative agency of a grammatical subject while relegating the feeding worm to a dependent clause: "Sweetest the fruit that the worm feeds on."

The deliberately awkward syntax makes available a reading that does not immediately take the worm as mere parasite. Blake avoids the much more fluidly idiomatic construction, "The worm feeds on the sweetest fruit." In this conventional rewriting, the meaning is clear enough: the worm identifies the "sweetest fruit" and *then* begins to feed. Oothoon's stranger formulation suggests a more ambiguous temporality, a crucial inversion that separates Oothoon's botanical argument from

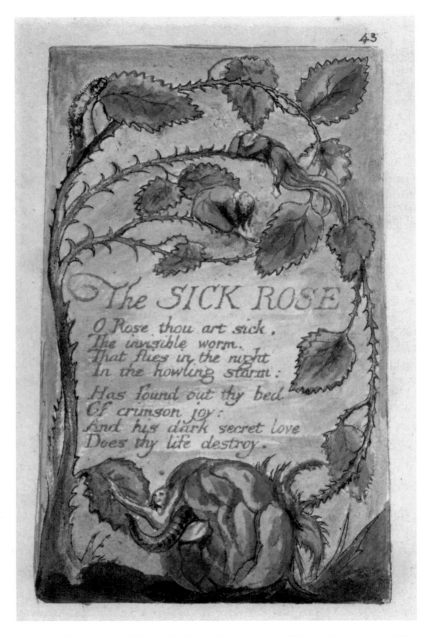

Figure 11. "The Sick Rose" from *The Songs of Experience* by William Blake, 1794. Call # 54039, The Huntington Library, San Marino, California.

the more legible ones of "Marriage" and "The Sick Rose." The metaphor has less to do with the discerning taste of a foul parasite than with a kind of symbiotic causality. Specifically, Blake's metaphor references Darwin's caprification in *The Loves of the Plants*, the fig tree's strange method of propagation that relies on the fig wasp's symbiotic predation.[15] In this Darwinian context, the worm's predation *engenders* the sweetness of the fruit in a kind of beneficial and botanical inoculation, making Oothoon's advocacy of free love infinitely more interesting and troubling. Through this invocation of botanical science, Blake struggles to imagine the exact form of forgiveness, its material conditions, its scientific plausibility, and its moral implications. I offer three preconditions for Blake's argument – Milton's "Comus," Darwin's *The Loves of the Plants*, and Montagu's *Turkish Embassy Letters* – not to apologize via contextualization for a violent and potentially misogynistic argument, but to begin to recover the medico-botanical research of a frequently nebulous Blakean poetics and to understand better the underestimated scope of Blake's radical and controversial reconfigurations of biological, sexual desire.

"Visions" begins where "Thel" ends. It even follows the exact sequence of Darwin's analogy about the "wonderful conformity" of nature: just as "Thel" borrows from Darwin's observation about the concurrence of the blooming pasqueflower and the "arrival of the swallow," "Visions" links the "marsh mary-gold, Caltha" with the singing cuckoo (figure 10). But whereas Thel merely observes the pasqueflowers at a distance, Oothoon, the female protagonist of "Visions," happily submits to the urging of the marigold/nymph in an intimate encounter:

> For the soft soul of America, Oothoon wanderd in woe,
> Along the vales of Leutha seeking flowers to comfort her;
> And thus she spoke to the bright Marygold of Leutha's vale
> Art thou a flower! art thou a nymph! I see thee now a flower;
> Now a nymph! I dare not pluck thee from thy dewy bed!
> The Golden nymph replied; pluck thou my flower Oothoon the mild
> Another flower shall spring, because the soul of sweet delight
> Can never pass away. she ceas'd & closd her golden shrine.
> Then Oothoon pluck'd the flower saying, I pluck thee from thy bed
> Sweet flower. and put thee here to glow between my breasts
> And thus I turn my face to where my whole soul seeks.   ("Visions" plate 4, 3–13)

If not for the replacement of the vales of Har with the vales of Leutha and the substitution of Oothoon's exclamation ("Art thou a flower!") for Thel's characteristic interrogative, these lines would hardly be out of place in the earlier poem. Like Thel, Oothoon begins her life happily in a world of constant regeneration – "the soul of sweet delight / Can never pass away" – and in the perfectly symmetrical cycles of life and death. The clothed Thel from the title plate, who eagerly awaits the opening of the pasqueflower bud becomes the nude Oothoon, who, in the argument plate, hastens her lips towards the desirous nymph while clutching the "Sweet flower" to her chest in a mildly sexual scene of botanical copulation. And Thel's "worm of the silent valley" reappears as Darwin's agent of caprification in Oothoon's paradoxical argument about sexual experience: "sweetest the fruit that the worm feeds on" ("Visions" plate 6, 17). Here, she exports the innocent image of the worm in "Thel" to the cruel world of experience in a forceful attempt to regenerate the decaying lives of repressed desire and enforced modesty. Blake offers this charged image of inoculation (via caprification) as Oothoon's solution to the problems of experience. Through this medico-botanical analogy, she makes the startling argument that virginal rape frees women from the bitterly repressive strictures of female modesty and introduces them to the "sweetest" liberated experience, unshackled from both Bromion's (her rapist) unitary law and Theotormon's (her rejecting lover) Enlightenment epistemology. Repressed heterosexual desire becomes the epidemic disease of this poem, and Blake's unlikely cure is Oothoon's botanical version of Montagu's famous Turkish inoculation, which the increasingly sickly Theotormon nevertheless rejects.

This organizing image of caprification as beneficial rape emerges in Oothoon's paradoxical discourse of purity:

> I call with holy voice! kings of the sounding air,
> Rend away this defiled bosom that I may reflect
> The image of Theotormon on my *pure* transparent breast.
> The Eagles at her call descend & rend their bleeding prey;
> Theotormon severely smiles. her soul reflects the smile;
> As the *clear* spring mudded with feet of beasts grows *pure* & smiles.
> ("Visions" plate 5, 14–19; emphasis mine)

Despite the misrecognition of this strange purity from both her lover Theotormon and her defiler Bromion, she persists in the inoculating language of Milton's tried virtue: her "defiled bosom" becomes the "pure transparent breast" and the "clear spring mudded with feet of beasts grows pure." Through this Promethean scene of purifying sacrifice, Oothoon brings the illuminating fire of violation to those who cower in the darkness of their secret desire. Her "transparent breast" and "clear spring" reflect not only the "image of Theotormon," but also the aggressive, "mudded" image of Bromion's violation. Oothoon successfully distills Theotormon's sadistic smile into the "clear spring" of her purified reflection. From the very beginning of her plaintive testimony, Oothoon's argument embarks upon the paradoxical logic of inoculation: the purification of Theotormon's sickly severity through the terrifying contamination of Oothoon's bloody violation.

Taking a Darwinian tack, Oothoon attempts to soften this paradox by sorting through some "looser analogies" about animal instinct – the chicken's fear of the hawk, the bee's hive mind, and the meekness of the camel – to naturalize her twisted logic until she arrives at the "stricter [analogies] which form the ratioci-nation of philosophy": her reference to caprification. The infant worm of "Thel" returns in this poem with "the secrets of the grave" ("Visions" plate 6, 10) and the pivotal analogy of Oothoon's counterintuitive "philosophy":

> Silent I hover all the night, and all day could be silent,
> If Theotormon once would turn his loved eyes upon me;
> How can I be defild when I reflect thy image pure?
> Sweetest the fruit that the worm feeds on & the soul preyed on by woe
> The new wash'd lamb ting'd with the village smoke & the bright swan
> By the red earth of our immortal river: I bathe my wings,
> And I am white and pure to hover round Theotormons breast.
>
> ("Visions" plate 6, 14–20; emphasis mine)

Armed with material evidence borrowed from Darwin's literary and botanical research, Oothoon reinvigorates her argument about her "image pure." Just as the worm-caprified fruit, the smoke-tinged lamb, and the clay-stained swan emerge sweeter, whiter, and purer, so too does Oothoon's sexual contamination and violation better prepare her for "happy copulation" ("Visions" plate 10, 1) with Theotormon. Purely metaphorical readings of this passage miscalculate this chain of causation: "The worm's assault *confirms* the sweetness of the fruit; the tinge of smoke *dramatizes* the whiteness of the lamb; and ... Oothoon's degrad-ing experience of sex *asserts* the holiness of her love" (Cox 113; emphasis mine). Caprification, however, transports Oothoon's argument to the botanical realm of natural law; consequently, the image of the worm is not merely Cox's "looser" correlation – confirmation, dramatization, and assertion – but rather "stricter" *causation*: the fruit's sweetness is not merely an independent property confirmed by the worm's interest, but is a necessary *product* of the process of caprification. These material precedents of Oothoon's rape insist on a return to this natural causality, to an instinctive love now blunted by the social construction of polite society. Thus, "the thoughts of man, that have been hid of old" ("Visions" plate 6, 13) must eventually re-emerge from their ancient hiding places to recontex-tualize Bromion's rape in the mitigating terms of caprification, of a fortifying botanical inoculation that erases from the sexually victimized body any poten-tial of corruption from "hypocrite modesty" ("Visions" plate 9, 16) or strained decorum. Oothoon appends botanical evidence to the theme of virtuous trial, transforming the Miltonic, literary appeal of "Thel" into Oothoon's Darwinian, scientific research.

Darwin's description of the wild fig tree and its unusual method of propagation entered Blake's metaphorical repertoire through their brief but formative collab-oration on *The Botanic Garden*. In an explanatory note to the fig tree, Darwin speculates:

Plumbs and pears punctured by some insect ripen sooner, and the part round the
puncture is sweeter. Is not the honey-dew produced by the puncture of insects? Will
not wounding the branch of a pear-tree, which is too vigorous, prevent the blossoms
from falling off; as from some fig-trees the fruit is said to fall off unless they are
wounded by caprification? ("The Botanic Garden" 408)

Here, Darwin takes several stabs at an explanation for caprification. The real
explanation is much simpler: the fig and the fig wasp participate in a unique symbiotic relationship in which the wasp pollinates the edible fig while the inedible
caprifig provides the wasps convenient receptacles for their eggs.[16] Darwin, however, prefers circuitous analogy to straightforward botanical explication. He imagines caprification as a type of beneficial inoculation that punctures and wounds
to produce the sweetness of various fruits. This insistently repeated language of
puncturing and wounding represents caprification as an enervating and preserving
penetration, a strikingly paradoxical account that nonetheless achieves a kind of
perverse cogency from its careful references to both botanical and medical science
(by this time Montagu had already popularized variolation in England). Consequently, Blake's rewriting of Darwin's assertion that "the part round the puncture
is sweeter" as "Sweetest the fruit that the worm feeds on" is not merely a throwaway line that blankly reconfirms the inherent holiness of Oothoon's sexuality;
instead, it affords her an increasingly misogynistic argument about generative violation some persuasive, medico-botanical evidence.

For Blake, mere Miltonic trial would prove rather quaint in the political tumult
of the 1790s. Both the Lady's test in "Comus" and Thel's final defiance ultimately
circumvent the problem of the fallen woman. The brothers rescue the Lady from
the lecherous Comus, and the question of violation never contaminates Milton's
discourse of virtue. Eighteenth-century literature would begin to deal with the
figure of the fallen woman according to a conventional pattern of what Roxanne Eberle has described as an "irremediable descent into first vice and then
death" (29). After Lovelace rapes Clarissa, for example, "the fallen woman cannot
imagine an alternate narrative script for her continued existence" (Eberle 29).
Just as Jacobin novels such as Mary Hays's The Victim of Prejudice (1799) began
to imagine this "alternate narrative script," Blake was similarly exploring the lived
experiences of alternative human sexuality. Milton, however, always seems uneasy
about the sexual dimensions of virtuous trial. After all, he deliberately deforms his
own argument in "Areopagitica" into the seductive strains of the villainous Comus
and the anti-heroic Satan. Blake does away with this sense of discomfort and
boldly rewrites the traditional plot of the fallen woman in the explicitly embodied terms of inoculation and violation. Unlike the Jacobin novels that chart the
fallen woman's "return to respectable society" (Eberle 95), though, Blake suggests
reforming "respectable society" itself with Oothoon's reclamation of virginal rape
as an expression of free love.

Oothoon's Experiment

This potentially anti-feminist rhetoric has produced a long critical history of confusion. Oothoon's problematic mimicry of patriarchal language, her resistance to Urizenic law, her tentatively abolitionist agenda, and her attack on global capitalism all seem to flounder in ideological incoherence. Consequently, her character has generated a curiously bifurcated history of criticism. On the one hand, feminist critics have taken Blake to task for his sexist, sadomasochistic fantasies of masculinist domination. On the other hand, Marxist critics have focused on the poem's triumphant denunciation of the language of commerce, particularly that of the slave trade.[17] The poem's sense of simultaneity and intersectionality, however, resists such dualistic parsing. Those "kings of the sounding air" are at once slave owners and avian rapists; the scene represents both the punishment of a disobedient slave and the rape of an already defiled woman. Towards the end of the poem, Oothoon's ironic lamentation, "Then is Oothoon a whore indeed! and all the virgin joys / Of life are harlots: and Theotormon is a sick mans dream / And Oothoon is the crafty slave of selfish holiness" ("Visions" plate 9, 18–20), finally makes impossible such compartmentalized and bifurcated readings; the poem's protagonist is both "whore" and "crafty slave," a doubly abject category that demands a more mixed account.

Perhaps anticipating an outraged reaction to his potentially anti-feminist rhetoric, Blake has Oothoon engage with not just her two male interlocutors (Theotormon and Bromion), but also two of the most learned literary women of the eighteenth century. First, he invokes the historic Mansfield judgment of 1772 and its relationship to the feminist politics of Mary Wollstonecraft. In the famous British court case, Lord Mansfield ruled that James Somerset, a Black slave in America who had escaped from his master in England, was indeed a free man, a landmark ruling that nominally made slavery illegal in England. Somerset's lawyer made his case by comparing slavery to marriage, a strictly legal institution that had no claim to universal rights or laws (Mellor, "Blake and Wollstonecraft" 345–70). Wollstonecraft capitalized on this analogy to link abolitionist and feminist causes: since marriage, like slavery, was a contractual arrangement of embodied property, taking a wife became tantamount to enslavement. Just a few years before the publication of "Visions," Blake encountered this nexus of ideas through his illustrations for Wollstonecraft's *Original Stories from Real Life* (1791), a collection of didactic tales about female rationality, proper education, and the ideal woman, liberated from the essentializing logic of slavery. Oothoon is not exactly Wollstonecraft's coolly rational and compassionate woman; she advocates instead a polyamorous free love in a passage that has proven to be the most shocking (and hardest to teach) moments in the poem:

But silken nets and traps of adamant will Oothoon spread,
And catch for thee girls of mild silver, or of furious gold;

I'll lie beside thee on a bank & view their wanton play
In lovely copulation bliss on bliss with Theotormon:
Red as the rosy morning, lustful as the first born beam,
Oothoon shall view his dear delight, nor e'er with jealous cloud
Come in the heaven of generous love; nor selfish blightings bring.

                                                ("Visions" plate 10, 23–9)

Here, Oothoon proposes to populate Theotormon's harem with various "girls of mild silver, or of furious gold." Her solution, "happy happy Love! free as the mountain wind" ("Visions" plate 10, 16), abolishes the contractual slavery of marriage in favour of ritualized virginal rape. In other words, her argument about the sweetness of caprified fruit threatens to reproduce, as Anne K. Mellor puts it, a heterosexual "male fantasy" of liberated sexuality ("Blake's Portrayal of Women" 148–55). If Blake's own views exactly coincide with Oothoon's speech, then "Visions" becomes an anti-feminist poem that unabashedly locates its advocacy of free love on the sacrificed body of Oothoon.

Whereas the influences of Milton, Darwin, and Wollstonecraft on Blake have been adequately documented, the possible balancing presence of Montagu – his riposte to the Wollestoncraftian concept of female rationality – has escaped critical scrutiny. Blake's oblique debt to Montagu's Turkish travels and her pioneering endorsement of variolation can be seen in at least two instances. First, Blake adds to his botanical reference an explicitly medical valence by alluding to Montagu's contraction of smallpox before her famous journey to Turkey, which occasioned her wistful poetic scene of lost innocence in her "Town Eclogues: Saturday; The Small-Pox" (1716):

Would pitying Heav'n restore my wonted mien,
Ye still might move unthought of and unseen:
But oh, how vain, how wretched is the boast
Of beauty faded, and of empire lost!
What now is left but, weeping, to deplore
My beauty fled, and empire now no more!   ("Saturday. The Small-Pox" 59–64)

Flavia, Montagu's poetic alter-ego, then calls upon Galen, the father of western medicine, and Machaon, the famed physician of the Trojan War, to cure her of her disfiguring and isolating disease. Like Oothoon, Flavia's marked body leaves her ostracized from an oppressively heteronormative, polite society that values women only for physical beauty. Second, Oothoon's much discussed offer to collect girls for Theotormon's harem of "lovely copulation" owes a debt to Montagu's detailed descriptions of seraglios in her *Turkish Embassy Letters* (1763), published widely in several languages after her death. Since Blake's friend Henry Fuseli had worked on the German translation of the letters, Blake would have been familiar with

Montagu's sympathetic accounts of exotic veiled women and of those Sultan's harem members whom she described provocatively as "the only *free* people in the [Ottoman] empire" (*Turkish Embassy Letters* 72; emphasis mine). Oothoon's version of "free" love, then, is not merely a "male fantasy" of unfettered polygamy, but simultaneously an orientalist fantasy filtered through early feminist politics. Blake's representation of Oothoon challenges what he perceived as Wollstone-craft's rational, sexless woman with his reading of Montagu's Turkish ideal of liber-ated, female sexuality. In these extremely selective (and hence distorting) citations of Wollstonecraft and Montagu, Blake boldly imagines Oothoon as an embodied site for sexual *and* medical experimentation, the "soft soul of America" ready to endure the painful inoculations of revolution.

Oothoon's argument thus becomes, in part, a literary experiment about the century-long debate over variolation. As historians of medicine have documented, this debate galvanized vociferous opposition from both the pulpit and the medical establishment. Theotormon, though, takes a more philosophical tack when he expresses his disdain for Oothoon's medico-botanical experiment. He begins with his version of book II of Locke's *Essay Concerning Human Understanding* (1690) in his niggling and joyless litany of epistemological questions: "Tell me what is the night or day to one oerflowd with woe? / Tell me what is a thought? & of what substance is it made? / Tell me what is a joy? & in what gardens do joys grow?" ("Visions" plate 6, 22–4). Locke defines "substance" somewhat recursively as a useful fiction that aggregates our ideas of substances: "not imagining how these simple *Ideas* can subsist by themselves, we accustom our selves, to suppose some *Substratum*, wherein they do subsist, and from which they do result, which there-fore we call *Substance*" (bk. 2, xiii, sec. 1, lines 13–16). Later, he admits that this definition is necessarily vague:

> because we cannot conceive, how [sensible Qualities] should subsist alone, nor one in another, we suppose them existing in, and supported by some common subject; *which Support we denote by the name Substance*, though it be certain, we have no clear, or distinct *Idea* of that *thing* we suppose a Support. (bk. 2, xxiii, sec. 4, 19–23)

Theotormon, though, futilely requires this "clear, or distinct *Idea* of that *thing*" and dully reduces human experience to empirically verifiable sense data. He ima-gines the solution for his "woe" as a ruthlessly rationalistic uncovering of the sen-sible qualities and ideas of "thought" and "substance." Instead of experiencing joys as joy, he seeks containment within some unspecified "gardens," or in some version of Locke's fictitious "substance" that conveniently aggregates sensible qual-ities into the discrete idea of a "thing."

Instead of finding a Boethian consolation of philosophy or a resolution to his doubts, he poses yet more questions about the nature of his increasingly medical-ized woe: "If thou returnest to the present moment of affliction / Wilt thou bring

comforts on thy wings, and dews and honey and balm; / Or poison from the desart
wilds, from the eyes of the envier?" ("Visions" plate 7, 9–11). Here, Theotormon's
medical rhetoric hastily divides itself into a false dilemma. His parsing of the solution
into the mutually exclusive qualities of cure ("dews and honey and balm") and "poison," willfully ignores, for example, Darwin's discussion in *The Loves of the Plants* of
poisonous flowers – Dictamnus (the burning bush), Mancinella (the little apple of
death), Urtica (the stinging nettle), and Lobelia (the pukeweed) – where he argues
assiduously for an interdependent ecology of predation and symbiosis, of "poison"
and "balm" ("The Botanic Garden" 362–4). In this way, Theotormon's Lockean
impasse not only misunderstands Oothoon's caprification and Darwin's pharmacological botany, but also the inoculating logic of Montagu's variolation. The "comforts"
that Theotormon desperately seeks need not arrive triumphantly on "wings" of "dews
and honey and balm"; Darwin's plants, Oothoon's "Sweetest" fruit, and Montagu's
variolation offer the stubbornly unhearing Theotormon much stranger comforts: the
contaminating yet curative balms of poison, violation, and inoculated disease.

Bromion proves no better at hearing Oothoon's illness narrative. His "infinite
microscope" ("Visions" plate 7, 16) strategically misunderstands Oothoon's argument concerning caprified fruit and variolous matter:

> Thou knowest that the ancient trees seen by thine eyes have fruit;
> But knowest thou that trees and fruits flourish upon the earth
> To gratify sense unknown? trees, beasts, and birds unknown:
> Unknown, not unperceivd, spread in the infinite microscope,
> In places yet unvisited by the voyager, and in worlds
> Over another kind of seas, and in atmospheres unknown?
>
> ("Visions" plate 7, 13–18)

Bromion's intense dissatisfaction with known quantities – the fruit of "ancient
trees seen by thine eyes" – and his preference for, and fetishistic repetition of, the
exotic "unknown" typify the slave owner's imperialist rhetoric. His world teems
with the anticipation of the "*un*known," the "*un*perceivd," and the "*un*visited," a
linguistic negativity that works hard to build positive momentum towards knowledge, enlightenment, and colonization. The caprified "trees and fruit" right in
front of his eyes are hardly enough. His conquering wanderlust must stake a claim
on the New World's undiscovered lands to gratify his increasingly ravenous senses,
to make known the unknown, and to make visible the invisible with his "infinite
microscope" and Newtonian law.[18] In Bromion's reductive monism, all experience
inevitably boils down to "one law for both the lion and the ox" ("Visions" plate 7,
22). Whereas Theotormon rejected Oothoon's caprification because of the distraction of his Lockean circumlocution, Bromion's objection emerges from a relentless
drive to satiate his wandering eye. Each infinitesimal particle of the natural world
awaits entry into Bromion's expanding empirical catalogue. He remains shackled

to the strict Linnaean taxonomies of botanical classification and to a rigidly scientific method that ultimately fails to grasp both the mixed ontology of caprification and the paradoxical logic of inoculation.

Oothoon's concluding rebuttal deals with both Theotormon's misapprehension of identity and Bromion's blindness to difference. While Theotormon brutally atomizes "thought" and "substance" to ever-finer heterogeneous conceptual particles, Bromion's microscopic eye furiously aggregates them into one universal law. After waiting "silent all the day, and all the night" ("Visions" plate 7, 25) – surely a sufficient interval to allow for a thoughtful response far beyond immediate, unthinking anger – Oothoon articulates her paradoxical thesis to break the ideological tension: "How can one joy absorb another? are not *different* joys / Holy, eternal, infinite! and *each* joy is a Love? ("Visions" plate 8, 5–6; emphasis mine).[19] She generously offers both the unitizing Bromion "different" joys that resist mutual annihilation and the particularizing Theotormon the promise of universal "Love." The long, final speech of the poem that follows unpacks this dense paradox through a final recapitulation of her caprification argument and of her successful cure for both Bromion and Theotormon's diseased, Enlightenment logic. To do this, she defines two models of "free" love: (1) Bromion's depraved cycle of generational rape and (2) her own idealized offer to institutionalize virginal rape in the accumulating contexts of virtuous trial (Milton), caprification (Darwin), and inoculation (Montagu). In the end, Oothoon's medico-botanical metaphor reconciles Theotormon's philosophical construction of abstract difference with Bromion's hard-headed insistence on coercive identity.

She first targets Bromion's argument with a list of incongruous images (a counsellor ape and a schoolmaster dog) to stir up trouble for his "one law for both the lion and the ox." Bromion's unitizing logic constructs a deterministic "wheel of false desire" in which his rape of Oothoon and his Newtonian penetration of the natural world initiate an unending cycle of diseased generation. In tracing this dysfunctional family tree, Oothoon finds herself

> … bound to hold a rod
> Over her shrinking shoulders all the day; & and all the night
> To turn the wheel of false desire: and longings that wake her womb
> To the abhorred birth of cherubs in the human form
> That live a pestilence & die a meteor & are no more.
> Till the child dwell with one he hates, and do the deed he loaths
> And the impure scourge force his seed into its unripe birth
> E'er yet his eyelids can behold the arrows of the day.   ("Visions" plate 8, 21–8)

The birth of Oothoon's bastard son with Bromion would represent a claustrophobic confinement of divinity to the limitations of a single "human form." As a result, the son will "live a pestilence & die a meteor"; his life will be nothing

but infectious disease and his death will produce yet another vector of miasmatic
contagion (here, "meteor" merely signifies any general atmospheric or meteor-
ological phenomenon). He shall rape another and start the vicious cycle anew
as "the impure scourge" eventually "force[s] his seed into its unripe birth." This
aggressively ironic return of Oothoon's discourse of purity ("impure scourge")
and of her caprified fruit ("unripe birth") underscores the disastrous results of
Bromion's failure to comprehend the complex nature of her healthful caprification. Oothoon's suggestive parody of Bromion's own negative language – his
"unknown," "unperceived," and "unvisited" are snidely rewritten as "impure" and
"unripe" – tracks this tragic history, from the idyllic health of Thel's vales of Har to
the perpetual disease of Bromion's "wheel of false desire." Oothoon's ever-insistent
solution remains the caprifying worm of the "Sweetest" fruit:

> Does not the *worm* erect a pillar in the mouldering church yard?
> And a palace of eternity in the jaws of the hungry grave
> Over his porch these words are written. Take thy bliss O Man!
> And *sweet* shall be thy taste & *sweet* thy infant joys renew!
> ("Visions" plate 8, 37; plate 9, 1–3; emphasis mine)

Here, Oothoon imagines optimistically that the worm's redoubled sweetness substitutes for Bromion's cycle of violation an eternal monument of mortal bliss.

Her subsequent counterargument against Theotormon again invokes both sickness and cure in its inoculating logic. Theotormon's disease remains his adamant
adherence to the ideal of "hypocrite modesty," and his persistent need to name
each thing as "Other" until differentiation ultimately becomes alienation. His
refusal to listen to Oothoon's lament highlights the conservative tenor of Enlightenment medicine, unable to accept an "Oriental" technique brought to England
by a woman outside the medical profession. As a result, images of sickness plague
the brooding Theotormon while Oothoon continues in her unrecognized health:
the jealous lover is associated with a "*sickly* charnel-house" ("Visions" plate 5, 36),
he becomes "a *sick* mans dream" ("Visions" plate 9, 19), and "his eyes *sicken* at the
fruit that hangs before his sight" ("Visions" plate 10, 20). He becomes chronically
ill despite the sweet cure of the caprified fruit that "hangs before his sight," and his
prophylactic refusal of Oothoon does nothing to prevent his eventual infection.
The stanza following Oothoon's Turkish proposition (her positive reclamation of
Bromion's "wheel of false desire") recapitulates her solution with a desperately
exclamatory force:

> Does the sun walk, in glorious raiment, on the secret floor
> Where the cold miser spreads his gold; or does the bright cloud drop
> On his stone threshold? Does his eye behold the beam that brings
> Expansion to the eye of pity; or will he bind himself

Beside the ox to thy hard furrow? Does not that mild beam blot
The bat, the owl, the glowing tiger, and the king of night?
The sea-fowl takes the wintry blast for a cov'ring to her limbs,
And the wild snake the pestilence to adorn him with gems and gold;
And trees, and birds, and beasts, and men behold their eternal joy.
Arise, you little glancing wings, and sing your infant joy!
Arise, and drink your bliss, for everything that lives is holy!

("Visions" plate 10, 30; plate 11, 1–10)

Oothoon organizes her last speech into three grammatical modes. She begins with
a version of Thel's interrogative structure that hovers uncertainly between the
repressive secrecy of the "cold miser" and the joyous expansion of the sun's "mild
beam." Her declarative second mode invokes the caprified rhetoric of paradox, yet
again, with the seafowl's freezing winter cloak and the wild snake's bejeweled "pestilence." Her "pestilence to adorn him with gems and gold" may even be a direct
allusion to Dryden's "gems sent to adorn his skin," that strangely decorative metaphor for his late friend Lord Hastings's smallpox pustules.[20] In the end, she arrives
at an exclamatory imperative – the anaphoric "Arise" – that celebrates a return to
the "infant joy" of Leutha's vale and the Darwinian utopia of bats, owls, tigers, sea-
fowls, snakes, trees, birds, beasts, and men in perfect communion. However, even
if Oothoon's exhortation reminds us of Darwin's idyllic and cosmopolitan conclusion in *The Temple of Nature*, it still fails to convince her ever-obdurate lover:
"Thus every morning wails Oothoon; but Theotormon sits / Upon the margin'd
ocean conversing with shadows dire" ("Visions" plate 11, 11–12), and the daughters of Albion can only "hear her woes, and echo back her sighs" ("Visions" plate
11, 13). Theotormon's unhearing chauvinism and the attenuating echo chamber
of Oothoon's lament challenge this stanza's triumphal trajectory, from the interrogative frame of the problem, to the declarative caprifying solution, and finally
to the exclamatory end.[21] The real-life history of smallpox inoculation met similar resistance despite its proven results, and Oothoon's selective ventriloquism of
Montagu points to how the unflagging conservatism of medical orthodoxy could
frequently mistake Birch's medical "experience" for wisdom.

Ultimately, Oothoon is neither Theotormon's discrete Lockean "substance"
nor an "unknown" quantity to be classified into Bromion's one law. Her admittedly repugnant solution of caprification or inoculation – virginal rape as virtuous
trial – nevertheless comes with a rigorously scientific gloss: it carefully measures,
as Darwin might put it, the precise dosage of M. de Thosse's turpentine to rid
the nectarine tree of infestation without killing the tree itself. The poem's alternative solutions of generational violence and vengeful abstinence both miscalculate
the solution at opposite extremes, leading to Bromion's wholly infected "wheel
of false desire" and Theotormon's sterile, "hypocrite modesty." Thus, Blake's
well-established aversion towards science is not the usual Keatsian complaint that

science "unweave[s] a rainbow" ("Lamia" II.237), or that a slavish adherence to scientism is bad for *literary* business. Instead, he levels a much more damaging charge against his Enlightenment bugbears: he mobilizes botanical and medical experiment to conclude that Bacon, Newton, and Locke – his favourite straw men of natural philosophy – are actually not even very good *scientists*. Instead of a naively literary backlash against a monolithic science, Blake shapes an informed medico-botanical corrective to empirical method, one that can acknowledge, understand, and implement radical techniques like variolation to the benefit of mankind. Bromion's Newtonian denial of ontological difference and Theotormon's Lockean reliance on philosophical hedging cannot hope to understand Oothoon's medico-literary illness narrative and her fierce advocacy of inoculated health. Blake would later cast Catherine as his real-life Oothoon, as a successful test case for Birch's radical electroshock therapy. His genuine excitement at his wife's rheumatism cure – "Electricity is the wonderful cause" – underscores his disappointment at the conservative medical establishment's inability to embrace new, effective (as Blake saw it) medical treatments. It is this context of medical and sexual radicalism that should inform readings of Oothoon's argument. The metaphor of caprification and variolation as rape stages a fertile encounter between innocence and experience, between virginal woman and desiring man, between English purity and Oriental disease, in order to articulate that dearly purchased yet joyous moment of universal health that punctuates Oothoon's final speech: "everything that lives is holy!" ("Visions" plate 11, 10).

Blake seems to take great pains to justify Oothoon's proposition through these various layers of literary, botanical, medical, and feminist contexts. Whereas Darwin skips over the inoculating means towards his cosmopolitan end, the indeterminacy of Blake's poem suspends the "drink your bliss" resolution, ending instead on the sombre note of Theotormon's continued refusal of Oothoon and the renewed sighs of the daughters of Albion. This indeterminacy suggests that Blake's voice never exactly coincides with Oothoon's, and her plan to collect sexual partners for Theotormon is not meant to be an ideal solution, but rather a disturbingly redemptive moment of a caprifying experiment that merely delays the congealing conservatism of political, medical, and literary systems. Dennis M. Welch suggests that we miss the point when we ask whether Oothoon's voice as a female slave succeeds in resisting her double oppression. Instead, he argues that the goal of the poem is "to present a strenuous voice of resistance against tyranny even if that voice may not succeed" (108); in other words, Blake's ideological stakes lie not in the utopian construction of a fully realized (and consequently hegemonic) radicalism, but in continuous resistance and revolution, guided by the central figures of caprification and emancipatory rape.[22] This indeterminacy, though, also threatens to become political and ethical irresponsibility. Mellor notes that if Blake "urges the reader to imagine an alternative to the slavery of modesty other than free love, the poem does not suggest what that alternative could be. As the creator of this poem and its designs, Blake must take responsibility for what the work does not say as well as for what it does say" ("Blake and Wollstonecraft" 368). What Blake "does not say" in the poem is exactly what Darwin *does* attempt to say in his brief treatment of the inoculation metaphor; that is, he hastily constructs a naive immunity-through-community that would transform Oothoon's plucked marigold and her unanswered prayer for "eternal joy" into a crystallized, cosmopolitan ideal. Blake's hesitation, however, is less a political blind spot than deliberate ideology; in his ponderous dwelling on revolution, resistance, and inoculation, he chooses to piece together his radicalism in the negative space of Theotormon's silence, in that arresting moment of perilous potentiality. Oothoon's inoculation models the continuous construction and destruction of the boundaries of self and other, of male and female, of human and non-human in order to reproduce, within the realm of sexual politics, the already proven botanical and medical successes of caprification and variolation. Even though Blake's medico-botanical metaphor is perhaps no less misogynistic, these various contexts might make it a bit less irresponsible. In this way, Blake reveals inoculation's true radical tenor, and its erstwhile ameliorative function, in the botanical work of Dryden, Burke, Bloomfield, and to a lesser extent Darwin, quickly becomes untenable.

The Experimental Results

Oothoon's increasingly problematic illness narrative about healthful violation rises to the level of our own modern conspiratorial stories of vaccine hesitancy and refusal. During the COVID-19 pandemic, for example, we saw outraged patients, holding pieces of metal to their bodies and arguing that the magnetic attraction confirmed that Bill Gates had embedded microscopic tracking chips or chemical sterilizers in the vaccine. As I mentioned before, Blake is not exactly endorsing these dangerous and outlandish tales or Oothoon's clearly appalling argument. He is, however, encouraging us and teaching us to take these illness narratives seriously. Instead of mere satiric targets of our rational, justified laughter and outrage, these narratives expose the systems and institutions that make these specious arguments possible in the first place. In the case of "Visions," they cast a light on Oothoon's condition of double abjection as both "whore" and "crafty slave." The subjugation of women and the enslavement of Africans produced these terrifying arguments. In the day-to-day business of the poem, Theotormon binds women with the marriage contract while Bromion captures Africans with his slaver's brand. Ironically, having two competing masters means having no master at all, leaving Oothoon momentarily free and able to argue for her continued freedom. But, as Frantz Fanon observed about the decolonized state, she must work through and understand her freedom independently lest she reproduce the unfreedoms of her colonizers. Instead of relying on an external system of prefabricated ethics, she tries out several escalating arguments throughout the poem. The poem's epigraph,

"The Eye sees more than the Heart knows," acknowledges that Oothoon is seeing too much too fast. Oothoon's boundlessly prolific argumentative energy about the suffering she sees before her may be too much to wrap up in just eleven plates.

After Bromion's vile speech in which he gives permission to Theotormon to marry Oothoon and to take care of a bastard child born of rage and rape, Theotormon summons the waves in anger to encircle Bromion and Oothoon, binding them back-to-back. Instead of weeping, Oothoon immediately begins to troubleshoot. She calls upon Theotormon's eagles to eat her filthy flesh away, and Theotormon briefly smiles at the eagles rending the ostensibly polluted flesh from her body. After this self-sacrificing show, Oothoon attempts that first argument to persuade her lover that the time of mourning has passed. "I am pure," she insists, "Because the night is gone that clos'd me in its deadly black" ("Visions" plate 5, 29–30). The trauma of her experience has awakened her, and she now realizes that she has been taught utter nonsense all her life: "They told me that the night and day were all that I could see / They told me that I had five senses to enclose me up / And they enclos'd my infinite brain into a narrow circle." ("Visions" plate 5, 31–3). While Oothoon is having her Wollstonecraftian awakening, Theotormon only sees her in the conventional context of a fallen woman: she is damaged goods and unacceptable to Theotormon's system of morality and ethics. This first half of the poem describes a graphic violation that highlights the sky-high stakes of this Revolutionary age. Just a few years earlier, Wollstonecraft had issued her call to action: "It is time to effect a revolution in female manners – time to restore them their lost dignity – and make them, as part of the human species, labour by reforming themselves to reform the world" (230). Oothoon, as a symbol of American freedom, is doubly violated: she is both a woman under the thumb of patriarchy and a slave in the shackles of imperial capitalism. Oothoon is that Wollstonecraftian reform in practice, struggling in fits and starts to find the means to reform herself to reform the world.

Because of this, Oothoon's arguments throughout the eleven plates are works in progress. Her increasingly creative arguments turn zoological. She looks to the natural world and the learned and instinctual behaviour of chickens, pigeons, bees, mice, frogs, wild asses, meek camels, wolves, tigers, worms, snakes, and eagles. As I have already detailed, her argument about her paradoxical purity then turns botanical and medical. Meanwhile, Theotormon's first reaction is all about his own woe, and Bromion just wants to move on with his imperial conquests. Oothoon's response to Theotormon's and Bromion's lazy arguments is redoubled argument, and this time she advocates for free love. She argues against Bromion's one law for the lion and the ox as well as Theotormon's "hypocrite modesty." Unlike her prudish lover, she is "Open to joy and to delight wherever beauty appears" ("Visions" plate 9, 22). By this point, the three had been debating this issue for so long that night had come; Blake's designs of sinewy nude figures are now draped in flowing folds to ward off the creeping transatlantic chill. Here, Oothoon's argument reaches that desperate pitch, from "Love! Love! Love! happy

happy Love! free as the mountain wind!" to her sex trafficking proposal ("Visions" plate 10, 16). In her desperation, she proposes her iniquitous scheme to appease the still brooding and impassable Theotormon. She learns from Bromion how to be a slaver herself, catching virgin girls for her lover's pleasure.

I mentioned parenthetically before that this is a supremely difficult moment in the poem to teach. There are other moments like this in *The Songs of Innocence* (1789) that are similarly tricky. In "The Chimney Sweeper," Tom Dacre learns the lesson from his dream that if he keeps doing his exploitative chimney sweeping duty, then he will never have to fear harm. In "The Little Black Boy," the titular boy recounts his lesson learned at his mother's knee that he should shield the little white boy from the sun until he himself turns white enough to be loved. And in "Holy Thursday," the poor folks learn to "cherish pity, lest you drive an angel from your door" (12). They learn that if you show insufficient gratitude, then that angel of charity might stop throwing ducats your way. In these three cases, as well as in Oothoon's, arguments go awry because of the very Wollstonecraftian problem of education. Tom Dacre, the "little black boy," the urban poor, and Oothoon are always on unequal footing in these debates. In a sense, these moments are not just difficult to teach because of these horribly offensive lines of argument, but also because they thematize bad teaching itself. Oothoon has learned only depraved lessons from Bromion's imperialism and Theotormon's misogyny, yet her very life depends on marshalling her prolific argumentative energy to arrive at a cogent argument. Her concluding idea that "everything that lives is holy" is a promising but uncertain sign that she can get there eventually. Throwing off the manacles of the mind is hard work, and Oothoon's illness narrative, from her base position of double abjection, demonstrates how much work that liberation entails. She wails every morning about a body that she insists is perfectly healthy, but Theotormon just talks to random shadows, convinced that her flesh is tainted. And even though the daughters of Albion are still listening at the end, they are left merely echoing back her still developing argument. "The Marriage of Heaven and Hell," the debate between the angel and the devil was a fair fight, and the devil won purely on the merits of his arguments. Oothoon, a woman and a slave, is instead Tom Dacre, the "little black boy," or the urban poor, developing from scratch an ideology of liberation, and that is much harder work. Unlike Darwin, Blake refuses to skip to the cosmopolitan, utopian end; rather, Oothoon's illness narrative dwells in the sick, distasteful, and errant revolutionary means.

Since neither Bromion nor Theotormon accepts Oothoon's unconventional inoculation story, Blake illustrates the results of this blanket refusal in his short but powerful medico-botanical meditation on disease, "The Sick Rose," reproduced here in full:

> O Rose, thou art sick!
> The invisible worm,

That flies in the night,
In the howling storm,
Has found out thy bed
Of crimson joy;
And his dark secret love
Does thy life destroy.   ("The Sick Rose" 1–8)

The "contrary states" of innocence and experience are here in full display (this poem is one of the most famous representatives of experience in the *Songs of Innocence and of Experience*): the rose's bright "crimson" contrasts with the worm's invisibility and darkness, the rooted plant with the flying parasite, and blushing "joy" with "dark secret love." Unlike Oothoon's caprification in Leutha's vale, the encounter between innocence and experience can now only be destructive, and that "dark secret love" engenders full-blown disease rather than purifying immunity. Theotormon's rejection of Oothoon's illness narrative and medical knowledge has made the mixed nature of inoculation impossible; the art of variolation is lost, which Blake underscores in this poem's mournful visual representation of a botched inoculation (figure 11). From the slumping rose emerges that repeated visual motif – the amorous couple from the pasqueflower in "Thel" and the nymph from the marigold in "Visions" – but instead of joyous, Darwinian intercourse with the expansive botanical world, a menacing worm lashes out to rein in the escaping female figure while the vermicular forms on the stem collapse in postures of lament.

The parasitic figure at the top left references that earlier analogy from Blake's "The Marriage of Heaven and Hell" – "As the catterpiller [*sic*] chooses the fairest leaves to lay her eggs on, so the priest lays his curse on the fairest joys" ("Marriage" plate 9, 16) – to reiterate visually the worm's "invisible" invasion of the Rose's "bed / Of crimson joy" with its "dark secret love," desire infected by oppressive sexual guilt and priestly curses. In a dark parody of the floral images of "Thel" and "Visions," the design of "The Sick Rose" refuses the Darwinian personification of botanical life; the worm – formerly the helpless infant of "Thel" and the sweetening agent of caprification in "Visions" – now restrains the very "life" of the rose into its "secret," Urizenic system of oppressive love. Inoculation is no longer effective in this world of hardened experience. In "The Clod and the Pebble," for example, the Clod feebly echoes the inoculating image of "Visions," "Trodden with the cattle's feet" ("Clod" 6), but instead of Oothoon's paradoxical "clear spring, muddied with the feet of beasts," the Pebble counters stridently with its infected definition of love: "To bind another to its delight, / Joys in another's loss of ease" ("Clod" 10–11). The Clod can only imagine making "a heaven in hell's despair" ("Clod" 4) and the Pebble a "hell in heaven's despite" ("Clod" 12); those moments of cosmopolitan intercourse now rely exclusively on an oppressive rhetoric of subordination rather than the radical and revolutionary language of inoculation. The worm, having progressed from its silent infancy ("Thel"), to its vocal participation in the economy of nature ("Visions"), and finally to a savage predator and destroyer of joy ("The Sick Rose"), is now fully responsible for the sickness of the rose. In suppressing the Darwinian ending in favour of radical potential of the illness narrative, Blake must also imagine the possible failures of revolution. Theotormon's rejection of Oothoon's inoculation narrative brings an incurable sickness upon the botanical world; whereas Darwin's flowers personified joyous intercourse, Blake represents a mirror universe of "dark secret love," slowly consumed by sickness.

This is not to say that Blake finally abandons his experiment with inoculated life entirely; after all, his work tends to reside in potential outcomes rather than final states. Due to the unique production process of his illuminated work, no single copy looks exactly like another, differing in "states, proofs, prints before letters, size and types of paper, and so on" (Viscomi 169). Indeed, Blake did not always make visible the "invisible worm" of "The Sick Rose," and the female figure's expression remains tantalizingly ambiguous, leaving the inoculation question uncomfortably open-ended. His treatment of the "Comus" illustrations also exemplifies this revisionist impulse: the multimedia rewriting of the story begins with "Thel," "Visions," and "The Sick Rose" and ends with his 1815 version of "Comus with His Revellers," his visual interpretation of Milton's scene of bacchanalian debauchery:

> Soon as the Potion works, their human count'nance,
> Th' express resemblance of the gods, is chang'd
> Into some brutish form of Wolf, or Bear,
> Or Ounce, or Tiger, Hog, or bearded Goat.　　　　　("Comus" 68–71)

In the image, Blake celebrates the assailed virtue of the Lady with exuberant animal-human hybrids who dance joyously above the seated figure of the Lady. Of note is that Blake retains both "Hog" and "Wolf" (the two figures on the left) from the 1801 image (figure 12), but in the 1815 version (figure 13), he replaces the "Ounce" (a lynx) with a strategically distorted version of a "bearded Goat."

The fourteen years that separate the two versions of "Comus with His Revellers" saw both Gillray's trenchant visual satire about the side effects of vaccination (figure 6) and Birch's medical pamphlet that strenuously objected to the new inoculating practice. Blake's "bearded Goat" is almost certainly not a goat but a bull-like figure in the same posture as one of Gillray's horned vaccination patients, further linking Blake's project to the ongoing debate about vaccination safety and efficacy. Unlike Gillray's caricature and Birch's pamphlet, though, Blake's "Comus" image revels in the effects of the transformative "Potion." And instead of Milton's chaste moralizing, Blake lingers on the trying of virtue rather than virtue itself, drawing attention to Comus's drunken revelry while visually subordinating the

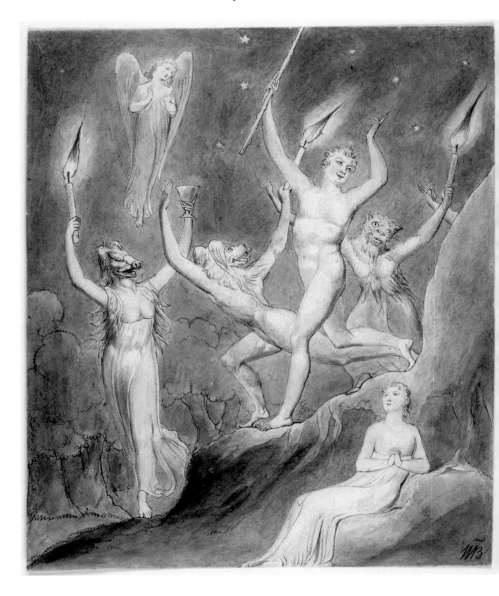

Figure 12. "Comus and His Revellers," commissioned from William Blake by Joseph Thomas, 1801. Call # 000.20, The Huntington Library, San Marino, California.

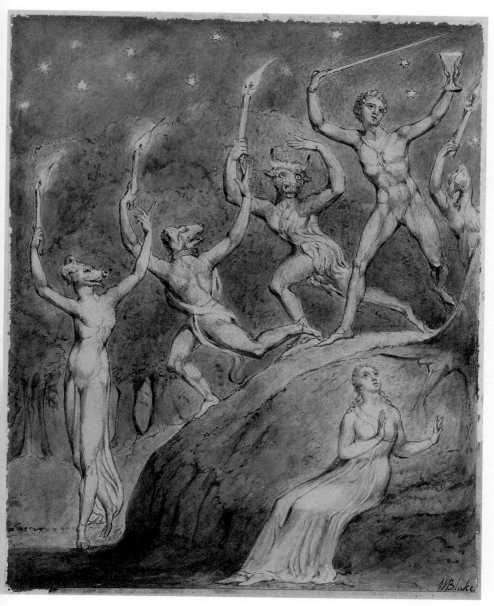

Figure 13. "Comus and His Revellers," commissioned from William Blake by Thomas
Butts, 1815. Accession # 90.119–126, The Museum of Fine Arts, Boston, Massachusetts.

Lady's stalwart decorum. Birch's turn from the radically experimental medicine of his early career must have disappointed Blake's long Comus-driven inoculation narrative, a disappointment that he registers in this celebratory, visual reclamation of Gillray's iconic bovine hybrids. In this way, Blake materializes Milton's more tentative argument in "Comus," "Areopagitica," and *Paradise Lost* about virtue into the medico-botanical metaphor of inoculation: he argues that "cloistered virtue" is nothing more than unthinking piety, and insists that innocent virtue must encounter the trial of experience – even if it leads to disastrous results such as Oothoon's rejection by Theotormon or the Rose's sickness – to inoculate the surprisingly porous body against the threatening infection of "Secresy," of Linnaean boundaries, and of the repressive systematization of an increasingly conservative medical science.[23]

In tracing the multiplying contexts of this single metaphor, I have suggested that Blakean imagery perhaps deserves a bit more patience. In recovering this scientific Blake, we might risk the loss of a sense of mythopoetic reverie, that famously iconoclastic, meandering, and freeing vision of love, holiness, and liberation. That Oothoon's argument may depend much less on the vatic vision of the daughters of Albion and more on exhaustive botanical and medical research does little to curtail the poet's stunningly prophetic reach. For example, contemporary debates about vaccination have echoed the medical controversies of "Visions" with eerie fidelity. Andrew Wakefield's infamous 1998 article in *The Lancet*, in which he alleged a link between MMR vaccination and autism, was apparently evidence enough for thousands of Theotormons to refuse the inoculating needle. Despite the study's flimsy evidence and questionable methodology, vaccination rates in the developed world plummeted, causing several outbreaks of otherwise preventable measles cases. So fragile is our relationship with the idea of inoculation that we accept any excuse to validate that creeping sense of discomfort and to tip the scale towards vaccine hesitancy or refusal. Blake offers Oothoon's solution not as a crystallized and fully endorsed ideal, but as a radical approach that, like Montagu's Turkish medicine, the MMR vaccine, and now the COVID-19 vaccines, brutally assaults our squeamishness, that viscerally ingrained sense of discomfort. With positive precedents in both nature (botanical caprification) and medicine (vaccination), Blake orchestrates this odd variation on the familiar Miltonic theme of uncomfortable trial: Oothoon's repugnant proposal to "collect" girls for Theotormon's harem is not merely Milton's abstractly metaphorical virtue that "sallies out and sees her adversary," but it is also a virtue that boldly registers trial in a localized and embodied violation that deliberately galvanizes discomfort, squeamishness, and outrage against diseased complacency. The material legibility of Blake's botanical verse, then, does not exchange a visionary poetics for "the same dull round" ("Natural Religion" 3) of empirical experience; rather, it strategically materializes radical ideology into a transgressively experimental practice based on the wild whims of the illness narrative. Thus, when Blake concludes in

"There Is No Natural Religion" (1788) that "If it were not for the Poetic or Prophetic character, the Philosophic & Experimental would soon be at the ratio of all things & stand still" ("Natural Religion" 3), he does not simply suggest that experiment should entirely give way to poetry. Theotormon's Lockean philosophy and Bromion's Newtonian experiment remain in continuous conversation with Oothoon's plaintive poetry, her illness narrative, and the prophetic daughters of Albion, suggesting instead a strikingly dynamic interplay between rational material and imaginative metaphor. In the end, Oothoon's medico-botanical metaphor – a painstakingly calculated "ratio" of Miltonic theology, Darwinian botany, and experimental medicine – does not "stand still."

Blake's botanical metaphor finally undoes Linnaean organization to amplify Darwinian personification into a revolutionary politics of embodiment. His attention to the actual, embodied process of inoculation rather than Darwin's Enlightenment timidity towards the inoculated body valorizes radical transgression in its potential to reshape both world and body. This brand of shaky cosmopolitanism, then, relies not on Darwin's hand-waving solution to the problem of revolution but on a sustained engagement with the particular units of the cosmopolitan encounter between self and other. The inoculation metaphor models revolutionary praxis with such fidelity that it must ultimately exceed its conservative, Burkean containment. As an inherently cosmopolitan metaphor that persistently erodes the coercive boundaries of body and state, inoculation provides both Darwin and Blake a figure from which to imagine that elusive Pythagorean ideal of the "transmigrating mass": an organic vision of variously interpenetrating life that entirely transcends the hierarchical logic of both Linnaean categories and Burkean purity. However, Blake's liberation of the inoculation metaphor also encourages a kind of experimental aggression in its problematic eagerness to rip apart bodies in the name of radical progress. After all, Oothoon's inoculation is purchased at a terrible cost: Bromion's violent rape, the eagles' purifying feast, and her outrageous offer to expand the practice of caprifying violation. Later Romantic authors – specifically John Keats and Mary Shelley – would have to find unique ways to deal with this troubling revolutionary legacy of the inoculation metaphor, a problem that Darwin was ultimately too squeamish to anticipate and Blake too eager to perceive. Blake centred the revolutionary human agent's illness narrative in healing sickness and reconfigured the idea of health itself. Oothoon's revolutionary interpretation of her own caprified body defiantly stands trial against Theotormon's Lockean epistemology and Bromion's Newtonian physics. As the daughters of Albion sigh back her lamentations, Oothoon emerges as the shaky voice of the new medicine. Even before Jenner's *Inquiry*, Darwin and Blake were already busy experimenting successfully and creatively with these narratives of inoculated life.

PART THREE

Interdisciplinarity

Chapter Four

Keats and the End of Disease

The New Medicine

The two versions of the Romantic illness narrative had coexisted up to the discovery of vaccination. Edward Jenner and William Wordsworth, armed with curiosity about the lived experiences of rural illnesses, shaped found narratives with their growing impulse to catalogue, classify, and standardize into a burgeoning professional medical archive. Rather than imagining the inoculation narrative as an occasion to authorize this kind of biopower, Erasmus Darwin and William Blake delighted in the unaccountable strangeness of the illness narrative. They listened even when (or especially when) it was hard. Darwin listened beyond the comfort of Linnaean classification, expanding the living world into a cosmopolitan universe of monstrous differences. And Blake listened even when the illness narratives turned repugnant, even when Oothoon decided that the ends of free love justified the means of ritualized rape. For Blake, even when illness narratives turned conspiratorial and dangerous, they were still crucial opportunities to listen. This next part on interdisciplinarity moves forward chronologically to the aftermath of vaccination. Even after vaccination had been normalized, professionalized, and institutionalized by Jenner's public health campaign, the Romantic illness narrative survived. In "Sleep and Poetry" (1816), one of John Keats's earliest published poems, the medically trained poet begins by wondering what is left for medicine in the aftermath of something like the unprecedented experimental success of vaccination. He sets the clinical scene with a Middle English epigraph (misattributed to Chaucer) in which the speaker puzzles through an inexplicable bout of insomnia:

> "As I lay in my bed slepe full unmete
> Was unto me, but why that I ne might
> Rest I ne wist, for there n'as erthly wight

[As I suppose] had more of hertis ese
Than I, for I n'ad sicknesse nor disese."   ("Sleep and Poetry" 58)

The body had become an empty signifier. The narrative of pain and suffering no longer depended on "erthly" concerns of either "hertis ese" or "disese," and the conventional vital signs of health had lost their explanatory force. This early scene of mysterious insomnia would continue to baffle and shape Keats's later poetry. Vaccination had promised a long life with neither "sicknesse nor disese," but a "slepe full unmete" would persist and fester in Keats's poetic practice. In imagining an objectively healthy future immune from disease, Keats concluded, like many medical theorists of the era supposed, that life itself might become the new diseased condition that eludes medical treatment. If we are forced to live, forced into the knowledge and sorrow of prolonged life, then the management of that potentially unending existence, according to Keats, must fall to the poets, not the professional physicians of his early career.

This is the unique premise of Keats's interdisciplinary pitch. By 1816, vaccination was old news, and medicine had begun to ponder new directions. As Nicholas Roe has documented, by the time Keats began his medical studies, vaccination had become a relatively routine procedure despite its residual taint of unnatural revulsion:

> His duties as apprentice would have given him an introduction to basic skills such as vaccination for smallpox, bleeding patients with a lancet or with leeches, dressing wounds, setting bones, pulling teeth, identifying the symptoms of illnesses, making up pills, ointments, poultices, laudanum, and other medicines. (167)

In charting medicine's next steps, Keats decided that the musty walls of Guy's Hospital were closing in, and Astley Cooper's surgical lectures were short on true inspiration. Keats's disciplinary transition from medicine to poetry reflected his belated arrival into a conflictual medical culture. Whereas Darwin and Blake had experimented with inoculation at the pivotal historical moment between variolation and vaccination, Keats found himself in the aftermath with different but equally hard questions to answer. What happens to the Romantic illness narrative after vaccination? After immunology, where was the new medicine to go?

The future of medicine was at stake, and the immediate reception of the cowpox vaccine in medical, scientific, and literary circles was understandably uneven. Ox-faced boys and anecdotal evidence of "quadrupedan sympathies" aside, Romantic medical experimentation flourished, emboldened by the successes of the new medicine. In *The Atmosphere of Heaven* (2009), Mike Jay has called attention to these "unnatural experiments" conducted by Romantic scientists such as Joseph Priestley, Thomas Beddoes, and Sir Humphry Davy.[1] Renegade science was in. Enlightenment historiography tends to fixate on these spectacular failures as a foil to the coherent and robust picture of the new professionalism. Even Roy Porter often suggests that vaccination was an Enlightenment triumph that succeeded despite the era's backwards culture of medical quackery. In his analysis of Jenner, he concedes that "elite medicine clearly had much to learn from folk tradition" (*The Greatest Benefit* 40) while still relying on a rigid binary that pits "elite" professionalism against "folk" healing. The success of vaccination, however, had already enlarged the role of "folk tradition" into a proper discourse. The mild derision of Porter's phrase underestimates the productive work of Romantic medicine and obscures vaccination's participation in a larger medical debate about radical experiment, appropriate care, and medical authority. Rewriting this marginalized "folk tradition" as what I referred to in the introduction as "a Romantic disease discourse" not only forces us to take more seriously a medical culture that produced one of the most significant epistemic breaks in the history of medicine, but it also grants us access to the vital literary dimension of Romantic disease management.

Keats's construction of the new medicine comes out of this peculiar interdisciplinary discourse. The later poetic work is much more capable of answering the pressing medical questions of the day than Porter might allow. As Alan Richardson rightly insists in his study of Romantic brain science, Keats's best work is "as much scientific as poetic" (124), and his move from the bustling anatomy theatre to the quiet bower of "Endymion" (1818) was less about poetic retirement than about disciplinary continuity. The later Keats realized that poetry can and should be the better medicine; it revitalizes the body beyond insular anatomical categories and towards a broader medical hermeneutics that acknowledges the real difficulties of symptomatic interpretation and the possibility of human progress beyond mere pathological knowledge. In this view, Romantic medicine cannot be written off as just a brief, embarrassing layover to the Enlightenment triumph of professional medicine. Keats did not simply abandon medicine for poetry when he left the institutional confines of Guy's Hospital; his decision to pursue poetry was instead a calculated move to preserve Romantic disease discourse and the genre of the Romantic illness narrative, even as the discipline of medicine was hurtling towards professional practice and rigid method. To pursue poetry, then, was no disciplinary break but a conscious decision to practise a different kind of medicine, one that could potentially replicate the proven success of vaccination.

Beyond Consumption

Keats started out, however, much more conventionally. His brief medical career continues to resist a definitively biographical accounting despite an extraordinarily well-mined trove of archival material.[2] Instead, several explanations remain in critical conflict, depending largely on the biographer's variable interest in Romantic medicine. All have in common, though, some form of abrupt disciplinary substitution – poetry for medicine – that either has the newly anointed poet writing with some residual medical influence or just abandoning rigidly medical pursuits altogether to achieve a more aesthetic, luxurious, and sensual poetics. I am interested in recovering a more medical Keats than either of these accounts allow, not, as one might expect, by rifling anew through the seemingly inexhaustible medical archive surrounding Keats, but by working to develop a sensitive, medico-literary perspective on his later poetic output, specifically in his letters, "La Belle Dame Sans Merci" (1819–20), and the *Hyperion* (1818–21) poems.

The most voluble of these biographical controversies must be that dramatic moment of disciplinary schism when Keats triumphantly declares, in an act of haughty rebellion against his stuffy guardian Richard Abbey, his bold intention to leave medicine for poetry. Questions of Keats's mental and physical investment in medicine continue to polarize his biographers. Did he merely skate by in medical school while dreaming longingly of his true poetic calling? In his transition from promising professional to penniless poet (1815–17), did he already begin neglecting his immediate medical duties? My reading of Keats does not claim to resolve these lingering questions of medical biography; instead, I focus on the later, more reflective Keats who writes wistfully about the scope and calibre of his intellectual progress:

> Were I to study physic or rather Medicine again, – I feel it would not make the least difference in my Poetry; when the Mind is in its infancy a Bias is in reality a Bias, but when we have acquired more strength, a Bias becomes no Bias. Every department of knowledge we see excellent and calculated towards a great whole. I am so convinced of this, that I am glad at not having given away my medical Books, which I shall again look over to keep alive the little I know thitherwards. (*Letters* 86–7)

In this well-known 3 May 1818 letter to John Reynolds, he eloquently sympathizes with his friend's struggle to balance literary and legal careers. Even though Keats had written just a few years earlier about his intense dissatisfaction with the medical profession, here he looks back at his education with mature, level-headed deliberation. The petulant "Bias" of his infant mind has given way to the "great whole" of comprehensive knowledge, suggesting that his early break from medicine was far from unequivocal apostasy. Understanding Keats's volatile relation to Romantic medicine sometimes means turning away from the young, rebellious medical student of Guy's Hospital and towards the tubercular, unbiased poet of "La Belle Dame Sans Merci," *Hyperion* (which he had begun writing in late autumn 1818 and abandoned in April 1819), and *The Fall of Hyperion* (which he had begun writing in late 1819 and worked on intermittently until his death in 1821), which were the final fragments of that "great whole" of Keats's brief yet prolific medico-literary production.

Donald Goellnicht has already begun to read the Hyperion poems productively within this medical frame: "although they are not concerned with medical themes in a strict or narrow sense, they do deal with the broad subject of a healthy or balanced life – a concept Keats developed from his medical training – both for the society and for the poet, and so deserve close analysis within the general context of Keats's medical knowledge" (212–13). Along the way in this "close analysis," he constructs a useful binary that begins to explain Keats's treatment of the medical metaphor. He argues that "states of health and disease often symbolize the imagination in periods of productivity and stagnation respectively" (172) and that "Keats realizes that, in order to become the poet-physician of society, he must first heal his own spirit of its violent vacillations between depression and fevered poetic trances" (212). Here, illness and health, neatly aligned with paralyzing depression and poetic activity respectively, divide the bodily condition into discrete "vacillations" between diseased and healthy states. Yet as Hermione de Almeida astutely points out, these two states were far from coherent for both Keats and his medical contemporaries: "Romantic medicine functioned upon the very energizing ambiguity that underlay all treatments, whether physiological or mental, specifically medical or largely philosophical" (138). Competing theories of health and disease abounded, and that "energizing ambiguity" eventually spilled across both disciplinary and national borders. In Scotland, John Brown tentatively theorized a continuum of health and disease according to various levels of nervous excitability, while his teacher, William Cullen, sought to differentiate and classify disease with Linnaean precision; on the continent, Novalis and Schelling were toying with the ideas of health as a perpetual state of disease and even of disease as a primary precondition for life. The healthful deliberation that Keats sought, then, is not merely a so-called fevered poetic trance that undergoes any kind of straightforward curing or healing; Keats could not have seen disease as simply a discrete exception to health. For him, disease was instead a condition inseparable from the very idea of the healthy body.

De Almeida, among other chroniclers of Romantic medicine, have significantly expanded our understanding of Romantic-era conceptualizations of disease, slowly moving that contested category away from the perils of negative definition: that disease is merely the absence of health. There remains, however, an important missing term in this argument. Just as the diseased body was, in a sense, already healthy, the Romantic concept of health deliberately maintained a selective access to disease. My account of Keats and his relationship to the concept of vaccination fills out this deconstruction of health and disease by emphasizing a carefully infected aspect of Romantic health.[3] With this more complete picture, the most challenging scenes of the Hyperion poems – Apollo's dying into life and those fevered encounters with Mnemosyne and Moneta – can be re-situated within their proper medico-literary context. The concluding Apollonian pains in *Hyperion* and the poet-dreamer's nauseating encounter with divinity in *The Fall of Hyperion* cannot be healed fully via conventional medicine but only with the help of the new preventive medicine of vaccination, the highly controversial practice that changed the very concept of health itself.

The innovative and effective treatment of smallpox, a key Romantic-era discovery, has not deterred most studies of Romantic medicine from focusing exclusively on two diseases that notoriously eluded treatment: consumption and cancer. With Keats, this pathological bias is understandable. After all, he lost both a mother and a brother to consumption before ultimately succumbing to the disease himself in 1821. However, the medical failures of the time – cancer and consumption were almost tantamount to death sentences – should not entirely shape our opinion of Romantic medicine. The extraordinary and enduring success of vaccination forces us at least to re-evaluate an era of medical practice that has been frequently dismissed as an embarrassment in the history of science. In Keats's time, cancer and consumption were common wasting diseases that unfortunately outpaced the progress of medical science; the acute illness of smallpox, however, spurred the positive movement towards a new paradigm of preventive medicine. As the example of vaccination strongly suggests, Romantic medicine thrived in this new paradigm's reliance on "half-knowledge" (*Letters* 42), as Keats might have put it. Its experimental and loosely structured methodology could handle dramatic epistemic shifts on the fly. Irritable states, nervous flare-ups, and other sparsely defined symptoms that resisted the clinical diagnosis and precise definition expected of modern medical practice were nevertheless treated successfully under this system of medical care. Unable to change with the times, the old Saturn of the Hyperion poems instead suffers from an enervating obsolescence, figured as an incurable wasting disease: "His old right hand lay nerveless, listless, dead, / Unsceptred; and his realmless eyes were closed" ("Hyperion" I.18–19; "The Fall" I.323–4). The Titan's already "dead" hands and "realmless eyes" contrast starkly with the regenerative vitality in the concluding vision of Apollo, god of both the new poetry and the new medicine, who spectacularly "die[s] into life" ("The Fall" III.130), inaugurating a new "Celestial" ("Hyperion" III.136) era of divine poetic inspiration and health.

Here, Keats envisions two competing medical practices: the old one that has failed to treat the Titans' degenerative diseases (cancer and consumption) and the new one that successfully produces an immunized community of fledgling gods, inoculated against the sting of death and the disfigurement of disease. The focus on the former has blocked our access to the idealism of the latter vision of perpetual health through the tightly controlled management of disease. The new gods' deathly inoculation – their dying into life – completes Keats's comprehensive poetic catalogue of disease. His work deals not only with the untreatable and unaccountable – cancer, consumption, melancholy – but also in the unprecedented medical success of smallpox treatment and the curative violence of inoculation. The poem ends with a movement towards more radical, effective care under the stewardship of the new gods. Through these medical tropes of his later poetry, Keats shows that he never really abandoned medicine. Rather, he followed a unique literary route towards what he considered the more effective medical practice: one that deliberately lingered in the multifarious experimentalism of vaccination, rather than pushing towards an increasingly professionalized and institutionalized medical practice. Keats never lost access to medical knowledge, and it is this medico-literary perspective of Romantic disease discourse that begins to explain the fraught encounter between physician and patient in "La Belle Dame Sans Merci" and the deathless worlds of the Hyperion poems. Beyond the stereotypical portrait of the consumptive poet is Keats's radical new health care proposal that reshapes our received history of biopolitics.

Vital Letters

Even in his casual correspondence, Keats pondered out loud to anyone who would listen about the shape of the new medicine. His letters often featured effortless forays into ongoing medical discussions about the material organization of the human body. He discussed anatomical theories and hypothesized about the vital principle within complex configurations of biological matter. For the many theorists in search of this elusive vital principle, William Harvey's watershed account of the systemic circulation of blood, through which the body regulates its "vital Spirits" (13), proved irresistibly suggestive. This vital principle – the fluid, current, or force that promised to expose life to the living – had acquired a provocative anatomical vocabulary that would fuel decades of bitter controversy.[4] A richly documented history has grown up around these nineteenth-century vitality debates, but here it suffices to measure their intellectual impact on Keats's medico-literary output. Several studies have enlisted his poetry – the "sixty-two" poetic images of "the life of blood" (de Almeida 90) or the excess of life in *Lamia* (Gigante 208–46), for example – but few have read the letters themselves as serious interventions in the vitality debate. Three letters in particular stand out in this respect: (1) the negative capability letter (December 1817) tentatively locates the vital principle within a "Penetralium of Mystery" of which we can only hope for "half-knowledge," (2) the "Mansion of Many Apartments" letter (May 1818) insists on further exploring the vital depths and branching complexities of human cognition, and (3) his February–May 1819 letter exchanges red blood for red wine in his medical meditation on the pharmacology of claret. With his literary participation in the medico-philosophical debate, Keats maintained a continuous interest in medical theory and practice far beyond an obsessive preoccupation with wasting diseases like consumption. In the end, he would find his own equivocal answer to the vitality question by abandoning fruitless Enlightenment enquiry for a more pragmatic focus on bodily health and proper medical care.

Keats's letter on perhaps his most famous turn of phrase – "*Negative Capability*, that is when man is capable of being in uncertainties, Mysteries, doubts, without any irritable reaching after fact & reason" (*Letters* 41–2) – attempts to express a philosophical concept through an anatomical metaphor. Instead of borrowing

Wordsworth's "burden of mystery" (his famous phrase from "Tintern Abbey") to describe the noumenal locus of truth, Keats concocts, in his uniquely mangled Latin, his own medical phrase: "the Penetralium of Mystery" (*Letters* 42). As Walter Jackson Bate has documented, Keats was no mere dabbler in Latin, so the singular back-formation of the plural *penetralia,* meaning "the innermost parts or recesses of a building" (OED), suggests deliberate distortion (the correct singular is *penetrale*).[5] The architectural metaphor anticipates the "Mansion of Many Apartments," but instead of that moody, sprawling design, he condenses the image into an inner sanctum, a central point from which his blueprint expands in exciting, unexpected, and mostly unknowable ways. The vital principle contracts with this centralizing metaphor, and the strange back-formation emphasizes singularity even at the expense of grammatical Latin. Keats imagines this centrality from which all worthwhile human knowledge derives, from which singular inspiration and individual creativity flourish. In this early version of his poetic ideal, the negatively capable poet extracts from this "Penetralium of Mystery" the half-knowledge that fills out the whole of human engagement with the noumenal world.

Keats's airiest epistemological reveries often find medical ground, and this "Penetralium of Mystery" does not disappoint. In the early eighteenth century, Thomas Fuller became quite famous for publishing hundreds of medical recipes for public consumption in his *Pharmacopoèia Extemporanea.* In the following excerpt from a 1761 English translation of the original Latin, he describes his "trusty" treatment for early stage consumption, "A Lohoch with Myrrh," with the disarmingly conversational tone of a home cook:

> Take Myrrh well powder'd 2 Drams; Saffron half a Scruple; Nutmeg half a Dram; Honey 2 Ounces; mix. This trusty Thoracic has the Privilege to be readily admitted (the Blood introducing it) into the inmost Penetralia of the Lungs, there to dissolve thick impacted Matter, deterge the Canals and Vesicles, dissipate Tubercles, heal Excoriations and little Breaches, imbue the whole Body of the Lungs with Balsam, impart Tone and Strength to its Fibres. In short, it's truly a most desirable and gallant Medicine for such a Consumption as is not yet gone beyond its first Stage. (274)

Jon Mee's note to Keats's Latin phrase acknowledges its strangeness but nevertheless casually dismisses its import: "*Penetralium*: as several editors and critics have pointed out, there is no such word in Latin. Keats means something like 'penetrating insights'" (*Letters* 383). During his constant care of consumptive relatives or his residency at Guy's Hospital, Keats may have come across Fuller's home remedy and his description of the "Penetralia of the Lungs," his phrase for the alveoli, or the grape-like sacs of the lung tissue, responsible for oxygenating carbon-dioxide-rich blood. This concoction, according to Fuller, reaches into the "inmost" recesses of the lungs to dissolve, deterge, dissipate, heal, imbue, and impart – a surprising range of action that suggests ample human access into the heart of an embodied mystery. Keats's "Penetralium," then, may not be merely "something like 'penetrating insights,'" but a medical intervention that locates inspiration in the body of the negatively capable poet, in the negative space of the alveolar sac, ready to breathe life and energizing creativity into depleted blood. This "most desirable and gallant Medicine" grants a tantalizing peek at this "inmost" mystery without any of the "Pain, Sickness, and oppression" (*Letters* 89–90) of the later "Mansion" letter.

According to this younger Keats, self-containing mystery and self-sufficient inspiration was enough. The older Keats would demand much more. The "Mansion" letter, with its interdisciplinary integration of poetry and medicine and its intertextual literature review of poetic masters, deliberately disperses knowledge across space, time, and discipline rather than localizing it in a singular, accessible unity. It is no coincidence, then, that this is the same letter in which he writes wistfully about the possibility of returning to medicine, of finding a painless way to integrate his two passions. He finds a solution to his disciplinary dilemma in a medically informed extension of the Lockean and Darwinian metaphor of the "mansion," newly renovated with the addition of "Many Apartments" (*Letters* 89).[6] He compares human life and what he calls the "grand march of intellect" (*Letters* 90) to a three-stage embodied, architectural exploration. Through the first door lies "the thoughtless chamber" (*Letters* 89) – a version of Locke's *tabula rasa* – in which the mind passively receives the various sense-experiences of the world without the burden of thought. The second is the "Chamber of Maiden-Thought" (*Letters* 89) where "we become intoxicated with the light and the atmosphere, we see nothing but pleasant wonders, and think of delaying there for ever in delight" (*Letters* 89). However, neither is ignorance bliss nor is knowledge exactly sorrow for Keats; rather, the third door both chides us against the blankness of maiden-thought and warns us of a knowable world "full of Misery and Heratbreak [*sic*], Pain, Sickness and oppression" (*Letters* 89–90). This door leads to dark passages, occluding mist, and Wordsworth's "burden of mystery." Wordsworth, who in Keats's linear account of literary history surpasses Milton, bravely explores these dim chambers to "make discoveries, and shed a light in them" (*Letters* 90). Such arduous work, he argues, belongs to the poets of his generation who sharpen their "vision into the heart and nature of Man" (*Letters* 89). He erects a new philosophical edifice that has progressed beyond Locke's claustrophobic metaphor of the architectural self. Like Darwin, Keats worries that the confining figure of the "mansion" inevitably bottlenecks the great progress of human knowledge. Instead, Keats's optimistic epistemology sees the "general and gregarious advance of intellect" (*Letters* 90) as linear expansion rather than as Locke's asymptotic limit. The spatial metaphor grows to capture all human experience; that darkness needs to be tamed, and Keats's metaphor attempts, though humbly and haltingly, to reclaim a small fragment of that space from human blindness.

The anatomical trajectory from lung (the "Penetralium of Mystery") to brain (the "Mansion of Many Apartments") plots Keats's evolving relationship to a simultaneously evolving institution of medicine. In the pulmonary metaphor, the "wise passiveness" (Wordsworth, "Expostulation and Reply" 24) of the negatively capable poet converts, with near-perfect efficiency, inspiration into creative production. This sense of imaginative mastery is not simply the residual voice of Hazlitt in Keats's poetics as some have suggested, but also is the lingering influence of his rigid training in pathology and anatomy.[7] The rise of pathology, as medical anthropologists like Georges Canguilhem and Michel Foucault have ably documented, depends precisely on this efficient absorption of bodily data into the authoritative diagnosis. Just as pathology had claimed to read the body with reassuring legibility, so does the negatively capable poet perfectly inhabit the wonders of the world – all while filtering out extraneous data, fact, and reason – with the picture-perfect fidelity of a "fine verisimilitude" (*Letters* 42). With the refined neurological metaphor, however, pathology begins to falter for Keats. He exchanges Wordsworth's "wise passiveness" for the considerably more excitable body of "Tintern Abbey." The speaker of Wordsworth's lyric poem shakily idealizes the "burden of mystery" with the material vocabulary of an anatomist only to end with a more spiritual conception of the body's relationship to the soul:

> Until, the breath of this corporeal frame
> And even the motion of our human blood
> Almost suspended, we are laid asleep
> In body, and become a living soul.   ("Tintern Abbey" 44–7)

The allusion to Harvey's seventeenth-century account of blood circulation lends medical substance to Wordsworth's turbulent and emotional representation of subjectivity. The speaker's near death experience and his body's functional suspension paradoxically grant a surprising and generous access to "the life of things" ("Tintern Abbey" 50), to the "living soul" of the temporarily suspended corpse. The body ceases to be the coolly capable force of pulmonary inspiration; rather, it becomes a tangle of neurological distress, excitable impulses, and unquantifiable sense data that the lyric speaker strains to interpret.

About a year later, Keats writes in a more light-hearted tone about these embodied "apartments" in a letter that clarifies the medical, anatomical, and pharmacological dimensions of the previous letter's philosophical point:

For really [claret] is so fine – it fills the mouth one's mouth with a gushing freshness – then goes down cool and feverless – then you do not feel it quarrelling with your liver – no it is rather a Peace maker and lies as quiet as it did in the grape – then it is as fragrant as the Queen Bee; and the more ethereal Part of it mounts into the brain, not assaulting the cerebral apartments like a bully in a bad house looking for his trul and hurrying from door to door bouncing against the waist-coat; but rather walks like Aladin about his own enchanted palace so gently that you do not feel his step. (*Letters* 201)

Here, those epistemological "Apartments" from the previous letter materialize dramatically into the "cerebral apartments" of the brain. William Lawrence, in his controversial vitality lectures, uses similar language to refute what he called the "immaterial principle," or the idea that human sentience, volition, and cognition all emerge from something external to the material parts, from a mysterious superadded force that escapes mechanical explanation. In his characteristic, politically charged tone, he pokes fun at this so-called vitalist position: "Physiologists have been much perplexed to find out a common centre in the nervous system, in which all sensations may meet, and from which all acts of volition may emanate; *a central apartment* for the superintendant of the human *panopticon*; or in its imposing Latin name, a *sensorium commune*" (*Letters* 81; first emphasis mine). Keats's metaphor of the "Mansion of Many Apartments" also rejects this central "*sensorium commune*" that ostensibly governs all sensation and volition. In a striking parallel to Darwin's argument in *The Loves of the Plants*, the expansive architecture of the mansion threatens to shrink into the panoptic prison. Relaxing his insistence on the singular experience of "the Penetralium of Mystery," Keats deliberately pluralizes "cerebral apartments" and avoids the frightening consolidation of coercive power in Jeremy Bentham's utilitarian vision of the Panopticon. Keats's materialism, like Lawrence's, insists on anatomical plurality, a neurological explanation of systemic cognition rather than a centralized "immaterial principle" that somehow breathes inspiration into the human mind. Each connection in the brain fires precisely to achieve the perfect thoughtfulness, and Keats's glass of claret provides exactly that material stimulation needed to energize the mind's creative process. No divine spark animates life; rather, a mindfulness of the body's architectural organization governs Keats's concept of health. His medical and literary interest, then, lies squarely within the pragmatics of health care – the human, rather than divine, management of the body – not in vitalism's fruitless speculation on the abstract principle of life.

   Keats's pharmacological experiment, then, must also warn against overdose and its consequences: fever, hepatic discomfort, and even brain damage. When the apartment doors are forced opened too quickly, the mind explores the mansion's dark passages with a heavy heart, burdened by noise, distraction, and paralyzing illness. Instead of a straightforward assault on the "cerebral apartments," Keats prefers the inoculating logic of carefully controlled, mind-altering substances to settle down into a cool "feverless" health. That potential fever recalls the darkness of his mansion's third door which leads to an apartment of world-weary knowledge and overwhelming sensation. The implicit trope of vaccination functions as the "Peace maker" of the body; the controlled infection, intoxication, and the charged interface of interior psychology with external stimulus successfully calms frayed nerves. Notably, he invokes a popular fable from the *Arabian Nights' Entertainments* to figure the otherness of infection. Here, Keats relates the management of the healthy body to cautious interracial contact, invoking the same model of Orientalized medicine that Montagu exploited in her advocacy of Turkish variolation.[8] In the popular story, an African magician relocates Aladdin's "enchanted palace" from China to Africa. Aladdin's task, then, is to travel to Africa, quietly sneaking around the palace, colluding with his captive princess, reclaiming the wish-granting genie, and purging the palace of its nefarious new owner. He arrives in the occupied palace cleverly disguised as an inconspicuous commoner; with gentle step, he passes through unnoticed and successfully reclaims the purloined palace. Keats fashions this tale into a fable of health: just as Aladdin infiltrates the palace while avoiding any outright "quarelling" with the magician, so too does the claret imperceptibly immunize the body against acute illness. All this is not to say that Keats explicitly alludes to vaccination here. Instead, the passage reflects Keats's ready access to a new preventive paradigm of healing while also expressing a simultaneous hesitation about its potential dangers: the side effects of overdose, inebriation, and loss of creative agency. Whereas Montagu turned to Turkey for the science of variolation, Keats turns to China and Africa for magical consolation to allay his worries about new medical territory. Despite lingering qualms, Keats would put his poetic faith in an immunized pantheon of new gods under the leadership of upstart Apollo, benefactor of the new poetry and avatar of the new medicine.

These three Keatses – the consumptive yet negatively capable poet (December 1817), the mansion-dwelling explorer (May 1818), and the medicating oenophile (February–May 1819) – all strive to represent a selective access to medical knowledge, yet end up troubling the notion of the healthy body. Romantic medicine's failures with consumption and cancer coupled with its success in productively challenging Lockean models of mind and body point to a deeply conflictual medical culture that struggled with the idea of proper care. Keats nonetheless remained optimistic. Even when faced with unanswerable questions about the vital principle and the prospect of incurable disease, he turned to Fuller's *Pharmacopoèia* for medical and poetic inspiration and to claret for thoughtful revitalization. And even when the "Mansion" letter confirmed that medicine might not always be so "desirable and gallant," Keats integrated medical and poetic knowledge to open the branching pathways of sensory experience to remain receptive to experimental treatment. In this way, Keats broke away from more conventional Enlightenment-era lines of inquiry. Instead of dwelling on the question of vitality, for example, he turned his attention to the pragmatics of health care. Consequently, his concern lies less in the motivating question of the vitality debates – what is life? – and more in the diligent maintenance of physical and psychological health. The letters' varied interests in anatomy, neurology, and pharmacology breathe life into the uninspired character and eases the overburdened mind rather than attempting to pin down an abstract philosophical principle. His equivocal answer to the vitality question, then, urges us to reconsider a medical orthodoxy increasingly in danger of abandoning the immediate needs of the patient for the dubious production of pathological and philosophical authority.

Keats's earlier metaphor draws from this compelling anatomical and pathological authority whereas the neurological metaphor begins to invoke a very different kind of medicine in its diagnostic uncertainty and its disavowal of the standardized nomenclature of pathology. Contemporary medicine would eventually gravitate towards the former. That the vaccination controversy led to government propaganda, compulsion, and finally pathology should not, however, diminish Keats's crucial tarrying with medical uncertainty during the vaccination controversy. Through the figure of inoculation, Keats's Romantic disease discourse develops novel medical experiments (what Hermione de Almeida describes as his relation to the *pharmakon*), anti-pathological interpretations, and new resources of medical knowledge making. He left behind an increasingly institutionalized medicine not because of some vague romantic impulse towards poetic retirement, but because he sought a means to resist a medical practice that systematically ruled out the unsystematic methods of Romantic medicine in favour of diagnostic expedience.

Inoculated Life

With a theory of Romantic disease discourse in mind, Keats turned to poetic praxis. The interdisciplinary experiment begins with one of his most well-known poems, "La Belle Dame Sans Merci." The poem's brevity and tight narrative structure have made it a perennial favourite of the literature classroom, albeit much to the dismay of the perceptive student. The poem's divergent critical responses quickly betray these deceptive trappings of easy legibility. As soon as one decides that the poem is a quest romance, for example, the poem's inconclusiveness frustrates proper generic accounting. As soon as one ascribes feminist agency to the belle dame's subjugation of her pining paramours, the nested narratives of male desire begin to assert their revisionist power. It is a ballad that paradoxically depends on the quirks of the written word, a lovesick knight's journey that ends in neither consummated love nor tragic death. The two extant versions of the poem introduce even more complications. What, for example, is the difference between "knight-at-arms" and "wretched wight"? How do the stanzas' sequencing determine the meaning of the narrator's ambiguous recollection of the belle dame's amorous speech: "And sure in language strange ... " ("La Belle Dame" 27)? Critics have paid especially close attention to that word "sure": it signifies either the knight's uneasy reassurance of his fading memory or his confidence in its retelling (Simpson 16–20). Alternatively, it might not even be about the knight at all. Andrew Bennett, for example, reads it as the belle dame's certainty in her proclamation of love (114). The poem's structure is at once multiple and spare, its presentation polished and extemporaneous, and its theme celebratory and mournful.

To clarify some of these challenging issues, I begin with the interlocutor's diagnostic question: "O WHAT can ail thee, knight-at-arms" ("La Belle Dame" 1)?[9] Foucault distinguishes between two versions of this question, separated by an epistemic shift in his history of clinical medicine:

> This new structure is indicated ... by the minute but decisive change, whereby the question: "What is the matter with you?", with which the eighteenth-century dialogue between doctor and patient began ... , was replaced by that other question: "Where does it hurt?", in which we recognize the operation of the clinic and the principle of its entire discourse. (*Clinic* xxi)

The clinical question ("Where does it hurt?") pragmatically reorganizes disease into pathological cause and observable effect whereas the older formulation ("What is the matter with you?") encourages a discursive notion of health and disease constructed at the agile interface of doctor and patient. The clinician chooses to close off access to that dialogue and imperiously maps disease onto the symptomatic body. The "principle of [the clinic's] entire discourse," then, is the apparent short-circuiting of the possibility of discourse itself and the subsequent erection of a monolithic medical archive from which illness can be easily isolated from local ("Where") rather than global ("What") cues.

Keats's interlocutor similarly bypasses the patient's narrative. After asking, "O WHAT can ail thee, knight-at-arms, / Alone and palely loitering?" ("La Belle Dame" 1–2), he turns his attention to possible environmental factors instead of waiting for an answer: "The sedge has wither'd from the lake, / And no birds sing" ("La Belle Dame" 3–4). The second stanza continues this pattern with minimal variation: "O what can ail thee, knight-at-arms, / So haggard and so woe-begone? / The squirrel's granary is full, / And the harvest's done" ("La Belle Dame" 5–8). In both cases, autumn has ended (the squirrel and the farmer have both made the appropriate preparations for a lifeless winter) and winter begun (the sedge has died off and the birds have migrated south). As Bewell has demonstrated in his *Romanticism and Colonial Disease*, early nineteenth-century epidemiology was well aware of the close relationship between climate and disease, and the interlocutor's diagnosis swiftly accesses that body of medical knowledge even without recourse to the particularities of the patient's narrative. Since winter had proven a historically reliable ward against the spread of disease, the knight's apparently symptomatic body unsettles this medical archive.[10] Stymied by this seemingly inexplicable symptomology, the interlocutor dully recapitulates pathology, relying only on the rote empiricism of an institutional medical education.

As several critics have surmised, he concludes his investigation with a particularly florid diagnosis of consumption.[11] The "lily" ("La Belle Dame" 9) and the "fading rose" ("La Belle Dame" 11) ostensibly represent respectively the knight's pallid complexion and his wasting health, both classic symptoms of the tubercular patient. What has been overlooked, however, is the interlocutor's subtle reference to pharmacological botany. His strange diagnostic construction, "fever dew" ("La Belle Dame" 10), embeds a floral pun on the feverfew, a flower that, according to the *materia medica* of the time, acts as "tonic, stomachic, resolvent, and emmenagogue [a menstrual stimulant]" (Woodville 74). William Woodville, physician and author of the well-known textbook *Medical Botany* (1810), goes on to say that "[Feverfew] has been given successfully as a vermifuge, and for the cure of intermittents; but its use is most celebrated in female disorders, especially in hysteria" (74). The knight's consumptive symptoms serve to satisfy an urge to link the poem with Keats's own struggles with disease, but the hysteria diagnosis much more accurately captures the two speakers' conversational dynamic. The well-worn consumptive reading of the poem largely derives its evidence from biographical contexts: since Keats wrote the poem after losing his brother Tom to consumption, the pale knight must surely be suffering from the same disease. The hysterical reading of the poem, however, resists that quick conflation of life and art and insists that biography meet textual evidence.

William Cullen, eminent British physician of the eighteenth century, struggled to classify the affliction known as hysteria (Cullen, "Hysteria" 153–8). The best he could do was to correlate the disease tentatively with nymphomania (*hysteria libidinosa*) while lamenting the difficulty in diagnosing such an amorphous disorder. Curiously, though, he also associates hysteria with widowhood, making the disease simultaneously a signifier of biological excess (the "plethoric habits" of nymphomaniacs) and sexual deprivation ("barren" wives left without a sexual partner). In a succinct summary of this oft-contradictory attitude towards hysteria, Rachel P. Maines concludes that "It is at … the beginning of the nineteenth century … that the nosological and etiological framework of hysteria become both confused and confusing" (34). Whether it manifested as libidinal overindulgence or pathological chastity, hysteria existed as some sort of "plethoric state" ostensibly caused by either menstruation or a vaguely defined "turgescence of blood in the uterus" (Cullen, "Hysteria" 157). Pooling fluids and unbounded surges of sexual energy insidiously supplanted feminine sensibility with "robust and masculine constitutions" (Cullen, "Hysteria" 155). Unlike consumption, then, hysteria was far from a wasting away of life but rather, as Denise Gigante might put it, a "monstrous surplus of the real" (237), or a dangerous excess of vital force that disrupts essential biological function. In other words, the knight is not dying as the consumptive reading presupposes, but his disease still lies just beyond conventional medical reckoning.

Even so, the confident interlocutor arrives at an authoritative answer that sets the knight on a carefully charted path from diagnosis to treatment. This masculine diagnosis of a hysterical patient recalls a long history of feminizing Keats consumptive fragility in general. Keats himself often participates in literary cross-dressing, which Margaret Homans unpacks as a "masculine appropriation of the feminine" (344). Anne K. Mellor similarly takes Keats to task for his treatment of the silenced belle dame (*Romanticism & Gender* 184) or, in Karen Swann's more extreme formulation, for the knight's "harassing the muse" with his decidedly biased retelling of the encounter (81–92). And more recently, Susan Wolfson has generously summarized Keats's rich and varied afterlife in relation to Victorian and contemporary notions of gender identity (*Borderlines* 205–84). In all these accounts, Keats only becomes open to femininity after anxiously reclaiming some tenable semblance of masculinity. In the specific case of "La Belle Dame," for example, he identifies with the hysterical knight only because he simultaneously claims membership in an exclusive men's club of lovelorn kings, princes and warriors ("La Belle Dame" 37–8) and because he frames the poem's action within the androcentric genre of the quest romance. Furthermore, Cullen helpfully reminds us that Romantic-era hysteria did not just affect women: "These affections have been supposed peculiar to the female sex; and indeed they most commonly appear in females: but they sometimes, though, rarely, attack also the male sex; never, however, that I have observed, in the same exquisite degree" ("Hysteria" 154). This strategy safely instrumentalizes femininity to convey the central concepts of Keats's poetics – negative capability, wise passiveness, and receptivity – as the feminine potential for creative (re)production. This gendered reading of Keats is now commonplace. My hysterical reading of "La Belle Dame," though, suggests that this richly documented Keatsian femininity also extends to a privileging of care over cure, a negative capability that can inhabit a diseased body that utterly baffles the medical lexicon. The knight's lingering on disease and disorder pits chaotic discourse against the interlocutor's clinical diagnosis. Even though this Foucauldian interlocutor efficiently communicates both disease and remedy within a claustrophobically compact pun – "fever dew"/feverfew – the feminized knight nevertheless persists in the uncertainties and doubts of his affliction without any irritable reaching after pathological diagnosis.

The interlocutor's introductory speech relies on the closed form of the tripartite syllogism.[12] The first stanza's premise announces winter's arrival (the withered sedge and songless birds), and the second describes autumn's end (both squirrel and farmer have concluded their seasonal labours). The third deduces from these environmental premises three possible conclusions, each attached to a floral medical trope: consumption ("a lily on thy brow"), hysteria ("anguish moist and fever dew") and smallpox ("on thy cheeks a fading rose"). The feverish lily's connection to consumption has been ably handled elsewhere, and I have already discussed the poem's hysterical context. For the interlocutor's third diagnosis, I again defer to David Shuttleton's book *Smallpox and the Literary Imagination* in which he traces the literary history of smallpox's rosy poetics, from Dryden's image of smallpox pustules as "Rose-buds, stuck i' th' Lilly-skin about" (58) in the late seventeenth century to Robert Bloomfield's redemptive "vaccine rose" in the early nineteenth. The interlocutor's syllogistic calculation can fathom only this finite set of possibil-ities. All that is left in his medical bag of tricks are the floral history of smallpox and the botanical repertoire of nineteenth-century pharmacology.[13] His medical gaze fixes on the legible, local symptoms of the brow, the skin, and the cheeks, finally directing the knight to answer the clinical question, "Where does it hurt?"

The knight, though, much prefers the older discourse of "What is the matter with you?" and deliberately eschews the clinical precision of the interlocutor's question in the narrative of his transformative encounter with the belle dame. When he finally deigns to acknowledge the original line of questioning, it is only to echo ironically the obtuseness of the initial diagnosis of "anguish moist and fever dew": "She found me roots of relish sweet, / And honey wild, and manna dew" ("La Belle Dame" 25–6). Feverfew can hardly compare to "manna dew," and the belle dame's remedies prove infinitely sweeter. The belle dame becomes a competing physician who bases her diagnosis not merely on unilateral access to a monolithic medical archive, but rather on a mutually constructed illness narrative. This sense of mutuality is the crux of Keats's revisions of the poem. In polishing the manuscript into the published 1820 "Indicator" version, Keats worked hard to balance the distribution of agency in the encounter. Stanzas V and VI of the man-uscript, for example, describes a courtship culminating in a passionate encounter:

> I made a garland for her head,
> And bracelets too, and fragrant zone;
> She look'd at me as she did love,
> And made sweet moan.
> I set her on my pacing steed,
> And nothing else saw all day long,
> For sidelong would she bend, and sing
> A fairy's song.   ("La Belle Dame" 17–24)

In the revised poem, Keats reverses the order of these stanzas, exchanging a scene of amorous courtship for one of forceful seduction. And later, when he re-writes "there she lulled me asleep" as "there we slumber'd on the moss" ("La Belle Dame" 33), he transforms the knightly victimhood of the earlier version into a pastoral portrait of mutual love. The manuscript presents a much more con-sistent narrative – the belle dame is indeed *sans merci* when she hastily declares her love, casts her soporific spell, and finally abandons the knight – while the "Indicator" version adds an odd counter-narrative in which the knight becomes an aggressive paramour who successfully seduces a beautiful woman before get-ting his comeuppance. The poem experiments with exchange and intercourse. It plays with the binaries of the seducer and the seduced, the narrator and the narrated, the victimizer and the victim. The dull opening encounter between the interlocutor and the knight, though, can never erupt in such uncertainty. Perhaps because of this, critics have ignored it or merely dismissed it as a convenient framing device for the poem's more interesting narrative. It is, however, an important medical foil, a diagnostic injunction against discourse, mutual understanding, and the patient narrative. The knight's tale is so enthralling because the diagnostician's question, "O what can ail thee, knight-at-arms?" ("La Belle Dame" 1), is so tedious.

Keats presents two competing medical systems in "La Belle Dame": the first depends on precise pathology, anatomical containment, diagnostic efficiency, and institutional knowledge whereas the second remains tied to pharmacological experiment, volatile discourse, and the illness narrative. Early nineteenth-century medicine struggled to work through this epistemic shift, but the knight seems to have his mind firmly made up. When the interlocutor asks the clinical question that cannot be disturbed by discourse, for example, the knight perversely provides a discursive answer and even pokes a little fun at the obtuse diagnosis. He mimes the interlocutor's tripartite structure in a mock-syllogistic explanation that recapitulates the first stanza with a deeply ironic difference:

> And this is why I sojourn here,
> Alone and palely loitering,
> Though the sedge is wither'd from the lake,
> And no birds sing.   ("La Belle Dame" 45–8)

He taunts the interlocutor's dependence on easy causal linkages with his enticing phrase "And this is why," a connective statement that purports to offer medical cause for symptomatic effect. Yet the interlocutor's telling silence at the end suggests another failure to comprehend. It cannot factor in a disease discourse that continues to resist the Foucauldian clinic. The knight's perspective dramatizes all three properties of Romantic disease discourse. First, the belle dame's experimental "manna dew" captures the negative image of the interlocutor's ingrained medical training and his institutional parsing of disease into syllogisms and binaries. The phrase "fever dew" condenses both problem (hysteria) and solution (feverfew) into the same clinical breath whereas the manna dew's soporific effect generously opens up the pharmacological discourse. Second, while the knight draws attention to the amorphous definitions of hysteria, the interlocutor anxiously tries to pin down a disease that notoriously frustrated nosological classification. Third, the poem ultimately refuses to assign unilateral medical authority. In a sense, all three characters fail to treat the illness: the interlocutor's diagnoses get him nowhere, the belle dame eventually abandons her patient, and the knight ends up aimlessly roaming the land still ailing and palely loitering. The belle dame, however, is certainly an improvement over the ineffectual clinician. The sense of mutuality in her medical discourse stands in stark contrast to the interlocutor's emergent professionalized, institutionalized, and pathologized medicine that seeks to neutralize any perceived threat of discourse. This is a poem about failure but not necessarily about defeatism. Dissatisfied with medicine's future directions, Keats continuously re-energized his advocacy of a different kind of medicine, of a Romantic disease discourse that could produce results like smallpox vaccination without the clinic's institutional trappings.

With the promise of vaccination, the end of disease was within Keats's sight. The knight is not dying; rather, he has survived beyond the thrill of the quest romance and persists in a life among ruins. The withered sedge and the songless sky chastise the knight's rote repetition of enduring life. The belle dame's "manna dew" has inoculated him against bodily ailment, and the "fading rose" – a symptom that the interlocutor misreads as deathly pallor – signifies the gradual return of bodily health through a conventional floral trope that figures the healing of smallpox pustules as withering rosebuds. This disjunction between the knight and his interlocutor underscores Keats's frustration with the direction of clinical medicine. The knight has become healthy beyond the clinician's reckoning. The clinician could hardly understand, for example, the similar description of Moneta's face in *The Fall of Hyperion*:

> Not pin'd by human sorrows, but bright blanch'd
> By an immortal sickness which kills not;
> It works a constant change, which happy death
> Can put no end to; deathwards progressing
> To no death was that visage, it had pass'd
> The lily and the snow   ("The Fall" I.257–62)

The "lily" reprises its role to describe Moneta's deathless fever, an oxymoronic diagnosis that necessarily eludes the interlocutor's method. The clinical archive surely has no account for an illness "deathwards progressing / To no death," so it comes to the poet-physician to untangle the paradox. In "La Belle Dame," this proves no easy task. Abandoned by the immortal "fairy's child," the knight is left to "sojourn" without purpose, unable to die, to ascend to heaven, or to fulfil the parameters of the typical quest romance. Instead of love or death, comedy or tragedy, he finds himself halfway between, in the sparse vignette of barely persisting life among the seasonal corpses of the natural scene. Keats's poetic experiment here is to reinvigorate the elegiac genre in the wake of a medical discovery that threatened to make it obsolete by materializing John Donne's pious prophecy: "Death, thou shalt die!" (14). The poems of *Lachrymae Musarum*, for example, invoke the nine muses to elevate the smallpox-ridden corpse of Lord Hastings into the preserving realm of art. The muse of "La Belle Dame" has no corpse to elegize. Keats's elegy does not presuppose death but instead depicts the perpetual, fevered existence of a life that passes the "lily and the snow." He proposes that in a world where medicine has finally triumphed, we must slowly learn how to mourn the living.

Keats eventually finds an elegiac teacher in Apollo, god of both medicine and poetry. In *Hyperion*, Keats introduces this divine figure at the end of his poetic fragment as the old gods give way to the new:

> Soon wild commotions shook him and made flush
> All the immortal fairness of his limbs;
> Most like the struggle at the gate of death;
> Or liker still to one who should take leave
> Of pale immortal death, and with a pang
> As hot as death's is chill, with fierce convulse
> Die into life: so young Apollo anguish'd:
> His very hair, his golden tresses famed,
> Kept undulation round his eager neck.
> During the pain Mnemosyne upheld
> Her arms as one who prophesied. – At length
> Apollo shriek'd; – and lo! from all his limbs
> Celestial ...   ("Hyperion" III.123–5)

Here, Keats scales up the knight's preserving encounter with the belle dame. Under the watchful eye of Mnemosyne, mother of the nine muses, Apollo dies his "immortal death" into painful life just as the knight is forcibly woken from the fevered dream into lifeless life. Even though the narrative components get some significant upgrades – the knight is recast as an emergent god and the belle dame becomes a Titanic original – Keats still refuses an entirely satisfying solution to the problem of elegy. He concludes the poem with a frustrating ellipsis that precludes such thematic closure. We are left wondering about Apollo's pained immortality, about a life without the chastising sting of death. The open problem persists in this fantastical story of Titans and fledgling gods. And the almost tautological "Celestial" moves the action just beyond human reach. Marjorie Levinson describes "Hyperion" as a "dependent fragment" because it is "an episode or exercise in the poet's career" (50) in which completion depends on a relationship to a larger canon. The fragment's completion depends not only on the later revision into *The Fall of Hyperion*, but also on the biopolitical themes of "La Belle Dame." Keats viewed "La Belle Dame" and *Hyperion* as partial failures that indulge too much in abstract "Miltonic inversions" or some noumenal realm of divinity.[14] In other words, instead of scaling up, Keats decided that it was time to scale down in the poet-speaker's encounter with Moneta in *The Fall*.

In this revision, the poet-speaker stands in for the similarly shrieking Apollo at the end of *Hyperion*: "I shriek'd; and the sharp anguish of my shriek / Stung my own ears" ("The Fall" I.26–7). Apollo's sublime divinity is rewritten in the later poem as a self-reflexive "I." And instead of Apollo's dying into life, Moneta tells the poet-speaker of *The Fall*: "Thou hast felt / What 'tis to *die and live* again before / Thy fated hour" ("The Fall" I.141–3; emphasis mine). The near total erasure of Apollo from the narrative brings the poet-speaker of *The Fall* much closer to the figure of the knight in "La Belle Dame." Moneta, though, proves more unambiguously sympathetic than the ballad's merciless female character. She acts as a paradoxical teacher that guides the dreamer away from guidance, a warning voice that tells the dreamer, in a dream, how to dream: "seek no wonder but the human face; / No music but a happy-noted voice" ("The Fall" I.163–4). Those knights who cloister themselves in nostalgic speculation and idle want forget the "wonder" and "music" of the human world. For this, Moneta at once criticizes and admires her enraptured listener – "Thou art a dreaming thing; / A fever of thyself" ("The Fall" I.168–9) – and ends up commanding him to "think of the earth" ("The Fall" I.169) as if he could, "Bearing more woe than all his sins deserve" ("The Fall" I.176), learn to take on the entirety of human suffering. She exhorts him to look beyond debilitating abstraction and solipsistic depression towards the primary medico-literary task of the poet: to heal Titanic loss and to "pour out a balm upon the world" ("The Fall" I.201).

Part of this burden requires that the poet-speaker decipher Moneta's face and "Part the veils" ("The Fall" I.256) that obscure her immortal visage. He fixates first on the visual field as the description teems with ocular phrases – "blanch'd," "visage," "planetary eyes," "benignant light," – and yet, the language of the eye almost immediately begins to compete with an embedded vocabulary of the mouth and the brain, sites of internalization rather than externalization:

> So at the view of sad Moneta's brow,
> I ached to see what things the hollow brain
> Behind enwombed: what high tragedy
> In the dark secret chambers of her skull
> Was acting, that could give so dread a stress
> To her cold lips ... ("The Fall" I.275–80)

The "view" of Moneta's face appears inadequate and the sexualized language of penetration – "enwombed," "cold lips," "dark secret chambers" – overreaches towards "high tragedy" and surgical discovery. Rather than giving in to these high Miltonic themes as he did in the earlier *Hyperion*, however, his volatile desire stagnates at the level of "I ached to see" and culminates "with act adorant at [Moneta's] feet" ("The Fall" I.283). Still prostrated, the dreamer asks of this "pale Omega of a wither'd race" ("The Fall" I.288):

'Let me behold, according as thou said'st,
What in thy brain so ferments to and fro.' –
No sooner had this conjuration pass'd
My devout lips, than side by side we stood,
(Like a stunt bramble by a solemn pine).   ("The Fall" I.289–93)

The passage from "the view of Moneta's brow" to "her cold lips" is mirrored in
the dreamer from "Let me behold" to "My devout lips," a parallel shift from eye
to mouth, from the dreamer's violent penetrative image of light shining through
Moneta's "dark secret chambers" to a more egalitarian model of conversation. By
the end, the strictly hierarchical image of prostration softens into the democratiz-
ing image of the two figures "side by side."

Hierarchical language persists, however, in the parenthetical comparison of the
speaker's "stunt bramble" to Moneta's "solemn pine," suggesting that the next section of the poem, lifted directly from the beginning of *Hyperion*, is less the words
of a Miltonic soothsayer and more a feeble vision of an epic tale. Even though we
hear this distortion and this "pain of feebleness" ("The Fall" I.429) through the repeated moans of the poet-speaker ("The Fall" I.412–29), he has seen "what things
the hollow brain / Behind enwombed" and finds himself in a privileged position
of a son ("stunt bramble") to Moneta's mother ("solemn pine") rather than a mortal slave to her untouchable divinity. Moneta, roughly this poem's equivalent of
Mnemosyne in *Hyperion*, becomes not only a mother to the nine muses but also to
the human poet. In exchanging the sexual encounter of "La Belle Dame" for this
(grand)mothering relationship, Keats tentatively moves away from the distracting
questions of hierarchy and violation. The two extant versions of "La Belle Dame,"
as I have noted previously, struggle with the sequencing of seduction ("I made a
garland for her head") and abduction ("I set her on my pacing steed"), while leaving the problem of authority open-ended and even, as the critical literature bears
out, endlessly debatable. The poet-speaker of *The Fall* eschews these questions by
turning away from the temptation of violation, of what Keats famously called
Wordsworth's "egotistical sublime," and instead "enjoys" both "light and shade"
without the eager intrusion of "self." Rather than assuming the role of the professional surgeon who brazenly explores the "dark secret chambers" of Moneta's skull,
the poet-speaker relies on a Romantic disease discourse that values imaginative experiment, diagnostic flexibility, and democratic conversation without the immediate assumption of arrogant authority and pathological certainty. He stands "side
by side" with Moneta in the undertaking of the hard task of poetry and finally
offers a solution to the pressing biopolitical problem of elegy. When faced with the
prospect of endless life, Keats insists that we must turn to compassion, receptivity,
and reciprocity, in a new medico-literary discourse that prioritizes life over mere
biological subsistence. Instead of elegizing the dead, Keats lingers on the state of
immunized life, "alone and palely loitering," cured of disease but not of the dark

melancholy of life itself. For Keats, Romantic disease discourse becomes not just a medical episteme, but a poetic project to manage a brave new world of biopolitical existence.

Romantic Biopolitics

At the core of this Keatsian biopolitics is the value of the illness narrative. When Keats imagined a knight, "Alone and palely loitering" while reporting his symptoms to a flabbergasted physician, he was previewing a bioethical debate that would erupt into the so-called right to die controversy of 1975. On 15 April of that year, Karen Ann Quinlan attended a friend's party at which she ingested a deadly combination of alcohol and Valium. After almost a decade-long persistent vegetative state, she died from respiratory failure. Through it all, Quinlan's parents confronted legal, religious, and philosophical challenges about the quality of their daughter's comatose life as she was, as Keats might have put it, "deathwards progressing / To no death." About a decade after Quinlan's prolonged death, Agamben mined the controversy for his book *Homo Sacer* (1998), a philosophical meditation on what he called sovereign power over bare life. "Karen Quinlan's body," he argued, "had, in fact, entered a zone of indetermination in which the words 'life' and 'death' had lost their meaning, and which, at least in this sense, is not unlike the space of exception inhabited by bare life" (164).[15] The state had to intervene within this "zone of indetermination"; advances in medical technology and life extension had made it abundantly clear that human life could not subsist as apolitical biology. Meanwhile, Keats's medical descriptions of the knight's unfulfilled quest romance and Moneta's deathless visage had anticipated both the Quinlan case and this ostensibly contemporary biopolitical insight by almost two centuries. For Keats's medico-literary mind, the human condition was never simply a discrete binary of life and death readily parsed into anatomical certainties. Two hundred years ago, the Romantic poet was already answering these hard questions of biopolitics.

According to Agamben, the crux of the "right to die" debate is what happens when "bare life" – his phrase for pure biology divorced from its social construction – necessarily comes within the purview of state power. Foucault's influential statement of the problem imagines a discontinuous archaeological shift from politics to biopolitics: "For millennia, man remained what he was for Aristotle: a living animal with the additional capacity for political existence; modern man is an animal whose politics places his existence as a living being into question" (*History of Sexuality* 143). In *Homo Sacer*, Agamben refines this contested condition of life by exploring its complementary Greek etymologies: "*zoē* ... expressed the simple fact of living common to all living beings (animals, men, or gods), and *bios* ... indicated the form or way of living proper to an individual or a group" (1). Unlike Foucault's dramatic and discontinuous archaeology, Agamben insists that *zoē* has always intruded upon the sphere of *bios* and that politics has always been biopolitics. His attention eventually evolves from this contested search for a historical origin story to an interdisciplinary effort to articulate a positive, non-degenerate biopolitics. The state must intervene in the Quinlan case, Agamben insists, but how? Foucault's conception of biopower remains cautiously and frustratingly value-neutral, but Agamben's more pragmatic approach attempts to imagine a "new politics" that can "construct the link between *zoē* and *bios*." He defines the "new politics" in a continuum with old, monarchical, and authoritarian forms of power: "Bare life remains included in politics in the form of the exception, that is, as something that is included solely through an exclusion" (11). The complex topological contortions of society's privileged inside and excluded outside are, for Agamben, the preconditions for thinking about this "new politics" of life.

Whereas Foucault and Agamben play coy about the shape of this "new politics," imagining it mainly in the negative (it is *not* about the outworn "form of the exception," for example), Keats turns to a more positive solution in his biopolitical poetry and his fanciful representations of the illness narrative. His reliance on a post-vaccination Romantic disease discourse shapes the contours of his good biopolitical life. Rather than Agamben's "new politics," Keats places his faith in a new *poetics* that cogently articulates the missing link between bare life and its political governance. Vaccination, for example, does not have to be immediately synonymous with biopower for Keats. Whereas Jenner and Wordsworth build up their case studies to rationalize the increasingly familiar compulsions of modern biopower, Keats imagines a very different biopolitical future. His epistolary answers to the vitality question, his discursive approach to disease, and his medico-poetic thought experiments in "La Belle Dame" and the Hyperion poems all work hard to forestall this kind of institutional power over human life. Rather than accede to the techno-optimism of early nineteenth-century compulsory vaccination programs and to professional medicine's well-intentioned intrusions into bare life, Keats's biopolitical poetry refuses to lead us down the garden path towards the compulsory eradication of disease. Instead of relentlessly and unthinkingly refining medicine's biopolitical efficiencies, Keats boldly leaves Guy's Hospital and proposes that poets stake their new claim as the unacknowledged physicians of the world.

I bring up the perhaps surprisingly contemporary case of Karen Ann Quinlan to illustrate how Keats anticipated one of the most famous contemporary touchstones of the right-to-die debate. Agamben's question about the bioethics of state intervention finds a strikingly pragmatic answer in Keats's poetics: he values the old form of the knight's illness narrative over the interlocutor's new paradigm of biopower. Without really listening to the knight, the interlocutor is all too ready to claim the knight's corpse. Similarly, the medical and legal system refused to listen to what it considered to be the backwards cruelty of the Quinlan family's request to remove the ventilator. In both cases, a top-down biopower insisted that it knew best: the knight should die and Karen Ann Quinlan should be forced to live; sacrificial and vegetative life are decided alike from on high. Keats, like Darwin and Blake before him, would instead urge us to listen earnestly to the knight's tale and do our best to honour the Quinlan parents' request. As Agamben observes, state intervention in these kinds of cases is inevitable and necessary, so it becomes all the more urgent to construct something like an alternative vision of a positive biopolitics. What Keats offers is a *bottom-up* vision of public health: listening to milkmaids' experiences with cowpox, caring for his brother Tom's fatal case of tuberculosis, valuing the request of the Quinlans, and taking seriously a ridiculous ballad of knights, fairies, and pale kings. Honouring illness narratives is, more than prescriptive biopower, the best the biopolitical state can and should hope to do.

This modest vision of the future of medicine is not as bizarre as it sounds at first blush. Recent work in medical and health humanities, narrative medicine, and disability studies has shown that biopower's clinical future can hardly boast of a great track record when deciding questions of human health. Iceland's professional medical community, for example, has sponsored an aggressive program of prenatal screening that has virtually eliminated the incidence of Down's syndrome births. Whether this is utilitarian biopolitics or the new eugenics has been hotly debated, but Keats's takeaway would have been modern professional medicine's startling efficiency in turning unvetted decision into unilateral action. This kind of modern biopower began in earnest at the beginning of the twentieth century with the first global effort to catalogue disease. The International System of Nomenclature of Diseases and Causes of Death – now abbreviated ICD-1 (1900) – sought to reduce human morbidity and mortality to an efficient list of discrete, accessible categories. Later, this ambitious effort expanded to include mental disorders in the first Diagnostic and Statistical Manual of Mental Disorders, now abbreviated DSM-I (1952). While diagnostic expedience has been strongly correlated with declining mortality rates, these statistical manuals were not without their critics.[16] Perhaps the most well-known of these controversies was the DSM's inclusion of homosexuality. Varying formulations of the homosexual "diagnosis" stubbornly persisted as late as 1986, when activist criticism and pioneering research on sexuality finally overwhelmed ingrained prejudices. Pathology had become a potential site of coercive normalization, a danger that did not escape the notice of a growing number of social historians of medicine. Canguilhem and Foucault, for example, both worked to expose pathology's social construction and to subvert its claim to scientific authority.[17] The nascent field of disability studies has continued further along these theoretical lines, undoing normative pathologies to reveal new ways to think about impairment and illness without recourse to essentialized and stigmatized models of disability. Yet there is still significant work to be done. In the attempts to reverse prejudicial exclusions, to recognize the costs of normativity, and to uncover the sociopolitical underpinnings of medical science, these studies have understandably depended on caustic reaction to produce their theories of the abnormal. Though Canguilhem and Foucault have been invaluable in exposing the structures of medical power, their conclusions remain bleak and their recommendations conspicuously sparse. Similarly, disability theory continues to struggle with dismantling pathology while often tabling the ultimate goal of social recognition.[18]

However, before these eruptions of modern biopower, Keats could sidestep this reactionary mode to theorize his positive poetic discourse of disease, disability, and abnormality. His knight-at-arms, not the myopic diagnostician of "La Belle Dame," quickly takes the biopolitical reins of the illness narrative. The towering historical roadblocks of the ICD and the DSM were yet unknown to Keats. Medical practitioners of the period could still resist the easy absorption of the abnormal body into an organizing gaze of institutionalized medicine because they did not yet rely on rigidly constructed borders between the normal and the pathological.[19] Romantic medicine and literature depended instead on a porous disease discourse that problematized the modern medical impulse to identify and rehabilitate the "defective" body. In the late twentieth century, however, Foucault could only shake his fist at the hypocrisy of a post-DSM clinic that selectively policed sexuality and non-normative embodiment. He observed, for example, that the state capriciously cast out lepers even as it held out a safety net for plague victims. The plague victim was granted immunity (both in the juridico-political and medical senses of the word) from ostracism and brought into the medical lexicon while the leper remained a lost cause, a hopelessly incompatible residue.[20] The plague victim's story could be told, heard, and valued; the leper's only ignored and eradicated. Foucault read these strangely selective immunities and exclusions – a leper, a gay man with AIDS, a child born with Down's syndrome – as the essential, immovable nature of arbitrary state power.

More recently, however, Roberto Esposito has used the metaphor of inoculation and immunity to model alternative communities free of Foucault's arbitrary governmentality. Esposito posits an "immunization paradigm" that reads the history of biopolitics as a *negative* history of eugenics, or what he calls – in a deathly opposition to the *bíos* of the more familiar term – "thanatopolitics." He surveys contemporary philosophy in his *Communitas* (1998), *Immunitas* (2002), and *Bíos* (2004) trilogy to find that immunity is almost always associated (at least implicitly) with a sense of sterility that purges "community" and the "extraindividual" from the immunized subject.[21] In the wake of this thanatopolitical history, then, he calls for a positive (contaminated or inoculated rather than eugenically purified) biopolitics. Esposito, however, seems like he is not fully invested in literary or medical history to search for this immunized biopolitics. Indeed, he even misspeaks about the smallpox vaccine when he refers to "the discovery of a *measles* vaccine by Jenner" (*Immunitas* 7; emphasis mine). For him, inoculation and immunity tend towards instrumental metaphors: they are useful insofar as they lead him to a better biopolitics. The tendency is to work through biopolitical notions of immunity as more or less a causeless effect; immunity is the abstract goal, but there is no deeply historical or material cause to ground the frequently intractable metaphor. The Romantic origins of immunity, especially Keats's medico-literary work, had already trialled this contaminated biopolitics and had already moved out of the leprous paradigm of quarantine and the quasi-eugenic purge of disease.[22] Keats, in the thick of the vaccination controversy's first wave, suggested that poets, not politicians or physicians, are the most qualified to immunize the non-normative body against social stigma and to talk through the true parameters of human flourishing.

Since Esposito, the now standard theoretical discussions of biopolitics have taken more care to preserve the link between the metaphor of immunity and medical historical reality. From a sociological perspective, Thomas Lemke's *Biopolitics: An Advanced Introduction* (2007, translated into English in 2011), has emphasized the messiness of the term itself. Lemke observes that biopolitics has come to mean very different things to different people: for some, it is sober, "rational decision-making and the democratic organization of social life," but to others it insidiously weaponizes rationality to justify "eugenics and racism" (1). And in *Systems of Life: Biopolitics, Economics, and Literature at the Cusp of Modernity* (2018), Richard A. Barney and Warren Montag assembled a group of distinguished authors to think about the historical formations of biopolitics at "the cusp of modernity" (around the Romantic era).[23] Esposito's immunitary logic is enormously helpful and generative, and his landmark work serves as both ally and foil in my own argument. Esposito, along with this more recent work in biopolitics, helps us to understand the profound strangeness of these Romantic writers: Darwin's caprification, Blake's violation, Keats's inoculating logic, and, as I will discuss in the next chapter, Shelley's contamination are all precursors to these biopolitical issues. These authors lived through and wrote about the birth of professional medicine. What the essays in *Systems of Life* demonstrate, for example, is that authors at "the cusp of modernity" might offer tighter links between a positive biopolitics and medical reality. Problems that seem utterly contemporary – end-of-life decisions, disabled access, and of course compulsory vaccination – find ready solutions in the Romantic illness narrative, and it is certainly worth going back to these earlier literary and poetic materializations of biopolitical thinking to reshape our own medical debates.

It is often difficult, though, to speak of Romantic poetry's slow luxury and the embodied urgency of diseased life in the same breath. Sontag's disapproving literary history of tuberculosis, for example, rails against the damaging and unrealistic metaphor of the consumptive poet in the Romantic period. In a more sympathetic account, Clark Lawlor has identified consumption with poetic agency in Percy Shelley's "Alastor": "Shelley's vision of the poet would therefore seem to be tragic: the sensitive poet is unable to survive his own burning desire. Only those lacking in sensibility can live long in the world" (147). In Lawlor's account, the difficulty persists in a different form; Romantic disease discourse threatens to become no more than a naively metaphorical appropriation of tuberculosis to aestheticize and idealize the consumptive and "sensitive poet." Even though consumption, for both Sontag and Lawlor, seems to reduce *Romantic* disease to *romanticized* disease, literary representation and medical reality need not always be at odds. With his mixed disciplinary background, Keats navigates the treacherous waters between Sontag's positivistic medicine and Lawlor's poetic idealization. Only recently, in the nascent field of narrative medicine, have we begun to take this kind of interdisciplinarity seriously. Rita Charon begins her book, *The Principles and Practices of Narrative Medicine*, with an instructive anecdote that pits an unfeeling physician (herself) against the suppressed narrative of a suffering patient, a telling picture of the state of contemporary medicine and an urgent call to action.[24] Yet we need not manufacture this theory of narrative medicine from thin air.[25] Keats's medico-literary work, as I have argued in this chapter, had already talked up the value of the patient narrative in psychological healing, in disease interpretation, and even in new directions for treatment and care.

When Ed Cohen, a scholar of modern biopolitics, searches for that sense of patient agency beyond the Foucauldian concept of a coercive and purifying bodily defence against leprous disease, he comes up short. In his concluding discussion of immunity, he wistfully fixates on modern medicine's missed opportunity to articulate such a contaminated biopolitics:

> When in the early 1880s Élie Metchnikoff characterizes a form of organismic activity as "defense," he gives the term "immunity" its modern biomedical valence. Imagine what might have happened if he had not been so focused on … the dynamics of aggression and response … He might then have described the dynamics through which complex organisms systematically mediate their relations with the others with whom they must concur by using immunity's etymological opposite, "*com*munity" … How might we have organized our care for the ill and our systems of healing … if we imagined that our ability to respond to corporeal challenge engages our ability *to commune* with others? … A silly thought experiment perhaps. Nevertheless, it does suggest that there may be more to immunity than we currently know, or are indeed even capable of knowing, so long as we remain infected by the biopolitical perspectives that it defensively defines as the apotheosis of the modern body. (281)

Romantic medicine's willingness to experiment, to suspend judgment on the abnormal, and to invite the broadest range of interdisciplinary perspectives all worked to redefine immunity in these generous terms. Immunity came from Romantic-era inoculation, in both the medical and metaphorical senses of the word, and Romantic disease discourse had already modelled Cohen's contaminated biopolitics. His "thought experiment" need not be "silly" because Romantic biopolitics offered a firm historical precedent for his wishful thinking. Indeed, Romantic medicine *required* this sense of biopolitical community to authorize its experimental mode, its nosological looseness, and its radical inclusiveness. Romantic literature and medicine confirm Cohen's hunch that "there may be more to immunity than we currently know."

It is quite telling that Cohen cites Metchnikoff's 1880 construction of the defensive body while ignoring Romantic medicine's alternative immunities. By the middle of the nineteenth century, medicine's more familiar narratives – institutionalization, disease classification, and professionalization – had begun to replace the radical experiments of Romantic medicine. Cohen's wistfulness starts to make much more sense: disease, disability, and illness converge with coercive pathology while health becomes more fully institutionalized, carefully policed, and meticulously defined as a defence against the non-normative. Within such a Victorian medical frame, biopolitics can indeed seem like the dead end of biopower or at best an occasion for Cohen's hypothetical "what might have happened." Romanticism frequently gets short shrift in medical histories because of its awkward disruption of Enlightenment genealogies, but it can offer a potent historical reconfiguration of modern biopolitics that offers medical humanities, disability theory, and narrative medicine at least two positive precedents. First, its stubborn resistance to pathology may bring us yet another step closer to a bioethical theory of non-normative embodiment. Second, its democratic inclusion of multiple perspectives – medical, literary, and lay – should motivate narrative medicine's push to place disciplines into productive conversation. As Cohen's elision demonstrates, we have lost this Romantic medico-literary history, and we have been working diligently ever since to recover it from scratch. Esposito and Cohen's search for a kind of immunity in community, disability theory's goal to find a place for the non-normative, and narrative medicine's work to forge a medico-literary language could all benefit from looking backward at Keats's model of Romantic disease discourse. Our focus on the Victorian case has obscured literature's role in representing the illness narrative and has blocked our access to a more generous biopolitical theory of immunity. The case of Keats and Romantic medicine instead reminds us that social justice and even medical efficacy are sometimes the casualties of contemporary medicine's brutal efficiency. This is not to discount the enormous gains we have made in the field, but modern medicine may be wise to reconsider brushing off Romantic medicine as a zany hiatus in the relentless drive towards Enlightenment progress. Instead, we should look more closely at a medico-literary culture that produced both vaccination, one of the most important and enduring discoveries in the history of medicine, and Keats, one of the most effortless and productive interdisciplinary poets in the history of literature.

Chapter Five

Shelley and Romantic Immunity

Biopolitics by Induction

As the previous chapter argues, John Keats imagines Romantic biopolitics in the sensuous terms of localized health: life and death felt on the pulse of his knight-at-arms, inspiration breathed into the lungs of the fever-dreaming poet, and knowledge distributed across branching neural pathways of the creative mind. What changes in this politics of embodiment, though, when Keats's one body problem divides in two? Mary Shelley's apocalyptic novel *The Last Man* (1826) enlarges the terms of Keats's local vision of health, imagining the end of disease not by peering inwardly to the regulation of the individual body, but by enforcing a cosmopolitan ethics in the geopolitical space *between* vulnerable bodies. To speak of humanity's triumph over disease in a novel that spectacularly stages epidemic annihilation against the futility of human endeavour might, at first glance, seem particularly perverse. To read the novel as any kind of biopolitical intervention, then, this chapter first recovers the radical utopian potential within the threateningly nihilistic plot to articulate precisely how Shelley hopes to leverage some hope of a Kantian cosmopolitanism against natural disaster. It is with this sense of controlled infection from otherness, an idealized cosmopolitanism that Kant calls "unsocial sociability," that Shelley arrives at not only the Keatsian concept of physical and mental well-being, but also at sociopolitical stability, with a cogent model of the healthy state and a medicine that finally values the unique, lived stories of illness. *The Last Man* incrementally compounds the biopolitical problem of health by piling on the stories of infected bodies; in this way, Shelley mobilizes a Romantic disease discourse to construct inductively a biopolitics by sheer numbers.[1]

This biopolitical induction depends on the presumption that the personal and political catastrophes that cluster around both author and novel *inform*, but do not determine, the ideological texture of Shelley's apocalyptic plague narrative. Despite charges of nihilism and anti-Romantic conservatism, Shelley offers several sites of social resistance to natural disaster that renovate, rather than reject, the philosophical and political idealism of the earlier generation of Romantic authors. Shelley's lifelong struggle with the ideal of androgyny, for example, demonstrates a staunch commitment to finding social solutions to ostensibly biological problems. Her evocation of Kant's cosmopolitanism of "unsocial sociability" similarly imagines strong moral checks to inevitable human conflict. Through a sustained focus on illness narratives of social resistance, Shelley employs a shrewdly revisionist strategy that continuously writes notions of human community and companionship – in the variable terms of gender, race, and even species – into nineteenth-century medical discourse. The central metaphor of inoculation manages these volatile terms by reference to a long material history of medical science, from Montagu's Turkish inoculation to Jenner's cowpox vaccine. In the end, Shelley models a cogent politics of possibility and articulates a mature medical evolution of the Romantic imagination's potentially transformative agency.

To this end, Shelley's novel reworks Burke's infamous warning against the radicalism of the French Revolution in which he associates the word "inoculate" with political contamination:

> We wished at the period of the Revolution, and do now wish, to derive all we possess as *an inheritance from our forefathers*. Upon that body and stock of inheritance we have taken care not to inoculate any cyon [*sic*] alien to the nature of the original plant. All the reformations we have hitherto made, have proceeded upon the principle of reference to antiquity; and I hope, nay I am persuaded, that all those which possibly may be made hereafter will be carefully formed upon analogical precedent, authority, and example. (*Reflections* 181)

Recall from the introduction that Burke uses the process of grafting a "cyon" (a scion or bud) onto a host plant as a metaphor for unjustifiable revolution. He elides two major details in his pursuit of rhetorical flourish at the expense of scientific precision: (1) botanists graft foreign buds onto plants to bolster resistance to diseases and to increase the health of the "body and stock" of the "original plant," and (2) by 1790, smallpox inoculation (variolation) had already proven to be a relatively effective deterrent to full-blown infection. Shelley, a meticulous and critical reader of Burke, must have noticed Burke's doubly poor choice of metaphor and capitalizes on his infelicitous turn of phrase in her own scene of inoculation in *The Last Man*. Since the novel is told from the perspective of Lionel Verney, the eponymous last man after a virulent plague sweeps across the world, the entire premise hinges upon his mysterious survival and the mechanism of his immunization. What saves Verney turns out to be his inoculating, cosmopolitan embrace of racial otherness and his inhalation of the "death-laden" breath of a "negro half clad."[2] By the end, though, Verney wanders the globe alone, his immunity seemingly a pyrrhic victory at best. Shelley's inductive step seems to falter here in the regression of biopolitics back to the base case of Keats's solitary body, "Alone and palely loitering." However, Shelley's novel works in much broader strokes in its careful manipulation of vaccination history, which complicates the medical register of the shaky conclusion. Shelley's failed induction is deliberate. She imagines an alternate – and hence avoidable – history of medicine in which the anti-vaccination movement has won and the illness narrative has been tossed aside, leaving humanity with the prospect of non-reproductive life, hopeless isolation, and even species extinction.

The third and final volume of the long novel abandons the search for a cure in favour of just reporting these illness narratives of plague victims. It is so important to Verney to tell these stories that he seems to shrug off the real possibility that there is no one left to read them. By this third volume, it certainly seems like the story is heading to that nihilistic conclusion:

> Plague is the companion of spring, of sunshine, and plenty. We no longer struggle with her. We have forgotten what we did when she was not. Of old navies used to stem the giant ocean-waves betwixt Indus and the Pole for slight articles of luxury. Men made perilous journies to possess themselves of earth's splendid trifles, gems and gold. Human labour was wasted – human life set at nought. Now life is all that we covet; that this automaton of flesh should, with joints and springs in order, perform its functions, that this dwelling of the soul should be capable of containing its dweller. Our minds, late spread abroad through countless spheres and endless combinations of thought, now retrenched themselves behind this wall of flesh, eager to preserve its well-being only. We were surely sufficiently degraded. (250)

Humanity had conquered the oceans to enrich itself with "articles of luxury" and to exploit "earth's splendid trifles," but all that human endeavour was "set at nought." Shelley evokes the language of materialism ("automaton of flesh") and vitalism ("the soul") to show how "mind" and the human mastery over nature had been reduced to mere body and degraded material. The mind, formerly expansive, boundless, and infinite, has now retreated to the mere "wall of flesh." And the rest of the novel is a dreary catalogue of these ample horrors of degradation, a tale that Verney compulsively records for no one.

Verney indefatigably continues his reporting of everyone's coping strategies: Ryland's every-man-for-himself plan (252), the "Black Spectre's" cling to sociability even as he dies from the plague (321), the Countess of Windsor's apology for opposing Idris's marriage (283), and the impostor-prophet's growing following of desperate believers (294). Verney remains a chatty witness to the horror but can offer no redress. Because of this, the long series of illness narratives can sound like impotent grievance, so what could possibly be the point in documenting this long chronicle of species extinction? Even Verney, the assiduous recorder of the end of days, seriously questions his writerly purpose:

Will not the reader tire, if I should minutely describe our long-drawn journey from Paris to Geneva? If, day by day, I should record, in the form of a journal, the throng-ing miseries of our lot, could my hand write, or language afford words to express, the variety of our woe; the hustling and crowding of one deplorable event upon an-other? Patience, oh reader! whoever thou art, wherever thou dwellest, whether of race spiritual, or, sprung from some surviving pair, thy nature will be human, thy habita-tion the earth; thou wilt here read of the acts of the extinct race, and wilt ask won-deringly, if they, who suffered what thou findest recorded, were of frail flesh and soft organization like thyself. Most true, they were – weep therefore; for surely, solitary being, thou wilt be of gentle disposition; shed compassionate tears; but the while lend thy attention to the tale, and learn the deeds and sufferings of thy predecessors. (312)

He has serious difficulties even imagining this "reader" now. His readership could be part of a purely spiritual race, a couple who survived in some unknown cor-ner of the earth, or just a solitary being like himself. Verney eventually clings to hope for some new human lineage and decides to continue the frontline report: "This tale, therefore, shall be rapidly unfolded. Images of destruction, pictures of despair, the procession of the last triumph of death, shall be drawn before thee, swift as the rack driven by the north wind along the blotted slendour of the sky" (311–12). And he does not disappoint with the rapid-fire illness narratives that follow, detailing every excruciating pain and nauseating cruelty. Margaret Atwood, in a recent *New York Times* essay on *The Handmaid's Tale* (1985) in the "Age of Trump," mentions that she is asked frequently about her novel's incredible prescience. "No, it isn't a prediction," she demurs, "because predict-ing the future isn't really possible: There are too many variables and unforeseen possibilities. Let's say it's an antiprediction: If this future can be described in detail, maybe it won't happen. But such wishful thinking cannot be depended on either."[3] Shelley's novel is Atwood's undependable but still powerful "antipre-diction": if we can imagine apocalypse in such fine detail, we can perhaps rob that future of its power. Detailing these sickening illness narratives, in a sense, inoculates us against catastrophe. Such prophylactic fiction seems hard to im-agine in the nearly nihilistic tale of *The Last Man*, but, as I will contend in this chapter, not impossible.

Genealogy

Shelley surely had cause for pessimism at this point in her life. By the time she published *The Last Man* (1826), her social and literary circles had disappeared, her husband had drowned, and the radical promises of the French Revolution had de-teriorated into Napoleonic violence and despotism.[4] Nevertheless, Lionel Verney, Shelley's narrator and eponymous last man, seems eager to recover from this sense of personal and political loss:

Hope beckons and sorrow urges us, the heart beats high with expectation, and this eager desire of change must be an omen of success. O come! Farewell to the dead! farewell to the tombs of those we loved! – farewell to giant London and the placid Thames, to river and mountain or fair district, birthplace of the wise and good, to Windsor Forest and its antique castle, farewell! themes for story alone are they, – *we must live elsewhere.* (*The Last Man* 326; emphasis mine)

The comforting cultural geography of Edmund Spenser's appeal to the Thames in *Prothalamion* (1596), Wordsworth's rustic paradise, and Alexander Pope's patriotic propaganda in *Windsor-Forest* (1712) vanish into the immense map of a plague-stricken globe. The "we" is no longer British, and the "elsewhere" appears nowhere on the redrawn map of the world. *The Last Man* is a novel of visions and revisions that strives with great difficulty to reconstruct both subject ("we") and place ("elsewhere") in a new framework of cosmopolitan community and political radicalism.[5] Before *The Last Man*, Shelley's career had relied upon varying degrees of collaboration to work through such nuances and revisions. She had a solicitous reader of *Frankenstein* (1818) in her husband Percy Shelley and an aggressive editor of *Valperga* (1823) in her father William Godwin. With *The Last Man*, she found herself completely alone, a feeling that she expresses in a frequently cited journal entry: "The last man! Yes I may well describe that solitary being's feelings, feeling myself as the last relic of a beloved race, my companions extinct before me" (*Journals* 476–7). Through Verney's "Hope," however, Shelley constructs several sites of effective social resistance to this ponderous sense of despair and alienation. She continuously rewrites redemptive narratives into *The Last Man* and gives shape to a politics of possibility that recovers the novel from charges of nihilism or anti-Romantic conservatism.

Many readers of *The Last Man* have emphasized this morbid pessimism. For example, Morton D. Paley has neatly classified readings of the novel into three categories that reflect its perceived reactionary posture: (1) a reaction against the violence of the French Revolution and Napoleonic despotism (Sterrenburg 324–47), (2) a reaction against Shelley's own ideal of the nuclear family in *Frankenstein* (Mellor, *Mary Shelley* 141–68), and (3) a reaction against the millenarianism of the "Romantic ethos" (Paley, "Apocalypse" 111).[6] If one reads the novel at all, it seems it must be read as a largely sterile *reaction* against the optimism of a bygone age, and any reading that locates a productive site of Romantic possibility seems to miss a "cruel joke by the author upon reader" ("Apocalypse" 119). Paley finds this joke in one of the novel's most poignantly ironic scenes: the organ performance of Haydn's "New-Created World" by an infected girl for her blind, dying father. In Anne K. Mellor's account, that joke is refashioned into a familiar axiom of deconstruction: "all conceptions of human history, all ideologies are grounded on metaphors or tropes which have no referent or authority outside of language" (*Mary Shelley* 164). The ideologies, metaphors, and tropes of the "New-Created

World" falter when the plague unapologetically claims both father and daughter, silencing any recuperative possibility of the girl's desperate hymn of praise. For this reason, Barbara Johnson, Mellor, and Audrey A. Fisch have all proleptically dubbed *The Last Man* an early – if not the first – novel of deconstruction.[7] In all these accounts, *The Last Man* reads as a novel out of time, a strange postmodern tribulation in an era of exuberant, Romantic prophecies about imagination, reform, and revolution.

Nevertheless, Mellor and Fisch also warn against the reductive "nihilism of a politically harmful deconstruction" in favour of a reading that credits Shelley for her tentative "roadmap for political change" (Fisch 274). For Fisch, the framing narrator (the authorial voice in Shelley's odd "Introduction") provides a model of political agency that at least partially rescues the novel from the deconstructive vacuum that Mellor describes. Jean de Palacio turns to three musical movements in the novel (the domestic drama in Windsor, the arrival of the plague in England, and the Haydn performance) to find "une période de concorde et de paix" (329) in the redemptive power of music to transcend its deconstructive containment. Sandra M. Gilbert, Susan Gubar, and Mary Poovey rely on Shelley's strategies of narrative indirection and her shrewdness about the status of the professional female writer to recover a sense of authorial agency amidst the stubborn nihilistic undercurrents of the plot (Gilbert and Gubar 95–104; Poovey 146–59). These critics argue quite reasonably that if "Shelley had staked her emotional and financial security on *The Last Man*" (Poovey 158), then eccentrically perverse nihilism hardly seems an appropriate strategy; instead, they struggle to resuscitate civilization from the life-denying force of the plague and conclude that Shelley participates in a liberal "politics of imperfection" (Fisch 278–81) or a dialectical "state of incompletion prolonged into eternity" (Poovey 153). These Romantic readings (as opposed to the more pessimistic readings of Paley and, to a lesser extent, Mellor) range from Hartley S. Spratt's triumphant proclamation that "Verney is prepared to confront the dream and win through to Romantic art" (535) to Robert Lance Snyder's more circumspect relegation of the novel to "the realm of the indeterminate," expressing a redemptive yet "chastened imagination" (451). This perceived personal and political "ambivalence" on Shelley's part prompts these various challenges against anti-political readings of the novel and articulates a hopeful reanimation of Romantic possibilities, no small feat in this decidedly dreary tale.[8]

My approach in this chapter continues this line of criticism but offers a more sustained narrative genealogy rather than isolated moments of authorial ambivalence. Neither Fisch's attention to the framing narrator nor Palacio's work on the musical episodes does sufficient justice to the novel's thematic unevenness. Any genealogy of the novel that relies on the severely flawed cast of main characters will incur some vexing residues. For example, when Paley invokes the division of power and knowledge in Percy Shelley's *Prometheus Unbound* (1820) as an evaluative standard for Adrian, Raymond, and Verney, he finds each of them lacking in some way or another, and quickly returns to his anti-Romantic reading ("Apocalypse" 112–15). Similarly, Fisch tracks Shelley's various portraits of male political leadership – "republicanism by Raymond; hereditary monarchy by Adrian; democracy by Ryland; theocracy by the 'imposter prophet'" (273) – and finally fails to find a viable political model which then leads to a somewhat hasty conclusion about the framing narrator's "nonhuman" alternative to limited humanistic politics. I have selected these two archetypal trajectories because they illustrate interpretive structures that have significantly overdetermined our readings of the novel: the former rejects human agency in favour of an anti-political, anti-Romantic, and even nihilistic conclusion while the latter replaces that elusive agency with a volatile ambivalence and a shaky faith in isolated redemptive episodes or characters.

Thus, instead of relying on a faltering genealogy of familiar faces – Adrian, Raymond, and Verney are more or less well-rehearsed portrayals of Percy Shelley, Byron, and Mary Shelley respectively – I will turn to the novel's buried genealogy of what Fisch would call "nonhumanness" (281) or what Spratt would refer to as the "more-than-natural" (534). My reading organizes the novel around Shelley's four unlikely attempts at pinning down both Verney's "we" and his fading "elsewhere": the much-discussed cave explorers of Shelley's introduction, the significantly under-theorized Evadne, Verney's embrace of the "negro half clad" (*The Last Man* 336), and Verney's canine companion. I argue that this sustained (yet admittedly somewhat obscure) genealogy evens out some of the ostensible ambivalences and indeterminacies of *The Last Man* and allows for not just a haltingly compensatory politics of imperfection or incompletion, but also for a mature evolution of the transformative agency of Romantic imagination and a surprisingly material and social basis for a reclaimed politics of possibility. In particular, I track Shelley's continuous revision of models of companionship and community from the ungendered creativity of the introductory pair, to the androgynous balancing act of Evadne, to the cosmopolitan embrace of racial alterity, and finally to the cross-species coupling at the novel's conclusion.[9] Even though the trajectory follows a gradual degeneration into farce, Shelley's revisionist strategy continuously invokes Verney's "Hope" through each iteration and finally recovers that politics of possibility despite the novel's tragic history of failure.

Gender and Agency

Like many of the other accounts that I have surveyed, my genealogy begins, quite predictably, at the beginning with Shelley's introduction. The framing tale is usually read as fictionalized autobiography; it tells the story of the Shelleys and their friend Claire Clairmont's exploration of the Cave of the Sibyl at Baiae on the Bay of Naples. Gilbert and Gubar take great pains to feminize this cavernous space and diagram a complex triangulation of agency involving Mary Shelley, Percy Shelley, and the Sibyl. Yet Shelley seems to take equally great pains to purge the feminine from this space. The framing narrator (not necessarily Shelley herself) maintains a Steinian aversion to gendered pronouns, the womb-like cave appears eerily sterile, and the divinely feminine Sibyl is conspicuously absent. If the unordered sibylline leaves indeed represent a lacuna of creative potentiality, it is not necessarily a feminine one. The epigraph from Adam's complaint to Michael in *Paradise Lost* (1667), "Let no man seek / Henceforth to be foretold what shall befall / Him or his children," does not immediately prompt an empowered Sibyl to claim, "But a woman can."[10] The two figures in the cave, neither women nor men, continually labour to rearrange the leaves into a coherent narrative. A narrowly autobiographical focus on this episode obscures the strangeness of this task and misses the unique, ungendered texture of Shelley's strategies of narrative deflection and disavowal. At least two critics have remarked upon Shelley's "lifelong concern with the psychological ideal of androgyny" (Veeder 2), but unfortunately they have mostly restricted this broad observation to readings of *Frankenstein*.[11] The genderless cave explorers in *The Last Man* propagate Shelley's lifelong theme with two crucial differences. The first is semantic: the pair is ungendered rather than simply androgynous. The second is thematic: in *Frankenstein*, androgyny materializes in efficient bifurcations (for example, the masculine Victor Frankenstein and the feminine Henry Clerval) whereas the genderless pair consistently resists easy psychological classifications, opening up several creative possibilities of sibylline revision in the erasure of restrictive gender differences. Shelley refines her search for the "psychological ideal of androgyny" into the ungendered cave explorers, which necessarily complicates any biographical reading that relies on fixed categories of masculine and feminine.

However, completely ignoring the autobiographical dimension of that sibylline labour also means glossing over important correlations in Shelley's *roman à clef*. She conceived the novel partially as an opportunity to exorcise her guilt over Percy Shelley's untimely death in 1822.[12] In the introduction, execution quickly catches up with conception when the framing narrator decides to share the task of deciphering the sibylline leaves with a companion who suddenly disappears: "For awhile my labours were not solitary; but that time is gone; and, with the selected and matchless companion of my toils, their dearest reward is also lost to me" (*The Last Man* 6). Just as Shelley's intellectual circle began to desert her, the framing narrator finds herself/himself alone with the sibylline prophecies. At this point, those "obscure and chaotic" (*The Last Man* 6) leaves come to represent not only the collaborative intellectual and literary work of the Shelley circle, but also the contested posthumous legacy of Percy Shelley's vast, unorganized body of visionary poetry. After his death, Shelley became an assiduous editor of her late husband's work despite the constant interference of Sir Timothy Shelley, her priggish and disapproving father-in-law. Through the framing narrator, Shelley imagines a way to circumvent the legal obstacles that stood between her and her husband's literary estate and claim the agency that she had been denied. As sole "decipherer" (*The Last Man* 6), the narrator takes up the task of not only preserving the ancient documents, but also of translating them into intelligibility: "Doubtless the leaves of the Cumaean Sibyl have suffered distortion and diminution of interest and excellence in my hands. My only excuse for thus transforming them, is that they were unintelligible in their pristine condition" (*The Last Man* 6–7). The narrator/Shelley boldly moves past mere translation to interpretive transformation and willful distortion, which not only mitigates the loss of the companion, but also provocatively suggests that the following tale of the last man might finally provide a satisfactory answer to Adam's lament.

Gender and agency are Shelley's twin preoccupations in the introduction; the ungendered narrator affords her the pragmatic means to articulate her idealistic ends: to renovate – not reject – the "Romantic ethos" of her late husband. Just as Michael confidently relates to Adam the redemptive martyrdom of the Son, the framing narrator offers (perhaps just as confidently) the story of the last man to the first. The impressive work on the novel's publication history has documented its participation in the increasingly hackneyed and "ridiculous" (Paley, "Apocalypse" 107) discourse of "Lastness" (several other last man narratives preceded Shelley's, including Byron's "Darkness"), but the novel's compensatory epigraphic handling of Edenic *firstness* remains underappreciated and under theorized.[13] Ungendered agency affords the framing narrator the transcendent objectivity to survey entire trajectories, from first to last, from airy prophecy to pragmatic interpretation, from masculine bluster to feminine revision. While Michael's quick answer skips over Noah's intervening last man narrative and moves directly to the *felix culpa* endpoint, Shelley expands the middle term and resists the easily redemptive conclusion. Because of this, her fixation on diluvial *middleness* has been misread as nihilistic *lastness*; in other words, Verney's story, like Noah's, does not necessarily fill out Shelley's expansive thematic trajectory. Her narrative strategy is both cautiously dialectical and consistently open-ended: firstness, middleness, and lastness are all constantly being shuffled into different permutations of the sibylline leaves. Thus, any gendered triangulation of creative agency underestimates the complexity of Shelley's narrative circumlocution and miscalculates the intersection between plot and autobiography. Instead, *The Last Man* is a novel of proliferating trajectories and frequently unwieldy potentialities that continuously revise Shelley's own discussions of gender, agency, and creativity.

As Shelley moves away from the cave and begins Verney's first-person narration, Evadne emerges as a calculated degeneration of the ungendered framing narrator into mere androgyny. At worst, critics have been content to discard her from the plot completely, and at best they have read her as a simple foil that exposes Raymond's critical flaws as a leader or a symbol of the plague itself.[14] However, the elaborate introductory setup for Evadne's sustained theme of androgyny and her long literary history suggest that Shelley put considerable thought into her own version of the character.[15] The two strongest literary antecedents are Beaumont and Fletcher's play *The Maid's Tragedy* (1619), where Evadne is mistress to the king and involved in a sham marriage to Amintor at the king's request, and Richard Sheil's play *Evadne; or, The Statue* (1819) where Evadne "Veil[s] all her charms in spotless chastity" and "Turn[s] strong temptations to the cause of Truth" (vi). The stage history of *The Maid's Tragedy* suggests that despite several popular performance runs in the seventeenth and eighteenth centuries, the play went silent until its Victorian revival. Shelley either encountered Beaumont and Fletcher's play via Sheil or from Charles Lamb's extracts in his *Specimens of English Dramatic Poets* (1808, 1813).[16] Despite the apparent correspondences (cross-dressing, adultery, and physical beauty), Shelley's Evadne departs significantly from both her dramatic forbears because of her uniquely subversive claim of authority and her rational, Wollstonecraftian mind: "she could subdue her sensible wants to her mental wishes, and suffer cold, hunger and misery, rather than concede to fortune a contested point," suggesting even a "disdainful negligence of nature itself" (*The Last Man* 116). The earlier play portrays Evadne as a mildly transgressive character who finally reasserts her "natural" femininity through tragic sacrifice, and Sheil's Evadne mobilizes feminine virtue to tame the masculine villainy of Ludovico's political scheming and the King's wild libido. Shelley's iteration of the character amplifies both the androgynous ambiguity and the emancipatory transgression of her literary antecedents. Through this amplification, Shelley revisits her critique of Victor Frankenstein's interventionist science as a "a rape of nature, a violent penetration and usurpation of the female's 'hiding places,' of the womb" (Mellor, *Mary Shelley* 122), which precariously aligns Evadne's "disdainful negligence of nature" with Victor's masculinist violation, a charge that most likely explains some of the critical disdain for her character.

However, Evadne escapes those interventionist indictments against Victor. Shelley's literary due diligence about the history of the character and the expanding theme of androgyny unbalance the gendered formulas of masculinized violence against a feminized Nature. Most readers of *The Last Man* can hardly suppress their disgust at Evadne's excesses, but a few cautious critics have resorted to some tactical hedging. Poovey argues that Evadne represents the author's frustration towards the repressive conditions of professional female authorship, and Bewell reluctantly acknowledges these biographical links even as he casts Evadne as a foul embodiment of the plague itself (Poovey 114–42; Bewell, *Colonial Disease* 299). Nevertheless, Evadne is not simply Shelley's sounding board to vent her dissatisfaction with her career; instead, she offers Evadne as the androgynous alternative that *Frankenstein* lacked. As several accounts of Shelley's earlier novel have established, *Frankenstein* is not a bitter tirade against science in general, but a more specific critique of Sir Humphry Davy's masculinist approach to science.[17] Nature does not emerge from the novel a sacrosanct, noumenal limit outside of human understanding, but rather as an object of study that requires empirical observation and reverent circumspection. In *The Last Man*, Shelley articulates more clearly this alternative relationship to nature through Evadne and a deft reversal of the didactic terms of *Frankenstein*: whereas her earlier novel encourages human endeavour to check its reach with natural delimitations, *The Last Man* constructs various ways for human social constructions to check nature itself. Evadne's "unnatural" qualities should not be mistaken for grotesque exaggeration; rather, her challenge to the "natural" via destabilized categories of gender, race, and class brings nature within human reach and complicates the already fragile economy of the social and the natural in *Frankenstein*. In this sense, *The Last Man* strives to complete the partial critique in *Frankenstein* with its positive substitution of Evadne's androgynous challenge to nature in place of Victor's criminal abomination.

Evadne voices (via Verney's narration) her preference for the social over the natural in her assessment of Adrian's radical yet impractical politics: "She thought he did well to assert his own will, but she wished that will to have been more intelligible to the multitude. She had none of the spirit of a martyr, and did not incline to share the shame and defeat of a fallen patriot" (*The Last Man* 44). This passage echoes both the Milton epigraph in its revision of the Son's martyrdom and the introduction in its insistence on the intelligibility of prophecy. Shelley mirrors her own scepticism about her husband's political and poetic projects through Evadne's coldness towards Adrian's system of reform. Scepticism, though, does not necessarily imply rejection; in the same language as the introduction, Shelley continues her efforts to ground those sibylline prophecies into something material and "intelligible" without dismissing them as fundamentally unworkable. Whether as Adrian's advisor, an anonymous architect, Raymond's mistress, or a cross-dressing soldier, Evadne always manages to find the appropriate practical means to achieve her ends. Yet this pragmatic opportunism also gets her killed in the very first chapter of the second volume. Verney finds Evadne, in well-worn military drag, dying on the Grecian battlefield. In her delirium, she curses Raymond, her former lover:

> By my death I purchase thee – lo! the instruments of war, fire, the plague are my servitors. I dared, I conquered them all, till now! I have sold myself to death, with the sole condition that thou shouldst follow me – Fire, and war, and plague, unite for thy destruction – O my Raymond, there is no safety for thee! (*The Last Man* 181)

Just as Nature ultimately triumphs against Victor's overreaching science, it seems that death wins out against Evadne's constructed human agency and has turned her into a bitter, vengeful, and cursing wretch, which potentially undercuts both her claim to the socially "intelligible" and her thoughtful rejection of martyrdom.

Out of context, the curse certainly legitimates some of that accumulated critical scorn directed against Evadne. However, Shelley's invocation of the curse must recall Percy Shelley's earlier tweaking of the same literary device in *The Cenci* (1819) and *Prometheus Unbound* (1820). In *The Cenci*, Beatrice is legally and morally condemned for her vengeful curse upon her incestuous and abusive father, whereas in *Prometheus Unbound*, Prometheus achieves his redemptive conclusion because he retracts his violent curse against the tyrannical Jupiter.[18] In Evadne's revision, Prometheus's four rewards – "Life, Joy, Empire, and Victory" (IV.578) – are snidely rewritten as fire, war, plague, and destruction. Percy Shelley's blatantly misogynistic schematization privileges Prometheus's masculine virtue of forgiveness and nonviolence over Beatrice's feminine hysterics of vengeance. Through Evadne, Shelley reclaims Beatrice's curse against Count Cenci and calls for worldly justice against worldly villains, recasting the curse as a material prophecy that sets up the subsequent plague narrative. Percy Shelley's "obscure and chaotic" idealism has no answer to Evadne's fourfold vision of apocalypse precisely because it fails Evadne's (and the framing narrator's) criterion of intelligibility. Evadne's early death does not erase her from the narrative; she survives as a reminder of human resistance to natural disaster and plague. Her immunity against disease (she is one of the few characters who recovers from illness), for example, suggests that her many social projects have inoculated her against natural threats, that the social has indeed triumphed over the natural.[19] Verney describes her recovery from illness in precisely those terms: "reflection returned with health" (*The Last Man* 146). Evadne's body becomes a contested site of human agency ("reflection") and natural contagion ("health"), and the surprising return of "reflection" in the face of debilitating illness suggests that civilization has some hope to survive well beyond Evadne's anti-Promethean vision.

Race and Species

Most of the novel's thirty-seven occurrences of the word "reflection" stage in some way or another the conflict between the viability of human social constructions and natural decay, disease, and disaster. Verney makes this connection explicit when he cites the most (in)famous reflection of the Romantic era:

> the mode of existence decreed to a permanent body composed of transitory parts; wherein, by the disposition of a stupendous wisdom, moulding together the great mysterious incorporation of the human race, the whole, at one time, is never old, or middle-aged, or young, but, in a condition of unchangeable constancy, moves on through the varied tenour of perpetual decay, fall, renovation, and progression. (*The Last Man* 228)

This passage, as Shelley herself documents in a contextual note, comes from Burke's *Reflections on the Revolution in France* (1790) in which he notoriously advocates the preservation of conservative political institutions because of their "just correspondence and symmetry with the order of the world" (184); in other words, Burke claims that the social whole is much more than its decomposing natural parts. When the language of Evadne's "reflection" reappears (almost verbatim) in

Verney's encounter with a diseased "negro half clad," the associated concerns with the social and natural composition of "the great mysterious incorporation of the human race" must also reappear:

> I lowered my lamp, and saw a negro half clad, writhing under the agony of disease, while he held me with a convulsive grasp. With mixed horror and impatience I strove to disengage myself, and fell on the sufferer; he wound his naked festering arms round me, his face was close to mine, and his breath, death-laden, entered my vitals. For a moment I was overcome, my head was bowed by aching nausea; till, *reflection return-ing*, I sprung up, threw the wretch from me, and darting up the staircase, entered the chamber usually inhabited by my family. A dim light shewed me Alfred on a couch; Clara trembling, and paler than whitest snow, had raised him on her arm, holding a cup of water to his lips. I saw full well that no spark of life existed in that ruined form, his features were rigid, his eyes glazed, his head had fallen back. I took him from her, I laid him softly down, kissed his cold little mouth, and turned to speak in a vain whisper, when loudest sound of thunderlike cannon could not have reached him in his immaterial abode. (*The Last Man* 336–7)

Halfway through the passage, Verney's "reflection" returns after the "aching nausea" of his infection by the diseased man, which provides another vital case study in Shelley's increasingly complex genealogy of inoculation and immunity. This time, though, she abandons the gendered apparatus of the framing narrator and Evadne in favour of an interracial encounter.

Verney's story of racialized immunity follows two parallel scenes, conveniently demarcated by Shelley's inoculating phrase "reflection returning": the grotesque yet redemptive cosmopolitanism of the embrace and what Mellor has referred to as Shelley's compensatory "ideal of the loving family" (*Mary Shelley* 44). One of the novel's few references to Blackness comes with an anxious reassertion of whiteness in the description of Clara as "paler than whitest snow." Both scenes begin with a light source illuminating the scene: "I lowered my lamp" in the first and "A dim light shewed me" in the second. Both scenes emphasize mouth-to-mouth communication: "his breath, death-laden, entered my vitals" in the first and "kissed his cold little mouth" in the second. With the diseased man no words are exchanged, and with Alfred, Verney vainly whispers to him even though the "sound of thunderlike cannon could not have reached him." The activity of the first scene and the passivity of the second highlights the distinction between the two competing ideals: whereas Verney actively lowers his own lamp to see the man, some off-stage lighting director casts the spotlight on Alfred. The scene of the "loving family" appears passive, hygienic, and automatic yet ultimately ineffective since Verney's kiss fails to save Alfred from death, and his whispered words are uttered in vain. In contrast, the active struggle of the first scene, what Kant would identify as an instance of "unsocial sociability" (*Universal History* 44), inoculates Verney against the plague while the easy *social* sociability of the "loving family" proves impotently tautological.[20]

The novel certainly questions conventional familial structures, but it does not, as some have suggested, reject outright the viability of Shelley's former ideal. *The Last Man* develops rather than repudiates the ideal of the loving family in *Frankenstein*; in the later novel, Shelley rewrites the De Lacey episodes with a provocative hypothetical: What if the De Laceys had warmly accepted the creature into their family? Verney's forced embrace of the ill man has several precursors that all offer tentative answers to this question. Early on, Verney, still wild from his Cumberland days, finds himself confronted with his ostensible persecutor, Adrian, only to be appeased a moment later by Adrian's angelic recognition of their former friendship. Similarly, when American and Irish invaders come to England, they fall under the beneficent powers of Adrian's persuasion, lay down their arms, and join their former enemies in the common purpose of survival. These moments of recognition and reconciliation stem from negative formulations of *mis*recognition and forced confrontation in *Frankenstein* and *Paradise Lost*. Just as the De Lacey family misreads the creature's kind intentions, the angel Ithuriel fails to recognize Satan in *Paradise Lost* when he asks, "Which of those rebel Spirits adjudg'd to Hell / Com'st thou, escap'd thy prison, and transform'd" (IV.823–4). Satan, hurt, replies, "Know ye not mee? ye knew me once" (IV.827). In the creature's despair, he commiserates with Milton's misrecognized and disfigured Satan: "Many times I considered Satan as the fitter emblem of my condition; for often, like him, when I viewed the bliss of my protectors, the bitter gall of envy rose within me" (*Frankenstein* 87). These failures of recognition infuriate both characters, leading to serial murders in the creature's case and the fall of humanity in Satan's. *The Last Man* eagerly attempts to expand its definition of familial recognition, yet the results seem significantly bleaker than either of its antecedents: the death toll dwarfs that of *Frankenstein*, and instead of a fortunate Fall that promises future redemption, the novel ends with a quasi-nihilistic scene of the last man, running around Rome with his dog and shouting in Italian at the ruins of civilization.

Verney's cosmopolitan inoculation is not only the culmination of this discourse of recognition and the increasingly plastic terms of familial sociability, but it is also a miserable failure in its willful rejection of Evadne's prophetic warning. It would be hasty, though, to dismiss this scene as an inevitable human failure against a deterministic nature. As Verney wanders through the Grecian battlefield, he surveys the scope of the human casualties and laments humanity's own social failures rather than natural disaster: "I turned to the corse-strewn earth; and felt ashamed of my species" (*The Last Man* 180). At this point, the plague cannot compete with the scale of human violence. Verney's failure is the inability to transform this species shame into a familial embrace of the diseased man or, in Kant's terms, to use the encounter of "unsocial sociability" to model a new cosmopolitan, "lawful order among men" (*Universal History* 44) and "universal community"

(*Perpetual Peace* 107). Since, as Peter Melville puts it, "Shelley's 'negro' is denied the chance to unburden himself of his miserable tale of suffering" (836), Verney loses this opportunity for a cosmopolitan discourse. Instead, the species discourse returns at the end of the novel with Verney's canine companion, a mocking reminder of Verney's social failure with the ill Black man. Species confusion replaces that emergent discourse of recognition in an evocation of eighteenth-century conflations of race and species. Several critics have studied the frequently shocking metaphorical registers of racial discourse and have tracked an extensive literary-historical trajectory that explains, for example, Gulliver's suckling at the teat of a female Yahoo and his futile conversations with horses.[21] In such scenes, authors register fears of miscegenation through cross-species plots and, just as frequently, the comical association of fashionable women with their lapdogs. Under all this laughter lies a stubborn scepticism about cosmopolitan possibilities and a conservative resistance to Kant's drive towards a "universal history." Shelley, however, strips the miscegenation story of its laughter and its cross-species metaphors and takes seriously the possibility of a redemptive cosmopolitanism. By the end of the novel, this optimistic history seems incomplete. The cross-species farce returns, and Verney, having failed to listen to the man's "miserable tale of suffering," nor having said anything of substance to him, now must converse with a dog, a situation that *would* be humorous if there were anyone left to laugh at it.

This disheartening conclusion unravels the narrative of *Robinson Crusoe* (1719) and Defoe's faith in the protagonist to reconstruct civilization. Verney reaches back almost four hundred years – the novel ends in the year 2100 – to find his literary companion: "For a moment I compared myself to that monarch of the waste – Robinson Crusoe. We had been both thrown companionless – he on the shore of a desolate island: I on that of a desolate world" (*The Last Man* 448). That moment of comparison quickly vanishes when Verney discovers his critical shortcomings. Whereas Crusoe single-handedly re-enacts the entire history of capitalist individualism – from his domestication of indigenous animals, to his colonialist conscription of Friday, and finally to his return to England as a successful entrepreneur – Verney follows the story almost exactly in reverse: he begins his narrative with the patriotic metaphor of England as a "well-manned ship" (*The Last Man* 9), fails to make use of his own Friday (the "negro half clad"), and finally discovers already domesticated animals wandering the depopulated world. Verney vainly pantomimes Crusoe's story through obsolete eighteenth-century stories of race and species, but instead he finds imagined savages and animals divested of both labour and utility that do very little to console the failures of his aborted rags-to-riches story.

These discoveries occur in two Friday-inspired scenes that underscore the lost opportunity of Verney's embrace with alterity. The first is the last man's wistfully subjunctive revision of the earlier scene with the "negro half clad":[22]

I *would* have knelt down and worshipped the same. The wild and cruel Caribbee, the merciles [*sic*] Cannibal – or worse than these, the uncouth, brute, and remorseless veteran in the vices of civilization, *would* have been to me a beloved companion, a treasure dearly prized – his nature *would* be kin to mine; his form cast in the same mould; human blood *would* flow in his veins; a human sympathy must link us for ever. (*The Last Man* 449; emphasis mine)

Crusoe's education of his own cannibal proceeds more smoothly: "I made him know his name should be *Friday* ... I likewise taught him to say *Master* ... *Yes,* and *No*" (Defoe 163). In Verney's case, the "wild and cruel Caribbee" remains strictly a colonial fantasy that cannot reproduce Crusoe's racist mastery; Verney's "would" replaces the hopeful future tense of Kant's cosmopolitan endpoint of perpetual peace with an irretrievable loss of human community and exchange. Even at this point, Verney still sees the man through his racist lens: the imagined savage is wild and cruel, a merciless cannibal, uncouth, brute, and remorseless. His acceptance sounds like mere condescension, but the broken parallelism of the final clause substitutes a more promising moral imperative ("must") for the ineffectual conditional. This grammatical and ontological shift becomes clearer in a second Friday-inspired scene when Verney comes to terms with his own savagery: "What wild-looking, unkempt, half-naked savage was that before me? The surprise was momentary. I perceived that it was I myself whom I beheld in a large mirror at the end of the hall" (*The Last Man* 455). Instead of finding Friday, Verney encounters his own degenerate humanity. Kinship, blood, and sympathy have finally been cast into the same human mould, but the victory remains solipsistically vacuous, wholly dependent on the mirrored subjectivity of "I myself"; the racial terms of difference and identity are crudely flattened into an unsignifying language of pure reflexivity.

Having failed to find his companion in either the imagined "Caribbee" or in his own savage reflection, Verney realizes that the eighteenth-century cross-species, miscegenation story has become his only recourse. In his desperation, he turns to a family of goats and an industrious sheepdog.[23] Both animal episodes parodically rehearse the novel's earlier concerns: the former serves as a painful reminder of Verney's family and the latter recalls the racial discourse of cosmopolitanism via the bestial metaphor. Verney discovers "two goats and a little kid" (*The Last Man* 459) feeding on a grass-covered hill and offers a handful of grass to the happy family. Just as the De Lacey family rejects the help of the creature, the male goat aggressively bares his horns at Verney's well-intentioned offering to protect his family against the perceived intruder. Unfortunately, the discourse of recognition ends with this parodic, bestial scene, a revision that recasts Verney, the last man, as Victor's monster, rejected again from the "ideal of the loving family." Nevertheless, at the very end, Verney manages to find a suitable (albeit quite absurd) companion:

My only companion was a dog, a shaggy fellow, half water and half shepherd's dog, whom I found tending sheep in the Campagna. His master was dead, but nevertheless he continued fulfilling his duties in expectation of his return … Riding in the Campagna I had come upon his sheep-walk, and for some time observed his repetition of lessons learned from man, now useless, though unforgotten. (*The Last Man* 468–9)

Here, Shelley retells the "cruel joke" of *The Last Man* through the dog's Sisyphean labour and his now worthless memory of "lessons learned from man." The deconstructive reading of the novel takes Shelley's annihilation of the human race as a categorical purge of all socially constructed metaphors, tropes, and ideologies, but it fails to account for the preservation of human memory in, for example, the dog's bestial labour. Everywhere, Verney finds human civilization embalmed in these painfully inaccessible alterities. Unlike the real-life 1818 outbreak of *cholera morbus* in Calcutta, Shelley's version of the plague cannot circulate across different species, which makes cross-species communication, in both senses of the word, impossible. Verney has no means to access bestial memory or the buried human narratives in the ruins of civilization. In an embarrassing travesty of the diseased man's inoculating embrace, Verney abjectly describes his new willingness to recognize alterity: "I embraced the vast columns of the temple of Jupiter Stator, which survives in the open space that was the Forum, and leaning my burning cheek against its cold durability" (*The Last Man* 461). This concluding cross-species farce does not immediately authorize the deconstructive erasure of human civilization; rather, it serves as an ironic lament for the several missed opportunities – androgynous, familial, racial, cosmopolitan – and as a warning against repeating Verney's apocalyptic history.

The Scale of Nature

I have suggested that through this buried genealogy of redemptive alterity and companionship – the framing narrator, Evadne, the Black man, and the dog – Shelley offers her version of an inoculated politics of possibility that persists even in conditions of war, scarcity, and plague. Admittedly, though, there is a conspicuous disparity in scale between these localized social resistances and the vastness of Shelley's plague. The novel's two orders of scale – the dizzyingly global and the claustrophobically embodied, and the natural and the social – must be placed into productive conversation. In her survey of anti-contagionist (communication of disease through miasmatic air) and contagionist (person-to-person communication of bodily infection) views of plague, Anne McWhir convincingly locates Shelley firmly in the anti-contagionist camp, which makes the plague an impossibly immense and intractable force that colonizes the globe.[24] Bewell offers another helpful estimation of the plague's overwhelming scale. When Verney writes, "I spread the whole earth out as a map before me. On no one spot of its surface could I put my finger and say, here is safety" (*The Last Man* 260), Bewell offers, in stark contrast, Tamburlaine's infinitely higher cartographical ambitions: "Give me a map: then let me see how much / Is left for me to conquer all the world" (Bewell, *Colonial Disease* 296–7). Tamburlaine scans the globe for a place to conquer while Verney merely seeks escape from a plague that does not respect national, racial, or ideological boundaries; the localized resistances of *The Last Man* seem ill-equipped to match Tamburlaine's imperial might and global reach. Malthus provides quite a sobering check to any aspiring Tamburlaines in his quintessentially anti-Romantic philosophy about the futility of human agency in the face of "positive checks to the population": "all unwholesome occupations, severe labour and exposure to the seasons, extreme poverty ... the whole train of common diseases and epidemics, wars, pestilence, plague, and famine" (23). For Malthus, the natural inevitably overwhelms the social, a conclusion that both political philosopher and writer William Godwin and Percy Shelley vehemently rejected with their more optimistic doctrine of social perfectibility.[25] In *The Last Man*, Mary Shelley departs significantly from both ideologies with a double agenda: to make sense of Malthus's famously half-hearted solution to catastrophic overpopulation – "moral restraint" (23) – and to ground dewy-eyed notions of Godwinian perfectibility with earnest research into medical science and material evidence.

As part of this ambitious project, Shelley pits two failures – the war between Greece and Turkey and the devastation of the plague – against the two successful inoculations (Evadne and Verney) to work out this thorny question of scale. I have partially staked my reading of Shelley's Romantic politics on cosmopolitan possibilities, so the novel's divisive war stands out as a particularly apposite case study. As Paley notes, it is the "sole international issue" ("Introduction" viii) that Shelley includes in her futuristic plot.[26] Some quick historical calculation reveals that Shelley imagines the war "continuing after more than two centuries, but now being fought in Turkey itself" ("Introduction" viii). Such protracted temporality unfavorably links the politics of Godwin and Percy Shelley to the insane prognosticating of Merrival, the novel's oblivious scientist who forever grasps at useless abstractions: "He was far too long sighted in his view of humanity to heed the casualties of the day, and lived in the midst of contagion unconscious of its existence" (*The Last Man* 289). Instead of merely tempering her idealistic radicalism after witnessing the reactionary, post-Revolutionary despotisms of Robespierre and Napoleon like most of her fellow surviving Romantics, Shelley takes it one step further and imagines a two-hundred-year timeline of continued violence. This is hardly the quick social upheaval that the French Revolution promised. After "Stamboul" finally falls after surely one of the longest wars in human history, the "Mahometans" seem to vanish unceremoniously from the novel without a clear explanation. After refusing to join Adrian's society in search of a safe haven from the plague, they disappear into the invisible margins of Verney's narration.

The east, represented by the Mahometans, stubbornly resists integration even to narrative extinction, and Verney's feeble last word on this cosmopolitan failure is shame for his species and despair at the persistence of violence.

Even plague fails to unite Mahometan and Christian under the common purpose of survival. The mysterious plague remains elusive through the politicians' various social programs, its mode of transmission is never exactly discovered, its virulence is never seriously assessed, and its origins are only anecdotally established. Verney's sister Perdita naively raises the question of origin to which he responds: "That word, as yet it was not more to her, was PLAGUE. This enemy to the human race had begun early in June to raise its serpent-head on the shores of the Nile" (*The Last Man* 175). The hurried modulation of these two sentences – from vague linguistic marker ("that word") to a carefully plotted vector of infection from the Nile, to China, to Constantinople – puts into doubt Verney's narrative certainty about the African origin of the plague; his information hinges on mere hearsay and anecdotal evidence. When he starts associating the plague with the "serpent-head" of Satan, tracing the plague's origin becomes nothing more than a futile exercise in fantastical abstraction and metaphorical excess. Each attempt to map the disease encounters socially erected barriers that prevent England from acknowledging the consequences of a global empire that refuses to act out her nationalist script. Similarly, Albert Camus's *La Peste* (1947) conspicuously avoids Arab and Muslim references despite being set in Oran, an Algerian town with a mixed Arab and French population. Just as the plague-devastated citizens of Oran cling to the increasingly insular Christian faith of Paneloux, the local Jesuit priest, the survivors of Shelley's plague forgo the opportunity to begin productive cosmopolitan community-building in favour of comforting, well-rehearsed Christian theodicies. Instead of questioning the national and ideological borders of the pre-plague globe, Verney stubbornly holds onto the "well-manned ship" of England until the very end when he frantically searches for any redemptive vestiges of western civilization.

Despite their local narrative scale, the inoculations of Evadne and Verney manage to temper these immense failures of war and plague through Shelley's mobilization of a fairly comprehensive medical history of inoculation and vaccination, from Montagu's experiments with smallpox in Turkey, to Jenner's study of the cowpox vaccine, and finally to early nineteenth-century efforts to popularize the practice of vaccination. In a 1717 letter, Montagu proudly announces her discovery to Sarah Chiswell: "A propos of distempers I am going to tell you a thing that I am sure will make you wish yourself here. The smallpox, so fatal and so general among us, is here entirely harmless by the invention of engrafting" (*Turkish Embassy Letters* 81). Not coincidentally, Shelley takes Turkey as the main national representative of her exotic East and suggests, like Montagu, that international travel, cultural exchange, and cosmopolitan understanding can render even disease "entirely harmless." Further, like the paradoxical agency of Montagu's veiled

Turkish women – "the only free people in the empire" (*Turkish Embassy Letters* 72) – Evadne's fluid transversals of national, cultural, and gendered borders make her one of the only "free" people in the novel. Her numerous veiled disguises allow her to circulate freely among the masculine architectural and military circles of England, Greece, and Turkey. Instead of a figure that "emblematizes [the East and the West's] epidemiological link" (*Colonial Disease* 299), as Bewell has claimed, Evadne "engrafts" her cosmopolitan experiences onto her infected body, inoculating herself against the diseased insularity of the British Empire.

The historical trajectory from Montagu's Turkish inoculation to Jenner's cross-species vaccination parallels Shelley's movement from the gendered and racial discourse of cosmopolitanism to the parodic eruption of species confusion in Verney's encounters with goats, dogs, and even columns. Vaccination was about the viability of the cross-species management of disease: "what renders the Cowpox virus so extremely singular, is, that the person who has been thus affected is for ever after secure from the infection of the Small Pox" (*Inquiry* 6). Whereas Jenner champions the curative effect of a bovine virus on the human immune system, Shelley deliberately elides the cross-species communicability of disease. Jenner frequently seems disgusted by cross-species fraternization because of his medical breakthrough: "The deviation of Man from the state in which he was originally placed by Nature seems to have proved to him a prolific source of Diseases ... he has familiarised himself with a great number of animals, which may not originally have been intended for his associates" (1). In a somewhat sardonic tone, he cites wolves that have become lapdogs, tigers that have become housecats, and the domestication of cows, pigs, sheep, and horses to illustrate his point about the unnatural and unhealthy environment of an industrial England. In Jenner's account, England has become a harmful breeding ground for cross-contamination and the circulation of new diseases, whereas at the end of Shelley's novel, the world has become a hopelessly sterile environment that precludes the circulation of both disease and humanistic discourse. Shelley selectively includes Montagu's discussions of inoculation and excludes Jenner's claim about cross-species contagion to reiterate her point that Verney's late embrace of alterity is not enough, that a cosmopolitan politics of species is a vacuous idealization, and that the degeneration of the discourse of gender and race into one of species is an irrecoverable loss.

This dire end point does not necessarily reproduce anti-Romantic, nihilistic readings of the novel; the narrative temporality authorized by Shelley's allegory of the cave permits – or perhaps even requires – continuous review and revision. Even in Verney's farcical Italian quest-romance, Shelley manages to recover at least the *form* of a redemptive cosmopolitan politics despite her conclusion's evacuation of all human *content*. Verney reverses the imperialist script by prostrating himself before the imagined savage, by rediscovering the ideal of familial structure in the goats, by finding companionship with a loyal dog, and, most absurdly and tragically, by simulating embodied human intercourse with the inanimate column of

Jupiter Stator. His newfound discourse of recognition finds no accessible target, but the form of his strangely cosmopolitan good behaviour recalls and revises the earlier failures in the novel. In subsequent arrangements of the framing narrator's sibylline leaves, Verney's substanceless shape of perfected cosmopolitanism can finally be filled out with material praxis.

The real history of vaccination, beginning with Montagu's importation of "engrafting" techniques from Turkish physicians, offers a brief glimpse of that ideal shape. After losing a brother to smallpox, she successfully inoculated her children against the disease and became an eager advocate of variolation in her aristocratic circle. By the end of the eighteenth century, her campaign was largely successful, and most believed that the benefits of inoculation far outweighed the risks. And in 1798, Jenner published his findings about the cowpox virus. He took his cue from country lore about milkmaids' unexpected immunity to smallpox and concluded that their exposure to the infected udders of lactating cows had inoculated them against the disease. The theory was met with immediate resistance because of its brazen crossing of species boundaries. By the time that Shelley published *The Last Man* in 1826, however, most of this vaccination anxiety had subsided, and by 1840, England had banned the practice of smallpox inoculation in favour of much safer vaccination procedures.

Shelley's novel recapitulates this century-long history of vaccination with some crucial differences. The episode with the "negro half clad," for example, fictionalizes Montagu's mediation of Anglo-Turkish medicine. Just as Montagu finds a potential cure for smallpox through her travels to the exotic East, Verney's immunity from the plague comes from his own charged encounter with racial otherness. Shelley later evokes Jenner's strange bovine experiments in the novel's equally strange interspecies conclusion. Unlike Jenner's *very* useful interaction with infected cows, however, Verney and his dog wander without purpose through an empty world. This ending raises a material question: Since Shelley sourced her plague from a real-life outbreak of cholera in Calcutta, a disease that *was* communicable across species boundaries, why is the fictionalized plague species-specific?[27] Why would she have us forget the lessons learned from this long history of vaccination? It was certainly not that Shelley was unaware of that vaccination history.[28] Indeed, in a discussion of the plague's virulence, Verney casually mentions that the smallpox vaccine had succeeded in eradicating the disease by the twenty-first century: "That the plague was not what is commonly called contagious, like the scarlet fever, or *extinct* small-pox, was proved" (*The Last Man* 231; emphasis mine). As her work in *Frankenstein* exemplifies, she always stayed sharply attuned to the most recent discoveries in the scientific community. And by the time *The Last Man* was published in 1826, just about everyone would have been familiar with Jenner because of his apotheosis as a national hero and as the triumphant conqueror of the eighteenth-century scourge.[29] As early as the 1818 *Frankenstein*, Shelley was depicting early nineteenth-century vaccination anxieties in the patchwork body of the creature.[30] Later, just as she was revising the novel for the final 1831 edition, she contracted a mild case of smallpox herself in 1828 and lamented that she was, like her creature, "a monster to look at" (*Journals* 508). For almost two decades of her life, smallpox was constantly on her mind.

The point in *The Last Man*, then, is that Verney somehow forgets. Shelley revives the corpse of early nineteenth-century vaccination anxieties to show how little her fictitious twenty-first century has learned. Verney relegates smallpox to a throwaway observation about its extinction, serving only to distinguish the new plague from the old. His failure to recognize his embrace of the "negro half clad" as his preserving inoculation powerfully presages our own twenty-first century in which a resurgent anti-vaccination movement has forgotten the lessons of not only smallpox, but also of polio, measles, mumps, rubella, and pertussis. Ever since Verney forcefully "threw the wretch" from his body – rather than actively fostering a generative experiment with cosmopolitan community to cope with the annihilating plague – he experiences nothing but loss and degeneration. Whereas, in *Frankenstein*, experiment exceeds bioethical bounds, in *The Last Man*, Shelley suggests that Verney's early cosmopolitan experiment falls short of its productive payoff. In this way, the novel interrupts the linear historical progress from variolation to vaccination. In this fictionalized account of medical history, the world eradicates smallpox but nevertheless forgets its legacy. As a result, the language of cross-species vaccination never enters the novel's medical discourse, and disease remains all too human: Verney's dog, the imagined "Caribee," and the columns of "Jupiter Stator" all remain inaccessible alterities with no regenerative potential. In this disastrous rewriting of the real-life history of smallpox, Shelley emphasizes the importance of sustained experiment and cosmopolitan conversation – without Turkish medicine, Montagu would not have popularized variolation, and without Montagu, Jenner would not have reported his results on cowpox. The novel's disavowal of Jenner, then, is certainly not an anti-vaccinationist indictment but a trenchant reminder of our debt to medical experiment and cultural exchange.

Thus, Shelley's answer to the question of scale is twofold: first, she retroactively magnifies the roles of Evadne and Verney into viable social resistances to the novel's vast scale of failure, and second, she documents the medical-historical precedents of her cosmopolitan solution. Godwin and Percy Shelley suggested vague notions about the palliative effects of social improvement and nebulous hints at the relationship between vegetarianism and reform, but *The Last Man* finally gives material shape to flighty social projects.[31] Critics' charges of Shelley's "ambivalence" and "indeterminacy" purchase cautious scepticism at the cost of missing Shelley's stunningly complex narrative temporality and her cogently empirical basis for the plague's socially constructed cure. By the end, Shelley's cosmopolitan politics is both consistently compensatory and remarkably lucid.

Alternatives to Extinction

Given Shelley's careful construction of a politics of possibility and her revisionist decoding of Romantic idealism, the central theme of *The Last Man* cannot be, as several critics have claimed in some form or another, the failure of the Romantic imagination in the face of natural disaster.[32] Since Jerome McGann's polemical warning against a damaging adherence to a unified, static "Romantic ideology," such anti-Romantic or pro-Romantic claims have lost some theoretical traction.[33] Nevertheless, this chapter has taken *The Last Man* as a sympathetic variation on a Romantic theme: Shelley's cosmopolitan politics reanimates the principles of a conventionally Romantic poetics in its belief in the vatic poet's infinite creativity, imaginative agency, and even, as Percy Shelley famously articulates in his *Defence of Poetry* (1821), world-shaping legislative power. The ideals of the novel – androgyny, family, cosmopolitanism – continue the familiar themes of *Frankenstein*, *The Cenci*, and *Prometheus Unbound* despite the apocalyptic devastation of the plague. This line of argument makes no claims for a unified Romanticism, but these specific ideological continuities remain crucial to any complete understanding of *The Last Man*. Evadne's anonymous foray into architecture, for example, models with great fidelity the raw poetics of the archetypal Romantic amateur, full of unrealized and perhaps unrealizable vision:

> The design was new and elegant, but faulty; so faulty, that although drawn with the hand and eye of taste, it was evidently the work of one who was not an architect. Raymond contemplated it with delight; the more he gazed, the more pleased he was; and yet the errors multiplied under inspection. He wrote to the address given, desiring to see the draughtsman [Evadne], that such alterations might be made, as should be suggested in a consultation between him and the original conceiver. (*The Last Man* 107)

The charm of Evadne's fanciful architectural project somehow offsets the multiplication of structural errors. She convincingly invokes a Romantic inexpressibility *topos* that delights in the brilliance of conception while bemoaning the inadequacy of execution. As Poovey has suggested, Evadne becomes a temporary stand-in for Shelley herself, a struggling Romantic artist whose conceptual reach exceeds her material grasp.

The love triangle of Raymond, Perdita, and Evadne hastily prioritizes the ideal of heterosexual love at the expense of Evadne's emergent androgynous poetics, a situation that closely mirrors Shelley's own turbulent balancing act between love and art.[34] Evadne's obdurate infatuation with Raymond clouds her "eye of taste" and pollutes her artistic vision. Shelley makes this conflict of interest explicit just after Raymond uncovers Evadne's disguise:

> When Raymond offered to clear her reputation, and demonstrate to the world her real patriotism, she declared that it was only through her present sufferings that she

hoped for any relief to the stings of conscience; that, in her state of mind, diseased as he might think it, the necessity of occupation was salutary medicine; she ended by extorting a promise that for the space of one month he would refrain from the discussion of her interests, engaging after that time to yield in part to his wishes. (*The Last Man* 116)

Even though her architectural "occupation was salutary medicine" (another socially constructed cure for the "diseased"), Evadne can only delay the inexorable force of the amatory plot "for the space of one month." Just as Verney defers to the familiarity of his dying son after the aborted intercourse with the diseased man Evadne abandons her androgynous critique and conscripts herself into Raymond's destructive war. Shelley's now twice-articulated claim – the first with Evadne's disavowal of her artistic pursuits and the second with Verney's turn from the man to Alfred – is that these Romantic ideals of heterosexual love and the nuclear family mean precious little when they come so easily.[35] To correct this, Shelley cleverly reclaims Beatrice's curse against Count Cenci in Evadne's dramatic final speech and offers a belated repudiation of her amorous heterosexual obsession. Evadne's curse – "Fire, and war, and plague, unite for thy destruction" – provides the necessary challenge with which to assess the practical viability of these untested Romantic notions. For this reason, readers of the novel have rightly noted that Shelley's narrative terrain is not particularly forgiving; Shelley's testing ground is a harsh battlefield of scarcity, disease, and death. Even though Evadne's curse materializes in some spectacular failures, war and plague do not emerge from the rubble entirely triumphant. Sheil's Evadne, for example, manages to turn rubble against tragedy. The second title of Sheil's play (*The Statue*) refers to Evadne's successful appeal to the lustful King's conscience through the figurative reanimation of her father's chastising statue. The actress who plays Olivia (Evadne's erstwhile friend) concludes in the epilogue:

> From that time forth, unwarmed by lover's breath,
> Statues, or bone, or stone, have slept in death.
> But if to-night, you bid *Evadne* thrive,
> We hope to see the miracle revive.
> To beauty's queen the Grecian poured his vow,
> Our poet bends to beauty's daughters now;
> Oh! May they waken his dramatic wife,
> And, smiling, warm his statue into life! (Epilogue 39–46)

Verney's strange intercourse with the sculptured columns of Jupiter Stator is neither farcical nor futile in Sheil's account. The "Statues, or bone, or stone" at the end of *The Last Man* do not necessarily signify the cold inanimate abjection of human endeavour against natural disaster; instead, through Evadne's (both Sheil's and Shelley's) relationship to art, it is possible to reclaim civilization from nihilistic lastness, to warm Verney's statue of Jupiter back into life. Reading the novel as a simple rehearsal of despair underestimates both Shelley's radical politics and her adaptive terms of autobiographical figuration. She recognizes the failures of the French Revolution, the rise of Napoleonic reaction, and the gradual disappearance of her literary and social circles, but she does not take them as occasions for idle hand-wringing or conservative retrenchment; instead, she revises these personal and political catastrophes into productive opportunities to round out Romantic prophecy and vision with material possibilities of cosmopolitan reform.

This revisionist strategy collects all those isolated redemptive moments that critics have identified and redeploys them into compensatory narratives that are continually returned to the cave of the Sibyl for redrafting. Melville's scepticism about Mellor and Bewell's readings of Shelley's Black man begins to account for this expansive narrative strategy. He notes that Mellor allows for a quickly extinguished "deconstructive spark of optimism" that encodes a cosmopolitan ethics and that Bewell "treats the appearance of Shelley's black man in a similarly brief fashion, leaving his thoughts on the matter to punctuate the final paragraph of his otherwise scrupulously patient book chapter on *The Last Man*" (829–30). However, after concluding that neither "gives sufficient consideration to the contexts of Lionel's encounter" (830), he goes on to offer yet another isolated "spark" in his alternative explanation for Verney's inoculation that just replaces the "negro half clad" with Verney's fevered dream in "Stamboul" (*The Last Man* 202). Those "contexts" are strangely absent both in the narrow focus on the "Stamboul" episode and in his erroneous observation about the narrative isolation of Shelley's Black man: "[Verney] will not return to, reflect on, or recollect the incident at any other moment either before or after its brief appearance in the text" (835). As I have documented, the scene has both "before" and "after": Evadne's recovery and her "occupation" as "salutary medicine" anticipate the scene of inoculation, and the "cruel Caribbee" echoes Verney's forced embrace of the diseased man. The narrative genealogy that I have offered reflects several of these continuous "contexts" and explains Shelley's penchant for recapitulation, which makes sense of Shelley's sustained trajectory of redemptive possibilities, from the introductory gender discourse, to the racialized problem of cosmopolitanism, and finally to the cautionary tale of Verney's cross-species plot.

Accusations of philosophical inconsistency and political fickleness have dogged Shelley because of these wildly variable modes of representation. On the one hand, Shelley celebrates a chastened version of Romantic science in *Frankenstein*, and on the other she seems to annihilate any trace of social agency in *The Last Man*. However, as I have argued, *The Last Man* strives to complete, not retract, the partial argument of *Frankenstein*. Vengeful nature punishes the overreaching masculinist science of Victor whereas, in *The Last Man*, Evadne and Verney's invocation of an alternate medical history of inoculation offers a successful social anodyne for the cruelties of nature. Social agency becomes properly commensurate to the awful sublimity of nature, and lofty Romantic prophecies achieve their proper material ground. The novel coherently models both a politics of cosmopolitan recognition and a Romantic poetics of androgynous agency. In this way, Verney's narration succeeds as Shelley's secular version of Michael's compensatory reassurance to Adam's postlapsarian despair. Through all this, Shelley emerges more ideologically articulate and philosophically coherent than most critical pronouncements would suggest. The unexpected compatibility between the youthful exuberance of *Frankenstein* and the mature reflection of *The Last Man* might mean that some earnest reassessments of her other works might be in order. The historical novels – *Valperga* and *Perkin Warbeck* (1830) – and the domestic dramas – *Mathilda* (1819), *Lodore* (1835), and *Falkner* (1837) – might reward some careful rereading in light of Shelley's intricate yet strikingly cogent weaving of political ideology with domestic ideals. More specifically, any evaluation of her literary career that attempts to track a steady trajectory towards conservative reaction must not take *The Last Man* as its exemplar because it is not a novel of anti-Romantic nihilism but a compensatory tale of level-headed reflection. Throughout, Shelley compellingly persists in her assurance that Romanticism can indeed survive the extreme crucible of Evadne's "Fire, and war, and plague."

For Shelley, why we should survive Evadne's curse eventually becomes just as important as the how. Like Keats, Shelley offers a biopolitical vision that weighs the possibilities of human survival into a post-vaccination future. Whereas Bewell describes Percy Shelley's inheritance of Godwin's doctrine of perfectibility as an ambitious claim "that human beings might attain perfect health" (*Colonial Disease* 206), Mary Shelley's speculative revision of medical history makes us earn it first. By short-circuiting the triumphal history from variolation to vaccination, Shelley bleakly imagines the end of humanity (the last man has no last woman to continue the species) due to the characters' stubborn reluctance to embrace the other in the novel's pivotal moments of cosmopolitan inoculation. Shelley, however, also hints at a cogent politics of possibility and articulates a mature evolution of the transformative agency of the Romantic imagination through her frame tale's strange narrative temporality. We are told that the story is just one possible arrangement of the cave's sibylline leaves, allowing for the infinite recombination and retelling of illness narratives in this dire tale of annihilation. Apocalypse may yet be averted if only the last man's cosmopolitan encounter could be the biopolitical rule rather than the grotesque exception.

PART FOUR

Modern Biopower

Chapter Six

The Case of Sherlock Holmes

The Veiled Prophet

By the middle of the nineteenth century, the efforts of Romantic-era authors and physicians to organize a new system of healing, care, and community had begun to unravel, and the more familiar post-Foucauldian narratives of Victorian medicine – institutionalization, disease classification, and professionalization – had begun to replace the radical experiments of Romantic medicine. In *Bleak House* (1852), for example, Charles Dickens begins with a premise similar to Mary Shelley's in *The Last Man* (1826): he rewrites the world-enshrouding plague as a London fog that insidiously reaches into "the eyes and throats" while "cruelly pinching the toes and fingers" (11). Miasmatic contagion stands in for the human corruption of the central Chancery plot of Jarndyce versus Jarndyce, a multi-generational legal battle over a hopelessly contested will. Esther Summerson's illness materializes the despair that arises from this world of poverty, filth, and injustice. Dickens ultimately manages to clean up all this corruption and filth with a tightly plotted comic ending in which the moonlight finally burns through the miasmatic fog, and the marks on Esther's face disappear to reveal her natural beauty (913–14). At the end, Dickens pairs patient (Esther) with physician (Allan Woodcourt) in a particularly *un*-Romantic yoking of disease and cure, sufferer and curer. The triumphal ending's neatly orchestrated marriage of patient and physician privileges a normative and rigidly defined diagnosis – Allan's final assessment that Esther is more beautiful than ever (914) – that takes the non-normative as defective, a blemish that stands in the way of perfect happiness and perfect integration into society. Dickens carefully bookends his story with references to disease and contagion to plot a normatively linear progress from illness to cure. In this account of medicine, there is little room for the experimentalism and definitional detours of Romantic disease discourse; indeed, Dickens would probably liken such a process to the deafening din of the aimless courtroom, to a fog, or to a ceaseless debate that stalls a medical practice that quickly pathologizes for the sake of expedient rehabilitation. The novel fixes medical authority in the consecrated union of Esther and Allan; the physician has cured the patient through efficient diagnosis and has purged the body of disease. Only then can Esther end her narrative (and the novel) mid-sentence with the abortive phrase "even supposing – " (914), abandoning her quibbles with Allan's claim – "you are prettier than you ever were" – in favour of contented silence. The patient can stop narrating her illness, the potential error of "supposing" can end, and Esther can finally stop writing her life in retrospect and start living it. In this case, Susan Sontag's famous warning about the pitfalls of illness metaphors starts to make a lot of sense. Within such a Victorian medical frame, literature's useless and ungrounded metaphors can indeed seem like Sontag's dead ends.

This is the dominant literary frame that has survived into contemporary discussions of literature and medicine. This chapter jumps to the late nineteenth century to feature Arthur Conan Doyle's failed struggle with Sontag's illness metaphor. Romantic disease discourse's open-ended experimentation, non-pathological language, and generous distribution of medical authority find a shrewd antagonist in Doyle's famous detective, Sherlock Holmes. Laura Otis even goes so far as to argue that Holmes's strange new method of medico-literary detection is not only a Dickensian privileging of pathological precision over the patient narrative, but also an aggressive form of imperial jingoism. She relies on the suggestive metaphor of a "national immune system" (91) to articulate Doyle's pitting of an infected outside (the imperial periphery and its colonial contagions) against a policed inside (the metropole and its nascent bacteriological investigations). Doyle's own keen interest in the swiftly developing science of bacteriology finds its way into the methods of his remarkable detective. In Otis's readings of the Sherlock Holmes stories, foreigners come to signify bacteria, and the nation comes into its role as the bacteriologist:

> ... disembodied faces abound in the Holmes stories not merely because the British fear of invasion of small, angry creatures, but because they fear for their own identity. Bodies in the imperial age exist as fragments, and Holmes's refusal to respect "the body's integrity as a living totality" reflects both cultural and medical changes. (118)

Infection becomes wholly synonymous with invasion (rather than controlled inoculation), and Holmes, perfectly assimilating the "cultural and medical changes" of the times, dons the uniform of the border patrol, keeping those "small, angry creatures" from overwhelming an insular sense of national "identity."

A medical man himself, Doyle made it a point to keep abreast of contemporary medical research. In 1892, having already established his literary fame, he wrote to Dr. Joseph Bell, his surgical professor at the University of Edinburgh, of his debt to his mentor's medical acumen:

It is most certainly to you that I owe Sherlock Holmes, and though in the stories I have the advantage of being able to place [the detective] in all sorts of dramatic positions, I do not think that his analytical work is in the least exaggeration of some effects which I have seen you produce in the out-patient ward. Round the centre of deduction and inference and observation which I have heard you inculcate, I have tried to build up a man who pushed the thing as far as it would go – further occasionally – and I am so glad that the result satisfied you, who are the critic with the most right to be severe. (qtd. in Liebow 172)

More than Erasmus Darwin and John Keats (who also balanced medical and literary careers), Doyle struggles to theorize and justify the relationship between his two trades. For Doyle, the literary assumes a subordinate role to medicine's "centre of deduction and inference." Those "dramatic positions" and the "exaggeration of some effects" are circumscribed by the humility of a "though" clause and a hedging "I do not think." He reaches towards a weak reconciliation of literature and medicine, finding in the former mere adornment around the "centre" of the latter. In his attempt to make literature matter to medicine, and vice versa, he makes a modest case for literature's productive intervention into medical matters. The fiction of Sherlock Holmes allows Doyle to push medical deduction and inference to an imaginative extreme, but only "occasionally." This strange condescension of the literary endeavour is neither satire nor false humility; rather, it is a sort of hero worship, a student's saintly portrait of his teacher. Doyle is Watson to Bell's Holmes, the sidekick literary humanist to the magisterial medical professional. The medical entirely absorbs the literary, a convergence that gives precedence to the peering ken of the medical gaze over the capricious "exaggeration" of the literary imagination.

This hero worship extended to other medical scientists of his day. Having discovered the microscopic organisms responsible for anthrax, tuberculosis, and cholera, Dr. Robert Koch had solidified his standing as celebrity bacteriologist by the time Doyle published *A Study in Scarlet* (1887). During his headline address at the International Medical Congress (4 August 1890), Koch announced triumphantly that he had discovered a viable remedy for tuberculosis. Three months later, after the result had been published and republished in several languages, the headline of the *New York Times* read "Koch's Great Triumph. The Discovery Called a Greater One Than Jenner's."[1] Here was the potential of mankind's dramatic second act in its centuries-long war against the traumas of infectious disease. Doyle, of course, followed the whole affair with great interest. With the enticing prospect of a live demonstration of the remedy by Koch's colleague Dr. Ernst Von Bergmann, Doyle headed to Germany even before securing an admission ticket. He explained this brash decision later in his 1924 autobiography:

A great urge came upon me that I should go to Berlin and see [Von Bergmann's demonstration of Koch's consumption cure]. I could give no clear reason for doing

this, but it was an irresistible impulse and I at once determined to go. Had I been a
well-known doctor or a specialist in consumption it would have been more intelligible, but I had, as a matter of fact, no great interest in the more recent developments
of my own profession, and a very strong belief that much of the so-called progress
was illusory. (*Memories* 87–8)

A no-brainer for the Romantic generalist, this "impulse" is hardly "intelligible" for
the modern "specialist." Unlike Wordsworth's medico-literary cases, Darwin's confident intervention in the Linnaean science of botanical mutation, Blake's boldly
sexualized botany, Keats's medical prophecy of disease eradication, and Shelley's
literary theory of contagion, Doyle's "very strong belief" would gain very little
medical traction. Medicine had sloughed off its literary affiliations, dividing even
further into its granular specialties. The professional specialist is, as Doyle would
describe suggestively, a "veiled prophet" (*Memories* 89), closed off to discourse and
dissent.

Doyle's arrival in Berlin was met with little fanfare, and his burgeoning literary
celebrity hardly impressed the German medical community. He had secured some
introductions and a medical article in the *Review of Reviews*, but he failed to get
in Dr. Von Bergmann's good graces. Neither Koch nor Von Bergmann would
speak to Doyle, but his trip was not entirely fruitless: an American physician who
attended Von Bergmann's demonstration took pity on the spurned author and
agreed to share his notes. With lecture notes in hand, Doyle had enough to write
his article for the *Review of Reviews*:

> I studied the lecture and the cases, and I had the temerity to disagree with every one
> and to come to the conclusion that the whole thing was experimental and premature.
> A wave of madness had seized the world and from all parts, notably from England,
> poor afflicted people were rushing to Berlin for a cure, some of them in such ad-
> vanced stages of the disease that they died in the train. (*Memories* 90)

Even though Doyle turned out to be right about the "experimental and premature" result, Koch, the "veiled prophet" who had foretold the end of tuberculosis, prevailed. No one would trust the objection of a non-specialist who had just
published a fantastical tale of Mormons and murder. Several months later, after
treatment failures, premature deaths, and botched inoculations, Koch finally had
to acknowledge his costly mistake. Romantic disease discourse had ceased to function; Doyle's literary-minded speculation had no access to the bustling and productive world of the professional physician. Doyle could only serve an ancillary
function, as an entertaining "exaggeration of some effects," a trivial adornment,
or a humble review of a much more significant work. Doyle's literary turn away
from medicine in his *Study in Scarlet* attempts to dismantle this emergent hierarchical disciplinarity with a balance of medical detection and literary delight, but

ultimately he fails to imagine any sort of reconciliation beyond subordination (his almost obsequious deference to his medical heroes) or opposition (his largely unheard quarrel with Koch and Von Bergmann).

The character of Sherlock Holmes perfectly embodies these discursive changes. Our first impression of Holmes comes second-hand from Stamford, one of Dr. Watson's former classmates from medical school. After learning that the detective beats "subjects in the dissecting-rooms with a stick … to verify how far bruises may be produced after death" ("Scarlet" 6), Watson overhears Holmes's triumphant first words: "I've found it!" ("Scarlet" 7). Doyle's "veiled prophet" solves the impossible case with impossible ease. By the late nineteenth century, that quintessentially Holmesian word "case" had evolved from the discursive exchanges of Wordsworth and Jenner to signify a narrow, diagnostic view of disease. This modern medical meaning suggests a metonymic substitution in which patients cease to be people and become merely cases to be solved: "an instance of disease, or other condition requiring medical treatment; 'a record of the progress of disease in an individual' (New Sydenham Soc. Lexicon). Also, (colloq.), a patient."[2] In the colloquial usage, the physician hides the "patient" behind the "case," a convenient metonymic abstraction ostensibly conducive to deductive objectivity. As an example, the OED cites the British Medical Journal from 1881, just a few years before A Study in Scarlet: "About two hundred cases of ulcerated legs pass through my wards annually." The medical "case" reflects the changing priorities of the medical culture. Instead of open-ended Romantic experiment, the Holmesian method flogs directed answers out of silent bodies. Instead of anti-normative language, the "science of deduction" ("Scarlet" 10–20) offers a meticulous, nosological approach to cataloguing poisons, botanical tinctures, and diseases. And instead of lay knowledge, medical authority consolidates into a singular mind, one masterful diagnostician who weaves connections effortlessly with recourse to neither patient narrative nor victim report. Susan Cannon Harris rightly describes Holmes as this generation's new breed of physician, "the medico-criminal expert" (447), who alone possesses the necessary competencies of the increasingly cosmopolitan world of exotic infections and unsolvable mysteries. In this reading, Holmes is the fictionalized avatar of Doyle's modern physician who glides effortlessly across national, disciplinary, and political borders to synthesize big data into compact solutions.

This is, however, hardly the whole picture. This first Holmes novel seeks to construct a composite portrait of the modern physician in tandem with Holmes's partner in detection, Dr. Watson. The elusive ideal for Doyle is one who possesses the penetrating acumen of Holmes and the humanistic generosity of Watson. Sylvia A. Pamboukian taps into this uncertainty of representation in her probing study of nineteenth-century quackery and literature. She argues that rationalism, deduction, and scientism are not wholly valorized; rather, Doyle lingers with the half-guesses and surmises about professional medicine: "Doyle encourages readers

to re-examine medicine not as a field of scientific certitude but as a field particularly invested in practices it theoretically deplores [namely, quackery]" (146). This
chapter pieces together these two conflicting readings of the Sherlock Holmes
stories. On the one hand, Doyle elevates Holmes as a "medico-criminal expert"
who privileges methodical science over illusory superstition. On the other, he
strategically acknowledges the medical as literary – error, doubt, estimation, and
misdirection – in his opaque dealings with the criminal world. I argue that Doyle
attempts, as Darwin and Keats did, to find a middle ground for his medical and
literary vocations. What he found, though, was that that ground was lost. Unlike
his predecessors, he can only claim literature's intervention as "exaggeration," as
a quiet objection to serious science, or as a sidekick in awe of the veiled prophet's
diagnostic detection. There is little left of Darwin's effortless interdisciplinarity in
Doyle's work. Medicine and literature had begun functioning as, in C.P. Snow's
famous formulation, "two cultures" (1–21) with mutually exclusive vocabularies
and specialized competencies. Unlike the Darwinian jack of all trades and the
Keatsian poet-physician, Holmes and Watson never cohere into Doyle's desired
composite portrait, remaining forever an odd couple of medical professionalism
and literary humanism.

Literary Dallying

It is no surprise, then, that Doyle's medico-literary mind works in oppositional
pairs. The first appearance of Sherlock Holmes in print, for example, is also a
curious disappearance. *Study in Scarlet* comes in two parts: the first is Watson's
fast-paced retelling of Holmes's exciting search for an elusive murderer, while the
second is a slow burn historical tale that indulges in the romance of love and revenge to detail the culprit's motive. In this second part, Holmes disappears almost
entirely as we gradually learn of Jefferson Hope's convoluted Mormon backstory.
Unlike Blake's progression through contraries, though, Doyle imagines the traffic
between this pairing as subordination rather than sublimation. First-time readers
of *Study in Scarlet* catch on to this awkward structural disjunction immediately.
And by modern critical standards, Doyle's fractured storytelling breaks almost
every cardinal rule of detective fiction. *Study in Scarlet* violates, to varying degrees,
sixteen of S.S. Van Dine's now famous "Twenty Rules for Writing Detective Stories" (1928). Most egregiously, the reader does not "have equal opportunity with
the detective for solving the mystery" (Van Dine 189) since Holmes points the
finger at Jefferson Hope well before we even know who he is. And in the story's
strange second act of Mormon melodrama and unrequited love, the reader must
patiently endure the injunction of rule sixteen:

> A detective novel should contain no long descriptive passages, no literary dally-
> ing with side-issues, no subtly worked-out character analyses, no "atmospheric"

preoccupations. Such matters have no vital place in a record of crime and deduction. They hold up the action and introduce issues irrelevant to the main purpose, which is to state a problem, analyze it, and bring it to a successful conclusion. To be sure, there must be a sufficient descriptiveness and character delineation to give the novel verisimilitude. (Van Dine 192)

Doyle's early stab at the genre of detective fiction wants it both ways: the first part's "successful conclusion" of a medico-criminal mystery solved and the second part's "literary dallying with side-issues." Critics of the story (and Doyle himself) finally decided that this was an aesthetic impossibility. And having learned his lesson, Doyle gradually abandoned this stilted storytelling to focus more squarely on Van Dine's ideal of a tightly organized structure of problem, analysis, and conclusion. His "literary dallying with side-issues" and the science of deduction proved entirely incompatible, and Doyle ultimately silenced the romance of faith, superstition, and ignorance in favour of the gripping reportage of Holmes's scientific detection.

Doyle would eventually apologize for the sprawling, literary exuberance of a messy story like *Study in Scarlet*. He was just a neophyte author who had yet to learn about the great importance of the editing process. If literature had anything to say, Doyle concluded, it was as a humble supplement to promote real men of science like Dr. Bell. This late nineteenth-century disciplinary reconfiguration would become a crucial precondition of modern biopower. This later Doyle came to sponsor an authoritative science that instrumentalized literature as biopolitical propaganda. Instead of Romantic disease discourse, Doyle consoled us with the magisterial healing power and imaginative fantasy of the detective-physician. Even though the early Doyle resisted the instrumentalization of the literary, he would eventually succumb. The inoculating logic of Romantic disease discourse had shifted away from Mary Shelley's cultivating, immunizing embrace of alterity to what Roberto Esposito describes provocatively as a purging exclusion of the infected part for the sake of the healthful whole.[3] The result was a disciplinary separation in which medicine finally freed itself from the errant dalliances of literature to embrace the mantle of monolithic authority.

Historians of science agree that the friction between these two cultures of the humanities and the sciences came to a head with the publication of Charles Darwin's *On the Origin of Species* (1859).[4] In *Dover Beach* (1867), Matthew Arnold registers this polarized landscape by nostalgically describing the world in terms of constant sea change: "The Sea of Faith / Was once, too, at the full, and round earth's shore / Lay like the folds of a bright girdle furled" ("Dover Beach" 21–3). He wistfully imagines post-Darwinian modernity as an abrupt encroachment, a new order in which there is "neither joy, nor love, nor light" ("Dover Beach" 25). According to Arnold's speaker, Darwin and Thomas Huxley's subsequent popularization of evolutionary theory had substituted a biological and ecological mechanism for the human comforts of religious "joy." Even when contemporary critic Gillian Beer tires to repair this disciplinary rift, she does so with eloquent idealism on the one hand and cautious understatement on the other:

> Encounter, whether between peoples, between disciplines, or answering a ring at the bell, braces attention. It does not guarantee understanding; it may emphasize first (or only) what's incommensurate. But it brings into active play unexamined assumptions and so may allow interpreters, if not always the principals, to tap into unexpressed incentives. Exchange, dialogue, misprision, fugitive understanding, are all crucial within disciplinary encounters as well as between peoples. Understanding askance, with your attention fixed elsewhere, or your expectations focused on a different outcome, is also a common enough event in such encounters and can produce effects as powerful, if stranger, than fixed attention. (2)

Interdisciplinarity, or "understanding askance" as Beer puts it, is at once "common" and "strange." It is as common as common sense: the dewy-eyed fantasy of cooperation, mutual understanding, and unconditional support. It is nevertheless strange: it stages an encounter that disrupts the disciplined focus, optimizations, and specializations of late capitalism. The two halves of *Study in Scarlet* exemplify this disciplinary double bind; scientific detection and literary romance had reached a palpable contradiction. Doyle's unquenchable desire to understand askance, to imagine his vocations in generative conversation, had brushed up against the limits of cold reality, of Von Bergmann's brutal rebuff and Koch's casual disregard.

Darwin, of course, was not solely responsible for this cultural schism. If Romantic-era science's defining moment was the public spectacle of the Lawrence-Abernethy vitality debates, then the Victorian era's analogous moment was surely the Wilberforce-Huxley debate on the question of evolution. In his seminal book, *Ever Since Darwin* (1973), Stephen Jay Gould gleefully animates the scene with the morbid language of combat and humiliation: "At the famous British Association meeting in 1860 (where Huxley creamed 'Soapy Sam' Wilberforce), the unbalanced Fitzroy stalked about, holding a Bible above his head and shouting, 'The Book, The Book.' Five years later, he slit his throat" (33). In Gould's sensationalistic retelling, Robert Fitzroy, Darwin's captain on the HMS *Beagle*, fatally expiates his guilt over his complicity in Darwin's heresy. Six years after Gould, though, J.R. Lucas casts some doubt on Wilberforce's "creaming" because of an inconsistent historical record. Even with this revisionist goal in mind, however, Lucas finds the appeal of Gould's triumphal rhetoric irresistible:

> The legend of the encounter between Wilberforce and Huxley is well established. Almost every scientist knows, and every viewer of the BBC's recent programme on Darwin was shown, how Samuel Wilberforce, bishop of Oxford, attempted to pour scorn on Darwin's *Origin of Species* at a meeting of the British Association in Oxford

on 30 June 1860, and had the tables turned on him by T.H. Huxley. In this memorable encounter Huxley's simple scientific sincerity humbled the prelatical insolence and clerical obscurantism of Soapy Sam; the pretension of the Church to dictate to scientists the conclusions they were allowed to reach were, for good and all, decisively defeated; the autonomy of science was established in Britain and the Western world; the claim of plain unvarnished truth on men's allegiance was vindicated, however unwelcome its implications for human vanity might be; and the flood tide of Victorian faith in all its fulsomeness was turned to an ebb, which has continued to our present day and will only end when religion and superstition have been finally eliminated from the minds of all enlightened men. (313)

Enlightenment science exposes and undoes the "literary dallying" of "clerical obscurantism," "pretension," "Victorian faith," and "superstition." Instead of the porous boundaries of Romantic disease discourse, Beer and Lucas both imagine cross-disciplinary dialogue as a violent, or at least awkward, "encounter" rather than as fluid exchange. It is into this world of hardened contraries that the character of Sherlock Holmes takes his first steps and is why my reading of this collection of detective stories leans on this fumbling, experimental first attempt. Otis's bacteriological reading, Harris's image of pathological empire, and Pamboukian's attention to the narratives of quackery all depend on the later work, the more tightly plotted affairs of, for example, "The Adventure of the Speckled Band" (1892) and *The Stark Munro Letters* (1895). The neophyte author of *Study in Scarlet*, however, has yet to work out his disciplinary loyalties. In this sense, my reading of this early Doyle casts him as a Romantic author born out of time, a pre-disciplinary mind conscripted into a post-disciplinary world.

In this awkward first tale, these disciplinary issues crop up even at the expense of narrative flow. Having investigated the grisly murder of Enoch Drebber, Doyle has Holmes and Watson pause to debate the connection between art and science. Upon returning from a concert, Holmes muses out loud:

> Do you remember what Darwin says about music? He claims that the power of producing and appreciating it existed among the human race long before the power of speech was arrived at. Perhaps that is why we are so subtly influenced by it. There are vague memories in our souls of those misty centuries when the world was in its childhood. ("Scarlet" 39)

Watson, playing Wilberforce to Holmes's Huxley, rebuts lazily with "That's rather a broad idea" ("Scarlet" 39).[5] This brief exchange re-enacts in extreme miniature the "creaming" of the 1860 Oxford evolution debate. The contest, though, is quickly dropped without a declared winner, and the two continue in their collegial spirit of collaboration. The Romantic doctor (Watson) goes on resisting the Darwinian thesis, and the Victorian pathologist (Holmes) continues to insist on radical materialism and biological mechanism. In this quick allusion to Darwin, Doyle stages an unresolved encounter between these two medical models of, as Lucas might put it, the humanistic "obscurantism" of Watson and the "plain unvarnished truth" of Holmes. In this inaugural tale of the Sherlock Holmes stories, Doyle yokes these heterogeneous ideas by violence together in a generative dialogue rather than a destructive encounter. Structurally, if not thematically, Holmes and Watson get equal billing in the two parts of *Study in Scarlet*. Doyle invokes the evolution controversy not to relive the thrilling spectacle of Huxley's trouncing victory over Soapy Sam, but to regulate the "turbid ebb and flow" (Arnold, "Dover Beach" 17) of the sea of faith's comforting anthropocentrism and science's encroachment into human life; a binary that Matthew Arnold would famously harden into the Swiftian battle of the books between the "sweetness and light" (*Culture and Anarchy* 42) of culture and the modern philistinism of anarchy.[6]

Part I, "BEING A REPRINT FROM THE REMINISCENCES OF JOHN H. WATSON, M.D., LATE OF THE ARMY MEDICAL DEPARTMENT," presents this divide first from the perspective of the cultured doctor. Holmes's exaggerated image of the Victorian specialist particularly confounds Dr. Watson:

> His ignorance was as remarkable as his knowledge. Of contemporary literature, philosophy and politics he appeared to know next to nothing. Upon my quoting Thomas Carlyle, he inquired in the naivest way who he might be and what he had done. My surprise reached a climax, however, when I found incidentally that he was ignorant of the Copernican Theory and of the composition of the Solar System. That any civilized human being in this nineteenth century should not be aware that the earth travelled round the sun appeared to me to be such an extraordinary fact that I could hardly realize it. ("Scarlet" 12)

Here, Watson is more Arnold than Wilberforce. He is baffled at the gaps in Holmes's knowledge and suggests that a liberal arts education in "contemporary literature, philosophy and politics" would bring his friend closer to a "civilized human being." The medical professional, according to Watson, should be well-versed in both Carlyle and astronomy. Watson's "reminiscences" are meant not only to record the exploits of the extraordinary detective, but also to civilize Holmes's Arnoldian philistinism. Holmes's efficient knowledge, admirable elsewhere in the story, is here utterly ridiculous. To be unfamiliar with Carlyle, "the Copernican Theory," or "the composition of the Solar System" would be utterly unthinkable in the late nineteenth century, and Doyle's dramatic irony squarely targets his oblivious detective. What is perhaps most surprising about this passage is that its sympathies seem to lie not with the magisterial anatomical knowledge of a Dr. Joseph Bell, but with the literary Watson, the Romantic jack of all trades who navigates the world equipped with the inefficient niceties of civilization and the meandering learning of culture.

Holmes's arrogant charisma, though, swiftly takes back the narrative reins. His section gets first billing, his name titles the first chapter, and his oblique disquisition on the case as "a study in scarlet" makes it to the title page:

> The ring, man, the ring: that was what he came back for. If we have no other way of catching him, we can always bait our line with the ring. I shall have him, Doctor – I'll lay you two to one that I have him. I must thank you for it all. I might not have gone but for you, and so have missed the finest study I ever came across: a study in scarlet, eh? Why shouldn't we use a little art jargon. There's the scarlet thread of murder running through the colourless skein of life, and our duty is to unravel it, and isolate it, and expose every inch of it. And now for lunch, and then for Norman Neruda. Her attack and her bowing are splendid. What's that little thing of Chopin's she plays so magnificently: Tra-la-la-lira-lira-lay. ("Scarlet" 37)

Holmes again theorizes the connection between art and science, this time without recourse to Darwinian allusion. And instead of taking Holmes to task for his "broad idea," Watson learns to keep his response to himself: "Leaning back in the cab, this amateur bloodhound carolled away like a lark while I meditated upon the many-sidedness of the human mind" ("Scarlet" 38). The disciplinary encounter loses a vital participant while the doctor dully ponders and the detective glides swiftly along from the case, to visual art, to lunch, and finally to music. Holmes's superhuman processing speed makes his deductive focus seem effortless, even trivial. Nonessential material immediately fades into the "colourless" background while he unravels, isolates, and exposes the scarlet thread. That scarlet centerpiece excites, and all else remains tightly shackled to the tedious clockwork mechanism of everyday life. The Darwinian hypothesis had laid bare life's grand plan, and our mysteries, the retreating waves of Arnold's "Sea of Faith," were fast drying up along "the vast edges drear / And naked shingles of the world" ("Dover Beach" 27–8). Holmes's task, then, is a form of cleanup, to deal with the few bloody, scarlet threads left over from that initial Darwinian purge of superstition and obscurantism.

In this mechanistic worldview, little room is left for art. Only after calculating, "two to one," that his immediate task had reached completion can he casually turn to an assessment of Wilma Norman-Neruda's violin performance. His carolling "Tra-la-la-lira-lira-lay" suffices as musical commentary, as a pretty afterthought to his ponderous metaphysics. Art is just a pleasant distraction from the more serious matters of scientific deduction. Watson settles into his role as a sidekick whose sole function seems to be to bring cases to Holmes's attention (Holmes "might not have gone but for" Watson) and to document his exploits. Thus, when Holmes zeroes in on both problem and solution, proudly fingering Jefferson Hope as the culprit, the story appears to have reached its timely conclusion. Watson, left "meditat[ing] upon the many-sidedness of the human mind" while Holmes has moved on to lunch, eventually catches up to Holmes's ever-proliferating chains of deduction, and the story seems to reach its logical end when sidekick and detective finally arrive on the same page.

Watson, however, decides the story could do with some "many-sidedness" after all. After the breathless pace and precision focus of the story's first half, Watson abruptly abandons the detective to relate a long-winded history of Jefferson Hope. Without any guiding preamble, we find ourselves on the Great Alkali Plain of Utah, in "an arid and repulsive desert, which for many a long year served as a barrier against the advance of civilization" ("Scarlet" 63). Watson does away with the dry, expository reportage of the first part and indulges in some uncharacteristically Byronic purple prose:

> From the Sierra Nevada to Nebraska, and from the Yellowstone River in the north to the Colorado upon the south, is a region of desolation and silence. Nor is Nature always in one mood throughout this grim district. It comprises snow-capped and lofty mountains, and dark and gloomy valleys. There are swift-flowing rivers which dash through jagged canons; and there are enormous plains, which in winter are white with snow, and in summer are gray with the saline alkali dust. They all preserve, however, the common characteristics of barrenness, inhospitality, and misery. ("Scarlet" 63)

Again, Watson's narrative task is to civilize. Just as he brings Arnoldian "culture" to Holmes's philistinism, he now imperiously proposes to usher in "the advance of civilization" to the barren, inhospitable, and miserable frontiers of the New World. Brigham Young's Latter-Day Saints and their violent policing of love and marriage meet Watson's disapproving narration as we gradually learn of Jefferson Hope's motive for revenge and his terrible mistreatment at the hands of Mormon fanatics. In this early tale (Doyle would later walk back his trenchant criticism of Mormonism), the Danites, or the secret police of the Latter-Day Saints, come to signify a perilous dogmatism, steeped in unnecessary mystery and unverified superstition rather than empirical observation and evidence-based knowledge. An erstwhile proponent of the "literary dallying" of Carlyle and Arnold, Watson discovers his miscalculation, and fully commits himself against what Lucas described as "clerical obscurantism." Here, Doyle as Watson finally takes a stance in the Wilberforce-Huxley debate, and becomes, like Huxley, "Darwin's bulldog."[7] He would later make the opposite choice. His late-in-life conversion to spiritualism and his odd insistence on the psychic traffic between the natural and supernatural led him astray from Watson, Holmes, Darwin, and Huxley. In either case, that fantasy of reconciliation briefly hinted at in Holmes and Watson's congenial conversation about Darwin becomes impossible. A clear disciplinary choice must be made between medicine and literature, science and faith, anarchy and culture. And Watson, after "meditat[ing] on the many-sidedness of the human mind," chooses Holmes over Brigham Young. Thus, in his very first appearance in the detective series, Watson willingly assumes his role as Holmes's bulldog.

This expansive scene of international crime – the American frontier, London back alleys, street Arabs, Mormons, Indians – demands a different kind of detective. Now that Watson has decided his loyalties, he gladly takes to his role as "bulldog" and names Holmes the man for the job. In contrast to local policemen like Inspectors Lestrade and Gregson, Holmes can more readily navigate the vast, dangerous world of "barrenness, inhospitality, and misery." These inspectors remain beholden to Old World forensics and cannot hope to locate that fine scarlet thread within the immense colourless skein. Here, Mary Shelley's idealized cosmopolitanism degenerates into a fearful paranoia of proliferating allegiances and indecipherable motives, and we are to put our faith in Holmes to decode the foreign ciphers of the modern world. Shelley pits the local, inoculated body against the global scale of plague, and ends with a hopeful politics of possibility. Doyle stages a similar encounter, but ends with almost the exact opposite, with Ed Cohen's conception of bodily defence and Otis's reading of the Holmes stories as a kind of thwarted bacterial invasion.[8] It makes sense, then, for Doyle to violate Van Dine's first rule of detective fiction – that the reader should "have equal opportunity with the detective for solving the mystery" (189) – because Doyle would have us defer to his detective to solve the mystery for us and to allay our xenophobic fears. This is the conclusion of Doyle's initial disciplinary experiment, beginning with collegial conversation, leading to generative opposition, and ending with utter subordination to the master detective, the romance to the detective story, the literary to the clinical, and the body to the regulation of biopower.

This trajectory is even clearer in the subsequent instalment, *The Sign of Four* (1890). In this second outing, there is decidedly more detection and less romance. In a wry moment of meta-narration, Watson narrates Holmes's evaluation of Watson's narration in *Study in Scarlet*:

> "I glanced over it," said he. "Honestly, I cannot congratulate you upon it. Detection is, or ought to be, an exact science and should be treated in the same cold and unemotional manner. You have attempted to tinge it with romanticism, which produces much the same effect as if you worked a love-story or an elopement into the fifth proposition of Euclid.
>
> "But the romance was there," I remonstrated. "I could not tamper with the facts."
>
> "Some facts should be suppressed, or, at least, a just sense of proportion should be observed in treating them. The only point in the case which deserved mention was the curious analytical reasoning from effects to causes, by which I succeeded unravelling it." ("Sign of Four" 125)

Holmes anticipates Van Dine's distaste for "literary dallying," and lays out his own rules of "proportion." By this point, we are meant to nod along with Holmes. The dramatic irony is no longer on Watson's side since Holmes's "cold and unemotional" method, even without the heliocentric model, is by now tried and true. The very idea of a "love-story or elopement" in Euclid's fifth proposition (that the base angles of an isosceles triangle are congruent) is surely absurd. Erasmus Darwin's *The Loves of the Plants*, then, becomes as unimaginable to Holmes as it was to the snide satirist of *The Anti-Jacobin* who penned *The Loves of the Triangles*.[9] Holmes's "sense of proportion" forbids the tinge of "romanticism" in Darwin's amorous plants, and consequently Watson must learn to edit his own literary digressions and defer to Holmes's "analytical reasoning from effects to causes." If the fact that the earth revolves around the sun does not immediately pertain to the case, then that fact "should be suppressed." Efficient detection mandates efficient storytelling, and Watson is only too happy to comply.

In this way, Doyle's Sherlock Holmes stories tend towards a *literary* justification of institutional biopower. Doyle offers Dr. Joseph Bell (via Holmes) as the image of the unflappable expert who alone can manage the big data of the modern world with the necessary diagnostic efficiency. Watson's "literary dallying" becomes almost synonymous with a kind of degenerate faith, a backwards superstition that prevents "the advance of civilization" by insisting on, for example, barbaric codes of revenge, marriage, and providence. Jefferson Hope represents the detective-physician's anti-type. He foolishly allows his targets a 50 per cent chance to live by choosing the correct pill: "Let the high God judge between us. Choose and eat. There is death in one and life in the other. I shall take what you leave. Let us see if there is justice upon earth, or if we are ruled by chance" ("Scarlet" 112). He leaves it to "the high God" to decide the guilt of his Mormon persecutors, Enoch Drebber (who chooses incorrectly) and Joseph Strangerson (who chooses instead to attack Hope). Hope fails twice: he is unable to convince Strangerson to play along, and he eventually gets caught by Holmes. Several materialist conclusions are meant to follow from this double failure: (1) that there exists no poetic or divine "justice upon earth," (2) that we are indeed "ruled by chance," (3) that Holmes's scientific deduction is our best bet to manage those odds, and (4) that literature, whether romance, revenge tragedy, or detective fiction, should merely undergird this clinical authority as delightful adornment. Even though Doyle begins the project in the medico-literary genres of Romantic disease, as unwilling as Keats to abandon medicine entirely for literature and as generous as Erasmus Darwin in his "literary dallying," he emerges a hardened clinician, unable to organize the roles of Holmes and Watson into a truly productive partnership.

Rediscovering Vaccination

By 1887, when *Study in Scarlet* first appeared in print, the vaccination debate had already sharpened into very familiar talking points. On the one hand, rationalists touted compulsory vaccination as a bulwark of public health, and on the other hand, irrational dissenters went on about religious exceptions, exaggerated side effects, and biopolitical tyranny. In that same year, Doyle himself entered the debate with open letters to his anti-vaccination sparring partner, a Colonel Wintle of Southsea. As early as 1840, and again in 1853, 1867, 1871, and 1873, England had passed vaccination acts that would outlaw the old variolation, require children to be vaccinated shortly after birth, criminalize unsafe inoculation procedures, and finally declare vaccination compulsory for all British citizens. Compulsion, at this point, was the new normal. Given the proven success of vaccination and the durability of these public health laws, Doyle initially feels that "the inherent weakness of [Col. Wintle's] position renders a reply superfluous" ("Vaccination" 6124). But he renders one anyway because the "interests at stake are so vital that an enormous responsibility rests with the men whose notion of progress is to revert to the condition of things which existed in the dark ages before the dawn of medical science" ("Vaccination" 6139). He educates these men of the "dark ages" in the ways of the modern world and demonstrates with statistics and mortality tables that anti-vaccinationists are "really opposing progress" and contributing to the "propagation of errors" ("Vaccination" 6247). Unlike Wordsworth's gradual evolution from illness narratives to biopower, Doyle arrived into a largely settled debate. Compulsion had won by purging malingering fictions from its construction of public health.

There is a kind of comfort in this story of pathology's inevitable triumph. The easy reassurance of the closed case in a locked room has fuelled a growing literary industry. A sprawling fandom has grown around Doyle's creation, and in the 2012 edition of the *Guinness World Records*, Holmes became "the most portrayed literary human character in film & TV," edging out Hamlet, the previous record holder.[10] Recently, Michael Saler has argued that Holmes stands apart from other eighteenth- and nineteenth-century literary creations and fandoms in the detective's ability to transcend historical context:

> Sherlock Holmes was the first fictional creation that adults openly embraced as real while deliberately minimizing or ignoring its creator, and this fetishization of Holmes has continued for over a century. The cult of Holmes focuses not just on a singular character, but on his entire world: fans of the "canon" obsess about every detail of the fictional universe Conan Doyle created, mentally inhabiting this geography of the imagination in a way that was never true for partisans of earlier characters. And the Holmesian phenomenon has continued for over a century, far longer than the intermittent eighteenth-century vogues for Samuel Richardson's Pamela, let alone the more restricted generational enthusiasms for Werther, Little Nell, and others. Sherlockian devotion is thus a departure from preceding public infatuations with fictional characters and a template for subsequent public infatuations for imaginary worlds and their protagonists. The popular fascination with Holmes commenced the

transformation of certain imaginary worlds into virtual worlds. The question is, why Holmes? (107)

Perhaps another more pertinent question for this book might be, why *not* Romantic-era creations like Victor Frankenstein, his creature, or Dracula (a character inspired by John William Polidori's *The Vampyre*)? Adaptations of these works have little care for an internally consistent "canon." Frankenstein and the creature have largely become interchangeable, and filmic representations of Dracula range from the murderous Count Orlok in *Nosferatu* (1922) to the vampire-possessed dog of *Zoltan, Hound of Dracula* (1978). Rather than momentarily entertaining one-offs, the detective's enduring appeal lies in an internally consistent world that operates under the attractive, comforting fantasy of biopower. No matter how global the scope or how complex the relationships become, Holmes is the man with the right solution. In exchange for a normatively defined and closely policed state of health, we gladly volunteer our bodies to the Holmesian detective-physician and place our faith in the ability of the biopolitcal "canon" to close the case.

This drive towards closure typifies modern adaptations of the Sherlock Holmes stories. The pilot episode of the BBC series *Sherlock* (2010) expunges the entire Mormon story from *Study in Scarlet* for a cleaner introduction to the primetime detective team. Gone is Doyle's disciplinary vacillation, and in its place, is a more coherent and reverent portrait of the master of deduction. In "minimizing or ignoring its creator," as Saler put it, the BBC incarnation of Holmes travels in the heavily regulated world of Sherlockiana. Authorial objections remain silent, leaving only the loud celebrity of the Kochian scientist who promises an unseen solution to our ills. In the television series *Star Trek: The Next Generation* (1987), Data, the crew's resident android, frequently cosplays as Holmes. Here, the detective is reimagined as an infallible machine capable of "60 trillion operations per second."[11] He becomes wholly synonymous with that "veiled prophet" or the all-seeing pathologist, promising his miracle cure if only we cease to see ourselves as patients and give our bodies over to the case study. Saler takes this as a kind of emergent secular faith. In the "absence of communal beliefs and higher ideals in an age that seemed dominated by positivism and materialism" (107), he argues, we build imagined worlds into virtual houses of worship. Biopolitical faith, then, means a slavish devotion to Dr. Bell or Dr. Koch's latest medical triumph, and Holmes's strictly curated afterlife becomes a sort of reassuring dogma that rewards its adherents with eventual salvation.

Even after trying to kill off Holmes in the famous "Reichenbach Falls" episode, public clamour brought the beloved character back. The stubborn desire to treat Holmes as real baffled even his creator who found it "incredible how realistic some people take [this imaginary character] to be" (Doyle qtd. in Saler 106). Doyle's hideous progeny generated unauthorized biographies of Holmes and Watson, speculation about Holmes's education, and fabricated documentation about Watson's marriages. Doyle would later try to disassociate himself from the empirical Holmes with his turn towards spiritualism, but this did little to dampen Holmes's popularity. Doyle's disciplinary struggle between Darwinian materialism and Arnoldian culture in *Study in Scarlet* had been resolved for him and had also claimed Holmes for the ordered taxonomies, nosologies, and internal consistency of the new evolutionary biology's clinical paradigm. Medico-literary fiction could no longer afford dalliances with the literary. The triumph of modern medicine found an enduring partner in the detective story, leaving behind Wordsworth's ambivalent cases of rustic life, Darwin's sprawling botanical epic, Blake's visionary poetics of violation, Keats's imaginative medicine of eternal life, and Shelley's cosmopolitan prophecy of global immunity. The thrill of detection – case and solution – filled out the medical narrative, and Jefferson Hope's romantic motive was forgotten or at best discarded as a trivial afterthought. Modern medicine had tightened into a closed, self-regulating system that could absorb Watson's literary-minded resistance and repurpose it as support. Doyle discovers this in *Study in Scarlet*; the Mormon romance of the second half, even as it complicates the mechanistic worldview of the first with mitigating motivations, only succeeds as propaganda for its real star. Any incongruence with the infallible science of deduction becomes frivolous filigree, mere "exaggeration of some effects" to be disciplined anew into the tightly ordered world of Sherlockiana.

In a sense, this book's disciplinary struggle has coincided with Doyle's botched effort to unite the two cultures. As I have claimed throughout, smallpox vaccination was as much a literary triumph as it was a medical one. It depended on Romantic medical writing that we have ceased to read as authentically medical: the careful balance of the individual illness narrative and the medical archive in Jenner's and Wordsworth's case studies, the radical and revolutionary experimentalism of Darwin and Blake, and the interdisciplinary biopolitics of Keats and Shelley. So, in this post-Victorian age of two discrete cultures, could something like the Romantic-era innovation of vaccination be rediscovered now? Could modern medicine reproduce the success of Romantic medical writing? If medicine remains beholden to the pathological siren call of Holmesian detection, then the answer is perhaps no. The story of the detective-physician does, however, produce a different *kind* of success. In 1854, for example, Dr. John Snow stopped an urban cholera outbreak by overlaying what Steven Johnson has called a "ghost map" onto the London streets. The detective-physician gradually followed the spectral trail of dead bodies to the contaminated Broad Street water pump.[12] The well-defined problem and Snow's singular solution have little need or patience for the literary dallying of the Romantic illness narrative. But what of the ill-defined problems and partial solutions of, for example, Wordsworth's encounter with an "idiot boy," Darwin's botanical storytellers, Blake's rethinking of sexuality through Oothoon's violated body, Keats's vegetative life, or Shelley's diseased embrace of a "negro half clad"? Romantic literature played a direct role in shaping medical outcomes, addressing the era's emergent bioethical problems, and anticipating the new ones. If modern medicine remains siloed in pathological and disciplinary knowledge, it will find itself unready to tackle the complex post-vaccination problems of the twenty-first century, including, just to name a few, reproductive technologies, gene editing, health disparities, and current and future pandemics. Romantic illness narratives, especially as they become increasingly illegible to us, demand a second look, if only for the mere possibility of rediscovering something like vaccination.

Conclusion

After several detours into Romantic literature and medicine, this book ends with the familiar Foucauldian narrative of the birth of the clinic and the fading of the illness narrative. The normal is now marked out against the pathological, and the medical gaze has subdued its docile bodies. Without the distraction of the strange classifications (Jenner and Wordsworth in part one), experiments (Darwin and Blake in part two), and interdisciplinarity (Keats and Shelley in part three) of Romantic medical writing, vaccination's afterlife has played out like the unruly legacy of Doyle's creation. It has become synonymous with an opaque biopower that legislates compulsory immunization at a distance. The close encounters of illness narratives, then, have had nowhere to go but rogue. Naturopaths, scientologists, evangelicals, faith healers, and "rogue" (Park) scientists like Dr. Andrew Wakefield have proven that contemporary vaccine hesitancy and refusal cuts across all the usual lines of class, gender, race, education, politics, and sexuality. The staged vaccination drive that led to the assassination of Osama bin Laden has stigmatized preventive medicine in the developing world. And Jenny McCarthy's national platform has brought her anti-vaccination agenda to affluent suburban neighborhoods in the United States. More than a decade after measles was declared eliminated in the United States, Texas reported twenty-one infections among members of the Eagle Mountain International Church near Fort Worth.[1] After hovering around zero for almost half a century, the reported cases of pertussis, or whooping cough, in the United States started to spike sporadically in the last two decades. Even Disneyland, the happiest place on earth, has failed to keep measles at bay. And the COVID-19 pandemic confirmed yet again that the happy story of Jenner's triumph is woefully incomplete.

The received medical history tells of a heroic physician who rose above the dark ages of medicine to find the pathological light of truth. When other physicians were busy with invasive prototypes of electromagnetic devices and laughable nitrous oxide experiments, Jenner was hard at work drafting the rubric for the new preventive medicine. In my hedging introductory remarks, I accused this account of being "not entirely accurate" and "not particularly useful." A conclusion deserves some plainer language: this story is both wrong and dangerous. First, the wrong. Milkmaids already knew from their daily labours that exposure to cowpox-infected udders would immunize them to the human smallpox virus. And there are scattered anecdotes of cowpox inoculation from as early as the 1770s. This is not a story of Jenner's miraculous discovery, then, but of the medical writing that made vaccination plausible, available, and desirable. It is a story about how disease and treatment were reported (hence the title, *The Smallpox Report*), and it is a story about what that reporting looked like (hence the subtitle, *Vaccination and the Romantic Illness Narrative*). Finding a truer account has meant rethinking Wordsworth's *Lyrical Ballads* as medical cases, Darwin's botanical fiction and Blake's visionary poetry as experimental research, and Keats's romances and Shelley's speculative fiction as interdisciplinary visions of post-vaccination public health.

Second, the conventional history of Jenner, vaccination, and biopower is not only wrong, but it has also turned into a dangerous fiction. In this fourth and final part of *The Smallpox Report*, the pathological certainty of the specialized physician-detective has prevailed, and compulsory vaccination has become the latest and best advertisement for a rational biopower. This should have been a winning argument. Smallpox was indeed eradicated in the late twentieth century, but other vaccine-preventable diseases continue to make periodic comebacks because of an adamant anti-vaccination movement that has slowly chipped away at herd immunity. The better argument is somehow on the losing side of history. If the argument is solely about rational biopower, it seems, then the movement marches on, and our dangerous exposure to vaccine-preventable diseases increases. In a sense, the four parts of this book have been four attempts to rescue the failing argument for vaccination. A catchier, public-facing subtitle of *The Smallpox Report* could have been something like "Four Ways to Talk to Your Anti-Vaxxer Friend." It is certainly a partial and ultimately inaccurate characterization of the book's overall approach, but it does provide a convenient way to talk about its contemporary implications.

If your anti-vaxxer friend privileges the personal anecdote over the established medical archive, then point her to the case studies in Jenner's *Inquiry* and Wordsworth's *Lyrical Ballads*. When Jenner listened to the anecdote of the milkmaid Sarah Nelmes, about her daily rounds, the thorn that scratched up her hand, and the subsequent cowpox inflammation, he recorded her story with a mix of respectful fidelity and medical invention. Jenner offers a composite portrait of Nelmes that preserves the pustules from her thorny labour while appending a fictitious, diagnostic pustule on her index finger (figure 3). His Romantic case study deliberately shifted between the individual and the universal, the patient narrative with a burgeoning medical archive. Similarly, when Wordsworth's census canvasser in "We Are Seven" tries to get an accurate household count from a little girl, he must weigh her stubborn refusal to omit her two dead siblings in her ghostly "seven" against his public need to enter the objective "five" into his ledger. Even if modern biopower has moved on from this Romantic ecology of private illness narrative and public good towards the exigencies of the latter, tell your anti-vaxxer friend that the smallpox vaccine was built from the ground up, from Wordsworth's and Jenner's rural anecdotes of embodied life. Her anecdotes and individual case presentation, in part, *are* vaccination's medical archive.

If your anti-vaxxer friend proudly hangs a print of Gillray's "Anti-Vaccine Society" caricature (figure 6) above her fireplace and argues that vaccine-preventable diseases are just not serious enough to justify the grotesque side effects of bovine matter leaking out of her ears, nose, and throat, ask her to glance away from the cross-species orgy on the right and towards the suffering on the left. The modern success of vaccination has allowed entire generations to forget the urgency of confluent smallpox pustules that blinded children for life and, much later, polio-infected legs withered to the bone. Darwin and Blake took great risks in their experimental research on the idea of inoculation to rise to what they saw as the vast scale of human suffering. Darwin boldly rewrote Linnaeus in heroic couplets, imagining a crossbreeding, inoculated "transmigrating mass" of biological life. In Blake's private life, he applauded his physician's electroshock treatments for his wife's rheumatism. And in his illuminated manuscripts he worked to detail Darwin's evolutionary vision with startlingly violent interpenetrations and inoculations of the human body. Romantic research's outrageous experimentalism is no occasion for your anti-vaxxer friend's supercilious laughter; rather, it is a trenchant reminder of a hidden history of suffering that she surely does not want to relive.

If your anti-vaxxer friend feels helpless in a sea of misinformation and can only retreat from unmanageable questions of herd immunity to her own individual vaccine refusal, then direct her to the interdisciplinary reach of the Romantic illness narrative. Just after the unprecedented success of the new preventive medicine, Keats felt a turning point towards a massifying biopolitics. But instead of retreat, he decided to leave his professional medical training to become a poet of the new medicine. For Keats, vaccination had promised the end of disease, and the real work left was not in Guy's Hospital but in the poetic task of shaping the new parameters of human flourishing. Shelley's novel *The Last Man* even predicts the eradication of smallpox, 154 years in advance of the WHO's official declaration in 1980. Again, rather than retreat into contented quietism, her novel speculates on the grandest scale about the new social and political challenges of human survival beyond the next extinction level event. Rather than leave medicine to the rising professional class, their speculative fictions took the lessons of Romantic disease discourse's non-normative embodiments, experimentalism, and interdisciplinarity and applied them to their positive visions of a biopolitical future that would, at last, value your anti-vaxxer friend's illness narrative. Ask her, then, to find her Romantic voice beyond the insularly negative critique.

If your anti-vaxxer friend is not merely content to retreat from the biopolitical arena and is itching for an activist fight against an intrusive government, then have her learn from the story of Doyle, the aspiring interdisciplinary storyteller who was nevertheless disciplined into pathological compliance. In his first Sherlock Holmes story, *A Study in Scarlet*, Doyle tries out Keats's disciplinary turn from medicine to literature, from his early pathology lectures to writing popular detective stories. In this early iteration, Doyle separates the story into two parts: the first features the whittling down of Holmes's suspect list to one, the culprit Jefferson Hope. The second part is a long, rambling backstory of Jefferson Hope's trek through Mormon country in the American west. Turn-of-the-century audiences, of course, preferred part one and did not bother to read after the murderer was identified. Pathological detection was in, and rambling discourse was out. In Doyle's second Holmes story, *The Sign of Four*, the backstory of Jonathan Small's involvement in the Indian Rebellion of 1857 shrinks into a brief flashback that quickly establishes motive. The more Doyle adhered to the formula of pathological detection, the more successful he became. This is the authoritarian backdrop for your anti-vaxxer friend's modern denialism, but she need not mould her reckless resistance from the chaotic void. The generic experiments of Romantic disease discourse offer a much more generative starting point for her developing health activism.[2]

Admittedly, these are hard lessons to glean from our inherited and overdetermined story about smallpox vaccination. And I am not, as I mentioned in the introduction, suggesting that these arguments will really work to change your anti-vaxxer friend's mind. The *real* work is in how we talk about illness and health and how we honour illness narratives in our biopolitical calculations. Contemporary history has a bad track record when it comes to doing this crucial work. For example, included in Metropolitan Life Insurance's *Health Heroes* pamphlet with the reverent portrait of Jenner (figure 7), is a two-page map (figure 14) that conveniently condenses the global human history of smallpox from its supposed origins in India, to its transmission through caravans and ships from east to west, and finally to its timely demise at Jenner's heroic hands.[3] Like Dr. John Snow's ghost map of cholera, the map reassures us with a straightforward epidemiological allegory of infectious cases. Illness narratives show up only in the cartographical shorthand of the crudest markers of race and ethnicity: the feathered headdress of the Native American, the spear of the African tribesman, the burdened camel of the Arabian nomad, and the turban of the Indian merchant. A cartoonish, personified smallpox looms over the world map, staining the dye of his red cloak first into the stylized "X" in India, then the Indian ox collar, then the dromedary saddle in Arabia, then the African blanket, then the flags and hulls of transatlantic ships, and finally into the Native American tunic. The "health hero" Jenner stands at the very end of this sponsored history in which the global scourge is "only checked at last, by VACCINATION." There is no pustule in sight, no eyes

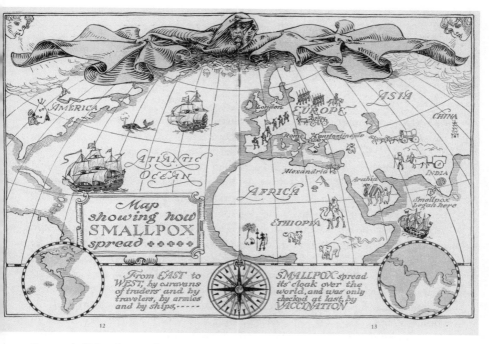

Figure 14. "Map showing how SMALLPOX spread" in *Health Heroes*, a series commissioned by the Metropolitan Life Insurance Company, 1926. Call # R489.J5 H3 1926, The Huntington Library, San Marino, California.

encrusted with healing tissue, no face scarred beyond recognition, not even Sarah Nelmes's hand covered in mild cowpox infections. Smallpox, in this view, was not about the sufferers; instead, it was about vectors of transmission – blankets, fabrics, building materials, cloaks – and the detective-physicians smart enough to catch the culprits.

The triumphal map efficiently conveys a comforting techno-optimism that exchanges patient agency, illness narrative, and embodied suffering for easy allegories of global health. Sarah Nelmes's hand unceremoniously disappears from the vaccination record, a forgotten trace of a hopelessly benighted age of medicine. *The Smallpox Report* instead has registered her pustule-ridden hand in its catalogue of Romantic medical writing. When Keats, for example, writes of his own precarious hand, he artfully fashions an unmappable medical knowledge:

> This living hand, now warm and capable
> Of earnest grasping, would, if it were cold

> And in the icy silence of the tomb,
> So haunt thy days and chill thy dreaming nights
> That thou wouldst wish thine own heart dry of blood
> So that in my veins red life might stream again,
> And thou be conscience-calm'd – see here it is –
> I hold it towards you.					("This Living Hand" 1–8)

In his latest and most desperate attempt to match the popularity of someone like Byron, Keats gave in to the urging of his friends to write a comic tale in the vein of *Don Juan*, which began appearing in 1819. *The Cap and Bells; or, The Jealousies* eventually became eighty-eight Spenserian stanzas that literary history would largely forget. In a 1911 *PMLA* article, Herbert E. Cory lovingly describes the work as a "pathetic attempt to play the motley with a cracked heart" (84). At this point, Keats already knew he was not long for this world and that his engagement to Fanny Brawne would never amount to anything. His "cracked heart" would not let his living hand finish the "motley" work of *The Cap and Bells*; instead, he scribbled these palliative lines right on the "pathetic" manuscript. He looked at his own hand, still "warm and capable / Of earnest grasping," and decided against spending these last moments of warmth, capability, and earnestness on some feeble attempt at Spenserian or Byronic imitation. The literary longevity of some popular comedy like *The Cap and Bells* might have survived the "icy silence of the tomb," but only through a conscience-shattering devil's bargain. Its long life would be so haunted by mediocrity that it would wish to transfuse its own blood to resurrect the hand of the true poet.

The strangeness of the fragment to a reader like Susan Wolfson is in the abrupt concluding gesture: "The parting shot issues an invitation, but to what? Does *it* refer to a warm living hand or a cold dead one? The reader has to imagine the present as past, the sensation of earnest grasping as the chilling grip of a nightmare, the actual as spectral, and the spectral as actual" ("Late Lyrics" 114). Even though, grammatically, we should expect a "living hand" – it is, after all, the subject of the long, compound sentence – Wolfson receives the speaker's hand in an uncertain state of superposition between life and death. What is to be done with this Schrödinger's hand? Is the speaker demanding transfused blood? Is it an invitation to bury the hand in the grave? In this arresting moment of ambiguity, Keats's fragment suddenly exposes our unreadiness to handle biopolitical questions of life, disease, or death. The speaker offers his objectively healthy hand and suddenly forces an inexplicably pronoun-shifted "you" to make an end-of-life decision. In the missing five syllables of the startling final line, the poem demands of the unready "you" a working theory of a healthy life worth living. And our lazy cartographical allegories are left without answers. *The Smallpox Report* preserves both Sarah Nelmes's immunized hand and Keats's living one in the vaccination record to remind us that our ideas of public health emerge not just from the state and corporate interests that narrowly define normative health, but also from these strange, forgotten Romantic illness narratives.

The Smallpox Report, in the end, exhorts us to engage critically with medical discourse, exposing the historical construction of arbitrary hegemony where relevant, and more productively, envisioning an inclusive medical establishment that acknowledges the diversity of our stories of human health. This, of course, does not mean legitimating anti-vaccination movements or giving them ideological cover. It does mean, however, changing the conversation. Much of the scientific literature on the loss of public trust in medical science has focused on top-down solutions: improving communication with the public, increasing understanding of how scientists work, and developing faith in the self-corrective processes of the scientific method. During the COVID-19 pandemic, this has meant flashing the graph of a flattened curve, patiently waiting for vaccine trials, creating a spectacle of public officials receiving the Pfizer and Moderna vaccines, and deifying NIAID director Anthony Fauci. This model pits the valiant, objective scientist against the stubbornly irrational layperson in the unproductive impasse of a zero-sum struggle. This categorical erasure of the Romantic illness narrative has invited distrust, misinformation, reckless denialism, and irresponsible protests of safer-at-home orders and mask mandates. What we can learn from Romantic medicine is that a unilateral biopower has never worked. Medical discourse does not solely belong to the chastising clinician who wags her impatient finger at an uncomprehending and irrational mass of misbehaving patients. This mode of medical paternalism gravely underestimates the contributions of writers, artists, anthropologists, historians, sociologists, and philosophers across national boundaries and medical traditions that have shaped and continue to shape our evolving stories of the healthy body.

Notes

Introduction

1 Foucault's descriptions of biopower are littered throughout his large body of work, but the recent collection of his lectures at the Collège de France (1978–9) is a convenient repository for this influential argument about the state's top-down control of docile bodies. Foucault's pre-modern state acts from moral, natural, or divine laws, the early modern state strives for a maximal top-down authority, and the modern state balances "between the maximum and minimum fixed … by the nature of things" (*Birth of Biopolitics* 19). Even in this late, more neoliberal Foucault, the modern state's biopolitical coercions must operate with this delicate balancing act between authority and consensus.

2 Here is Hardt and Negri's useful definition of the common from *Commonwealth*: "The notion of the common does not position humanity separate from nature, as either its exploiter or its custodian, but focuses rather on the practices of interaction, care, and cohabitation in a common world, promoting the beneficial and limiting the detrimental forms of the common. In the era of globalization, issues of the maintenance, production and distribution of the common in both these senses and in both ecological and socioeconomic frameworks become increasingly central" (viii).

3 In Richard A. Barney and Warren Montag's edited collection *Systems of Life: Biopolitics, Economics, and Literature on the Cusp of Modernity* (2018), the editors and contributors offer a rich discussion around the Enlightenment-era emergence of biopolitical thought out of the political and economic culture of incredible scientific and industrial progress. They take the emergence of the Enlightenment idea of "system" as an occasion to reflect on why contemporary biopolitical theorists like Michel Foucault, Giorgio Agamben, and Roberto Esposito pay such close attention to this historical period at the "cusp of modernity" (1–33).

4 See my entry on Meeke's novel in the forthcoming *Cambridge Guide to the Eighteenth-Century Novel* edited by April London. The smallpox plot serves only as a convenient device for the protagonist to discover his true aristocratic heritage.

5 Throughout this study, I will make a clear distinction between biopower and biopolitics. I take "biopower" to mean top-down solutions that prefer institutional control of docile bodies whereas "biopolitics" encompasses the full range of solutions to the problem of public health.

6 Several critics have given short shrift to Romantic disease and privileged instead the period's heated vitality debates. At stake was the vital principle, the spark of life that animated dead matter into sentience. Radical materialists such as John Thelwall and William Lawrence rejected the vitalist position, exemplified by John Abernethy's theory (by way of Jenner's mentor John Hunter) of a mysterious "invisible substance, superadded to the evident structure of muscles" (39). These spectacular debates and charismatic personalities have made the principles of life and death central to our discussions of Romantic medicine. For example, Sharon Ruston, in *Shelley and Vitality*, has tracked the language of vitalism through Percy Shelley's poetic career, and Denise Gigante, in *Life: Organic Form and Romanticism*, has meticulously documented the period's investment in locating the vital principle. In James Robert Allard's *Romanticism, Medicine, and the Poet's Body*, he flips the terms of the vitality debates in his discussion of Thomas Lovell Beddoes's fascination with death: "that essence lay in death … in the moment of disjunction, at the moment of death, when both our mortality and immortality are most called into question and most visibly apparent" (119). This polarized critical discourse of Romantic medicine – Gigante's investigation of the "excess of … electric life" (230) on the one hand and Allard's deathly "disjunction" on the other – excludes the crucial middle term of disease, a category that, in many ways, proves even more theoretically intractable than either life or death.

7 Here, I refer to Cullen's work on nosology where he sets out his grand purpose: "But as diseases, different in their nature, require not only different, but even contrary remedies, it is of the utmost consequence to the medical practitioner to be able, with certainty, to distinguish any disease from every other (*Nosology* i). For a very different perspective on the medical practice, see Brown (81–98). For Continental contexts about vitality, materialism, and disease, see Elizabeth A. Williams's treatment on the conflicting semiotics of the encyclopedic medicine of Diderot and Cullen and the pragmatic medicine of vitalist physicians in the treatment of smallpox (215–54).

8 Again, this is reflected in our scholarship. In addition to de Almeida and Allard's work, Alan Bewell's *Romanticism and Colonial Disease* has opened up the discussion by directing us to read disease in its colonial context and understand its threateningly vast geographical reach – the "dangerous disease environments that colonial contact had brought into being" (12). The "medical metaphor" (Allard 64) of disease also appears in the language of the Revolutionary controversies of the 1790s: Burke and Mary Wollstonecraft, for example, famously use – at cross purposes – figures of disease and plague to diagnose the health of the body politic. Burkean conservatives would cast revolutionary ideas as a dangerous contagion from the continent while Paineite radicals would turn aristocratic privilege and political despotism into distemper, plague, and even, in Wollstonecraft's case, digestive trouble.

9 This anxiety has an even longer history. Even before Jenner, inoculation was seen as a terribly threatening procedure. See the discussion of eighteenth-century fears of smallpox inoculation in Felicity Nussbaum's *The Limits of the Human* (109–34).

10 See Wakefield (144) for the infamous article. Every author (except Wakefield himself) has retracted their contribution since the 1998 publication.

11 As I have mentioned, Tim Fulford and Debbie Lee's wonderful article on Jenner contains an efficient summary of vaccination's conservative afterlife (139–65). For a more thorough historical account of vaccination politics in the nineteenth century and the emergence of interventionist state power in matters of health, see Deborah Brunton's historical study *The Politics of Vaccination: Practice and Policy in England, Wales, Ireland, and Scotland, 1800–1874* (2008). Brunton goes even further to describe the public issue of vaccination as "the relationship of medical practitioners to the state" (4), leaving the vaccinated body increasingly out of the equation.

12 It is strange that, in a work that seeks to reclaim Romantic medicine from critical obscurity, there is no mention of vaccination – an idea that has saved more lives than almost any other scientific innovation in history.

13 When I talk about "inoculation as narrative," I am partially relying on the already robust construct of "narrative medicine," as described by interdisciplinary medical practitioners like Rita Charon. Her work since the early 2000s has culminated recently in a supremely useful edited collection *The Principles and Practices of Narrative Medicine*. Of particular interest for my argument in this book is the discussion of the practice of close reading and its importance to narrative medicine and thinking about medical ethics (157–205).

14 The battle for vaccination gained its primacy through some remarkably sensationalistic images. See Haslam (235–44) on the connection between vaccination and its visual culture in *From Hogarth to Rowlandson: Medicine in Art in Eighteenth-Century Britain* (1996). See also Ron Broglio's chapter "Cattle and Human Animality" (187–208) in which he discusses bovine images in vaccination propaganda.

15 Indeed, recent historians of science have theorized cogently about the value of error and failure in some of humanity's greatest scientific discoveries. In Tamara Horowitz and Allen Janis's edited collection of essays on scientific failure, the editors begin, "There are indeed many instances where an examination of the failures of science sheds light on its development or, in the case of contemporary failures, provides insights that help one see one's way out of the morass" (1). Romantic medicine, I argue, thrives under these conditions.

16 For the history of medical professionalization, Porter has the authoritative account. Porter's reading of vaccination is not unique, however. See also Erwin Ackerknecht's *A Short History of Medicine* in which he also conscripts vaccination into the familiar Enlightenment story (142–4).

17 My account of the paradoxical and "capricious age" of Romantic medicine will fall far short of a comprehensive history of inoculation; such an expansive project would be both impractical and counterproductive. Especially for non-Romantic medicine,

there is already a large body of work in the history of science and medicine. For Classical, medieval, and early modern medicine, de Almeida's work, Ian Maclean's *Logic, Signs and Nature*, and Suzanne E. Hatty and James Hatty's *The Disordered Body* represent just a few of the seminal texts. This study's literary historical archive focuses instead on Romantic medicine's critical slipperiness. Its awkwardness and its ideological inconsistencies frustrate both Foucauldian master narratives and teleological histories of scientific progress. Because of this, some unusual suspects emerge to fill out the radical literary history of vaccination. Historians of science prefer to discuss "proper" scientists: Jan Golinski has emphasized the public spectacle of Romantic science by charting Sir Humphry Davy's rise to fame (188–235), while Lynn Hunt and Margaret Jacob have linked Davy's bodily experimentation with nitrous oxide (laughing gas) to a culture of political radicalism (505). Literary critics, however, hover around the ambiguous figure of the "poet-physician." James Allard, for example, turns to authors who had both medical training and literary talent. He even goes so far as to establish a strict, twofold rubric for admittance into the category of "poet-physician": (1) he must have spent an "extended term as a registered student at a recognized medical school" (12) and (2) he "must have explicitly addressed the interconnections between poetry and medicine" (13). The interdisciplinary approach of this book will strive for a bit more flexibility. I privilege neither the institutionalization of medical and scientific knowledge nor the theorizer of medico-literary hybridity. Erasmus Darwin's unselfconscious interdisciplinarity, for example, is no immediate cause for exclusion. My approach does not depend upon a robust theorization of the "poet-physician"; such a study would indeed be worthwhile but also outside the scope of my argument about Romantic inoculation and disease. Instead, I rely on a less proscriptive mode of interdisciplinarity, an approach that can admit Jenner – a man who was alternately country bumpkin and scientific genius, clumsy poet and medical hero – into an uneven, paradoxical, novel, and capricious literary history of Romantic inoculation.

18 Hermione de Almeida has helped us think about Romantic medicine more seriously, especially in the context of Keats's poetry. Even since her groundbreaking study, though, we still tend to view Romantic medicine as a minor embarrassment in Enlightenment histories of scientific progress.

19 Grinnell describes hypochondria as a malady that resists the legibility of the body, requiring both physician and patient to produce diagnostic accounts of illness: "hypochondria embodies an anxiety troubling disciplinary formations that would produce the body as an object of knowledge" (3).

20 For a concise summary of these changes in "medical cosmology," see the two diagrams in Jewson (228).

21 My insistence on these radical dimensions of inoculation is motivated by several payoffs. First, it rewrites the undeserved reputation of Romantic medicine as merely an entertaining misstep in the magisterial march of medical progress. Second, it opens a space in Foucault's restrictive history for non-institutional medical practices. Third, it restores the importance of literature to the history of inoculation beyond reactionary

propaganda campaigns for compulsory vaccination. Fourth, it values an enduring ethic of care for diseased and non-normative embodiment and not just a relentless race for the cure. Fifth, it explains how radical patient agency has survived into the modern age of biopower.

1 Wordsworth's Romantic Path to Biopower

1 Jerome McGann's influential polemic in *Romantic Ideology* (1983) announces the collapse of honest, historical investigation because of a slavish adherence to some mythically unified and comprehensive idea of Romanticism.

2 This is the exclamatory opening statement of *The Political Unconscious* (Jameson 9).

3 For this classic treatment of Wordsworth's early career, see Geoffrey Hartman's *Wordsworth's Poetry 1787–1814* (1964). In particular, he reads the girl's misunderstanding as a kind of epistemological failure (143–5). For Wordsworth's telling but largely ignored commentary on the little cottage girl's error in "We Are Seven," see Wordsworth's "Preface" (1802), 598.

4 Here, I deliberately invoke Foucault's original coinage: "the sudden emergence of the problem of the naturalness of the human species within an artificial milieu. It seems to me that this sudden emergence of the naturalness of the human species within the political artifice of a power relation is something fundamental ... what we would call biopolitics, biopower" (*Security, Territory, Population* 22). This biopower, he explains later, emerges in the obsessive monitoring of birth and population rates in eighteenth-century France. By using the word "biopower," I mean to express Foucault's concept of this artificial power exercised over biological processes.

5 This comprehensively Romantic reading could easily extend to a novel like Mary Shelley's *Frankenstein* (1818) in which sympathies inevitably align with the abandoned creature. Indeed, it has been convincingly argued that Victor Frankenstein represents a monstrous version of Mary Shelley's husband Percy while the creature is a mere victim of Promethean ambition. See in particular Mellor's *Mary Shelley: Her Life, Her Fiction, Her Monsters*.

6 In addition to Aaron Fogel's work on the anti-census genre, Charlotte Sussman has argued for the importance of demography in Mary Shelley's apocalyptic novel *The Last Man* (1826). Despite nominally being about the last man's struggle with his loneliness, the novel actually "devotes much of its energy to representing human aggregates, to imagining populations" (286).

7 Robbins provides the most exhaustive account of the census debate's relation to Wordsworth's poem. Her comprehensive history starts from early eighteenth-century missteps to the triumph of the British census in the early nineteenth century (202–8).

8 Jonathan Swift's *The Battle of the Books* (1704), for example, famously weighs in this notable debate by portraying the "*Antients*" as noble citizens of Parnassus and the opportunistic "*Moderns*" as petty morons who start a war over "a small spot of ground" (3).

9 For a concisely expressed timeline of Foucault's history of power, especially the transitional moment between eighteenth- and nineteenth-century "discipline" to modern
   biopower, see the chart in Jeffrey Nealon's *Foucault Beyond Foucault: Power and Its
   Intensifications since 1984* (2007), 45.

10 Smith enjoyed a reputation as the poetic voice of the age, so these remarks can more
   or less be safely taken as representative of the era's most contentious political issues.
   In Stuart Curran's introduction to Smith's collected poetry, he goes so far as to say
   "Charlotte Smith was the first poet in England whom in retrospect we would call
   Romantic" (xix). Unfortunately, Wordsworth's words turned prophetic, and Smith's
   body of poetic work certainly has failed to equal the robust afterlife of Wordsworth's.
   Curran tells a compelling story of Wordsworth's begrudging respect for his poetic pre-
   decessor (xix–xx).

11 Here, I suggest that Keats's famous critique of Wordsworth's "egotistical sublime"
   applies not only to the intensely autobiographical language of later work like *The Prel-
   ude*, but also to Wordsworth's earlier work in *Lyrical Ballads*. See John Keats, *Selected
   Letters*, edited by Robert Gittings and Jon Mee (2002), 147.

12 For more historical detail and precise figures on the historical populations of England,
   see E.A. Wrigley and R.S. Schofield's *The Population History of England 1541–1871*
   (1989), 209. Wrigley and Schofield have painstakingly reconstructed best estimates
   about these populations based on available census data and much cruder data before
   1801.

13 The seminal account of this history of secularization can be found in Keith Thomas's
   Religion and the Decline of Magic (1997).

14 After enquiring about the knight's condition, Keats's speaker begins establishing the
   poem's timeline: "The sedge is withered from the lake / And no birds sing" and "The
   squirrel's granary is full / And the harvest's done" ("La Belle Dame" 1–8). The withering sedge, the silent birds, the hoarding squirrel, and the finished harvest all indicate
   the imminent approach of a potentially harsh winter.

15 More on these wild guesses in the Keats chapter. Chapter 4 discusses the poem in
   greater depth.

16 In "Visions of the Daughters of Albion" (1793), Blake paints an idealistic world
   of liberated sexuality, "free love," and "happy copulation" ("Visions" 142–52).
   Wordsworth, I argue, prefers an abstracted notion of population growth over embodied images of procreation.

17 For an extended discussion of the particular case of Down's syndrome and the questionable eugenic ethics of prenatal testing, see Michael Bérubé's moving account
   of his own son in *Life as We Know It: A Father, a Family, and an Exceptional Child*
   (1998). In particular, he argues that genetic conditions like DS are certainly not obstacles to human flourishing. "What does it mean," he asks provocatively, "that we
   have developed a society in which people with Down's syndrome can flourish as never
   before (thanks to antibiotics, modern surgery, and/or early intervention programs),
   but in which they are too often denied the chance to flourish?" (52). In the accounts

of disability theorists, biopower's coercions are never automatic or necessary sacrifices to the greater public good.

18 Agamben argues that in "Placing biological life at the center of its calculations, the modern State therefore does nothing other than bring to light the secret tie uniting power and bare life" (6).

19 My reading of Keats's poem will be further developed in chapter 4.

20 Examples include "The Mad Mother," "The Thorn," and "The Idiot Boy." See Emily Stanback's book *The Wordsworth-Coleridge Circle and the Aesthetics of Disability*.

2 Darwin's Evolutionary Metaphor

1 See Jenner's letter to William Clement, 3.

2 In Jacob's distinction, "the engineer works according to a preconceived plan in that he foresees the products of his efforts ... he has at his disposal both material specially prepared to that end and machines designed solely for that task" (1163), while the tinkerer "does not know exactly what he is going to produce but uses whatever he finds around him whether it be pieces of string, fragments of wood, or old cardboards" (1163). Evolution is a tinkerer rather than an engineer as we can see most clearly in the sheer number of extinct species. In Jacob's estimation, there are only a few million extant species whereas there have been five hundred million extinct species in the history of biological life. Engineered perfection is neither the method nor the goal of evolution.

3 See the discussion in the introduction about Burke's use of botanical inoculation as a metaphor for foreign contamination. Donald C. Goellnicht has documented botany's close connection to chemistry and medicine in his work on Keats's medical contexts (84–119), but few, if any, have tracked the literary and political uses of botanical inoculation as a *medical* metaphor.

4 The Oxford English Dictionary's first definition of "inoculate" is "To set or insert (an 'eye', bud, or scion) in a plant for propagation; to subject (a plant) to the operation of budding; to propagate by inoculation; to bud (one plant) *into, on,* or *upon* (another)." It gives as an example Dryden's translation of Virgil's *Georgics*: "Various are the ways to change the state of Plants, to Bud, to Graff, t' Inoculate." See "Inoculate." Def. 1. *Oxford English Dictionary Online*, Oxford UP, n.d. Web. 28 June 2013.

5 These are just a few recent approaches to Darwin's eccentric verse. Jenny Uglow has written a very thorough and entertaining account of Darwin's participation in the innovative society of "lunar men" that included Matthew Boulton, James Watt, Josiah Wedgwood, among others (3–14). Alan Bewell teaches us about his cosmopolitan conception of nature ("Cosmopolitan Nature" 19–48), Devin Griffiths takes apart his analogical rhetoric (645–65), and Julia List intervenes in the discussion of female sexuality in Darwin's botanical world (199–218).

6 For more a more detailed biographical account of Linnaeus, see Wilfrid Blunt's account of the man's genius in *Linnaeus: The Compleat Naturalist*. In a 2002 reprinting

of this magisterial 1971 biography, William Stearn sums up, by way of introduction, Linnaeus's contribution to the systematization of biology: "These two remarkable works, the *Systema Plantarum* (1753) and *Systema Naturae* (10th edition, 1758), which gave binomial names to all the organisms then known, fully justify Linnaeus being regarded by the Swedes as a great national hero" (8).

7   For the collection as a "covert attempt to mourn the death of Charles I," see Clarke (113). For more about the poem's connection to royalist causes, see Loxley (196–201).

8   It is important to note here that Dryden had access to the inoculating metaphor even before smallpox had been connected to inoculation. His poem somehow uses the language of vaccination even before Jenner. As I will continue to argue throughout, this is no mere coincidence but a material connection between literature and medicine and a striking example of a literary precedent to a medical cure.

9   For more about the poem's conservative bid for patronage and the politicization of vaccination in the early nineteenth century, see Fulford and Lee (139–65) and Shuttleton (182–205).

10   See Bewell ("Cosmopolitan Nature" 19–48) and Sha (16–50).

11   See Jon Mee's *Conversable Worlds* (2011) for his robust theorization of conversation both as polite exchange and as Samuel Johnson's model of "talking for victory" (qtd. in Mee 84).

12   This approach rests on the assumption that metaphors matter. Susan Sontag has claimed that metaphors of illness tend to divorce disease from medical reality, a dangerous consequence that leads to irrational rejections of treatment, blatant misinformation about modes of transmission, and general misunderstanding about the "real" nature of illness. In this account, metaphor is perilously out of place in the field of medicine. My argument resists this powerful and influential rejection of metaphor in representing illness. The literary and medical history of smallpox, from the representations of physical and emotional scars to vaccination's unprecedented triumph over the disease, must give us pause before casting off the significant role of metaphor in managing both mental and physical manifestations of disease. Shuttleton, for example, helpfully reminds us that smallpox was a disease that never exceeded representation. As early as the tenth century, the Arabian physician Muhammad ibn Zakariyā Rāzī (better known to the West as Rhazes) was already describing the disease through analogy: he claimed that smallpox pustules were external manifestations of fermented blood. Dryden was elegizing the pustular body of Lord Hastings, and Montagu was popularizing smallpox inoculation in England with metaphors of sensibility. In all these cases, metaphor functions as a productive and expressive outlet that effectively manages both the social perception and the medical reality of the disease. Nevertheless, representation could also turn into insensitive caricature as in the case of Gillray's outrageous image of cartoonish smallpox victims. Lennard J. Davis has warned about the nineteenth- and twentieth-century novel's unfortunate tendency to endorse social constructions of normalcy, as in his reading of Esther Summerson's miraculously vanishing smallpox scars in *Bleak House*. Sontag's point gains traction in these cases,

but it still does not obscure the positive role that metaphor has played in Romantic medicine and the crucial influence it had in the eventual disappearance of smallpox; a disease that still retains the vaunted distinction of being the only infectious human disease to have been eradicated by man. This chapter presents a case study of what happens when an imaginative metaphor (botanical inoculation) meets a material disease (smallpox) all while insisting on a positive role for literary representation in the traumas of illness. Still, this does not materialize completely in this chapter because of Darwin's political ambivalence and figurative hedging. In later chapters, I track the development from the botanical metaphor to a Romantic disease discourse that has learned how metaphors create recognition for disease, aid its legibility, and even model a cure in the specific case of Jenner's vaccination.

13 References to the prose sections will be cited parenthetically by the image number of the facsimile copy from *Eighteenth Century Collections Online*. References to the verse will be cited by volume, canto, and line number. Volume I refers to *The Economy of Vegetation* and Volume II refers to *The Loves of the Plants*.

14 In the 16 April 1798 issue, the editor includes this didactic poem by the fictitious Mr. Higgins. In a direct parody of Darwin's language, Higgins claims to "enlist the IMAGINATION under the banners of GEOMETRY" (111).

15 Such an undertaking requires a certain level of scientific authority. Desmond King-Hele, Darwin's most reverent biographer, argues that the Lichfield poet-physician did indeed merit such scientific currency: "No one since Darwin has bestridden so easily and effectively the fields of science, poetry and medicine, and now that science has expanded so vastly it is safe to say that no one ever will again" (*Erasmus Darwin* 172). In addition to being one of the most popular poets of the 1790s, he was a prolific inventor, founder of the Lunar Society, a well-respected and dedicated physician, an innovator of industry, and a diligent Linnaean botanist. Among these incredibly varied achievements, his most enduring remains his early theorization of biological evolution, which his grandson Charles Darwin later developed empirically with his more well-known observations on the finches of the Galapagos Islands. His contemporary legacy, though, tends to understate these significant contributions to both science and literature. In recent years, we have begun to recover from Darwin's mysterious vanishing act from history, perhaps because of growing sympathy towards interdisciplinary studies or heightened interest in the history of Romantic science. Now, instead of being forced to see Darwin as a mere dilettante who dabbled in poetry only when he lost interest in science or medicine, we appreciate his easy and productive crossings of disciplinary borders. In this more sympathetic reading, Darwin manages to write a coherent poem that simultaneously delights with "poetic ornament" and instructs with the scientific authority of "eloquent orations," a balancing act that Burke mishandles with his bungled botanical metaphor.

16 Despite being rather harsh about Darwin's ornate style, Coleridge admitted that Darwin was "the first *literary* character in Europe, and the most original-minded man" (215). For the full discussion, see his letter in Coleridge (216, 305).

17 See Stuart Harris's short treatment on form in which he claims Darwin's epic poems are first and foremost Enlightenment "philosophical discourses" (1). In describing Darwin's excitement about Enlightenment progress, Donald M. Hassler argues that the poet insisted that "the only human thing to do is to give up the old illusions about an anthropocentric universe" (91). And Jenny Uglow associates Darwin closely with the principles of the Scottish Enlightenment (26–34).

18 Locke's phrase appears several times in his *Essay Concerning Human Understanding* (1690). Each time, the phrase stands in for a kind of classificatory containment. For example, he uses "our mansion" to refer to a divinely ordained ontology, a carefully regulated sensation, and a perfectly ordered cosmos. For these instances see Locke (45, 87, 120, 302, 555, 665).

19 For the purposes of this botanical argument, two plants belong to the same species if, and only if, they are able to produce non-sterile progeny.

20 That correct solution would use Mendel's law of segregation to explain the probabilistic phenotypical expression of a plant's genotype. It would also depend on an explanation of genetic mutation as a mechanism of evolutionary development.

21 See "Caprification." Def. 1. *Oxford English Dictionary Online*, Oxford UP, n.d. Web. 13 July 2013.

22 For a few representative radical and Revolutionary readings of Darwin's poem, see Teute (319–45), Kelley (193–203), and Bewell ("Cosmopolitan Nature" 19–48). For a more politically sceptical perspective, see List (199–218). Overall, the history of Darwin scholarship has proven that his politics remain difficult to pin down.

23 Even though Darwin's temple represents a somewhat awkward juncture of science and religion, the Romantic divide between empirical knowledge and religious faith should not be overstated. It was not until the publication of Charles Darwin's *On the Origin of Species* (1859) and Thomas Henry Huxley's famous advocacy of evolution did these divisions crystallize into near incompatibilities.

24 For a clearer picture of Darwin's relationship to the discourse of cosmopolitanism, see Bewell ("Cosmopolitan Nature" 19–48).

25 In 1794, between the publications of *The Botanic Garden* and *The Temple of Nature*, Darwin soberly attempted to pin down disease into well-defined empirical categories with his long prose piece *Zoonomia*, a largely unsuccessful stab at Linnaean preservation that nonetheless resulted in the eventual turn towards his impossibly ambitious final poem. Darwin struggled with the Cullen-Brown divide in medicine, whether to participate in Cullen's obsession with nosological classification (*Zoonomia*) or to subscribe to Brown's more loosely defined theory of excitability (*The Temple of Nature*). With the benefit of hindsight, we can conclude, perhaps unexpectedly, that the *Temple of Nature* and its enduring (yet highly conjectural) evolutionary insights were far more successful than the awkward (and mostly wrong) nosological precision of *Zoonomia*. For an extremely thorough account of Darwin's work in *Zoonomia*, see King-Hele (*Doctor of Revolution* 234–63).

3 Blake's Revolutionary Metaphor

1 For a discussion of Darwin's interpretation of and involvement in Josiah Wedgwood's reproduction of the Portland Vase, see Brooks (149–56).

2 It remains unclear if Darwin and Blake ever physically met each other.

3 There are several readings of Blake that attempt to pit him against Darwin's Enlightenment commitments. Desmond King-Hele, for example, says that "Blake was drawn towards Darwin in the 1790s, but later developed what could be called a distaste … produced mainly by Darwin's evangelism for science and technology: the burning of the Albion Mill pleased Blake and dismayed Darwin" ("Disenchanted Darwinians" 116).

4 For Darwin's participation in the Lunar Society and his extensive network of industrialists, scientists, and inventors, I continue to use Jenny Uglow's book *Lunar Men* as a reference.

5 See "Secret." Etymology. *Oxford English Dictionary Online*, Oxford UP, n.d. Web. 6 July 2013.

6 For a representative study that connects "Thel" with "Comus," see Levitt (72–83).

7 Citations of Blake's poems will be made parenthetically in the text, and, when available, I will cite with the plate number and line number.

8 See Northrop Frye's foundational (1947) but largely outdated reading of the poem as "the failure to make it" (232).

9 See Anne Mellor's discussion of Thel's ambiguous shriek (*Blake's Human Form Divine* 20–39).

10 For an extremely focused study of the Romantic figure of the worm, see Janelle Schwartz's *Worm Work: Recasting Romanticism* (2012). In particular, see chapters 2 and 4 on Darwin and Blake respectively (27–70, 113–48).

11 All citations of "Auguries" come from the Morgan Library and Museum copy of *The Pickering Manuscript* available online from *The William Blake Archive*. The commentary is from the website's introduction to *The Pickering Manuscript*. See especially Blake's introductory paradoxes: "A robin redbreast in a cage / Puts all heaven in a rage. / A dove-house filled with doves and pigeons / Shudders hell through all its regions" ("Auguries" objects 13–14). "Auguries" can be fit into Morton Paley's influential division of Blake's career into early and late. Here, Blake ostensibly has moved beyond "the liberation of energy through the interplay of contraries" (Paley, *Energy* 10) and towards a more mature, transformative "imagination."

12 Michael Ferber, for example, remains unconvinced of the viability of Oothoon's paradoxical argument: "Oothoon's exuberant defense of unique individuality may have carried her too far" (81). He concludes that "Blake means to do justice to the real difficulties, but he does not relax his demand for forgiveness and self-sacrifice, even on behalf of Satan" (82). I suggest that Blake's strange botanical metaphor gets closer to doing "justice to the real difficulties" than Ferber allows.

13 Donald Ault's explanation of Blake's scientific imagery in his *Visionary Physics: Blake's Response to Newton* (1976) remains foundational in any discussion of Blake and science (24–56). Stuart Peterfreund has continued to mine Blake's reading of Newton to develop a larger cultural sense of the poet's counter-Enlightenment critique (38–57). Neither Ault nor Peterfreund casts Newton as purely villainous, though. Instead, both rightly assume that "Blake's assimilation of 'scientific imagery,' involves both critical and positive functions" (Ault 52). These "positive functions" of science have been explored more recently by Mark Lussier's description of Blake's anticipation of quantum physics and Richard Sha's reading of Blake in the scientific context of sexual perversity (Lussier, "Scientific Objects" 120–2; Sha 183–240).

14 Lussier has provided an extremely helpful and comprehensive historical background on the subject of Blake and science ("Blake and Science Studies" 186–213) in which he documents how the opening lines of Blake's "Auguries" became the unlikely rallying cry of the new science.

15 For more on Darwin's treatment of caprification, see the previous chapter.

16 For a more detailed explanation of this strange method of fecundation, see the introductory paragraphs of Kislev, Hartmann, and Bar-Yosef (1372) and the botanical discussion of Darwin in the previous chapter.

17 In the seminal work on Blake's anti-imperialist ideology, *Blake: Prophet Against Empire* (1954), David Erdman reads "Visions" as "a dramatized treatise on the related questions of moral, economic, and sexual freedom and an indictment of the 'mistaken Demon' whose code separates bodies from souls and reduces women and children, nations and lands, to possessions" (228). More recently, Saree Makdisi's book *William Blake and the Impossible History of the 1790s* (2003) has argued similarly that Oothoon strives against that reduction of "women and children ... to possessions," or in Makdisi's more specific formulation, the "reduction into a single subjective selfhood" (96) produced by institutionalized slavery and patriarchal constructions of female sexuality.

18 Donald Ault's *Visionary Physics* and Stuart Peterfreund's *William Blake in a Newtonian World* have already meticulously documented Blake's informed reception of Newton's *Opticks* and the *Principia*.

19 Oothoon's careful response recalls the role of "Female Philosophers" in the radical debates of the 1790s. Blake's evocation (and even endorsement) of Wollstonecraft and Montagu in Oothoon's rhetoric reinforces the rise of a "public political role for women with international ambitions" (Craciun 27). For a thorough historicizing of this emergent agency, see Craciun (27–59).

20 See the discussion of Dryden's smallpox elegy in chapter 2.

21 The futility of Oothoon's caprifying solution continues into Blake's later work. Her character briefly reappears in "Europe" (1794), chastised by her mother Enitharmon for giving up "womans secrecy" ("Europe" plate 14, 22). And in the "Africa" section of "The Song of Los" (1795), Jesus deigns to hear Oothoon's complaint but accepts only the "Gospel from the wretched Theotormon" ("Los" plate 3, 22). In these works, Oothoon's story is subjugated to Blake's increasing interest in Biblical typology, a

trajectory that is ably handled elsewhere (Tannenbaum 154, 188). This essay, however, focuses primarily on the material, embodied argument of "Visions" that has frequently escaped critical notice.

22 Saree Makdisi helpfully distinguishes Blake's more subversive radicalism from the "hegemonic" radicalism of Thomas Paine and Mary Wollstonecraft. It is from this agile and contingent call for socio-economic "levelling" rather than the hegemonic, "liberal-radical position" that we should situate the politics of Oothoon's call for sexual liberation (Makdisi 16–77).

23 It is worth noting that Blake makes an earlier attempt to articulate this argument in "The Marriage of Heaven and Hell" (1790) but without the much more troubling issue of sexual violence in "Visions" (1793). In a famous account of his unique etching process, Blake describes "printing in the infernal method, by corrosives, which in Hell are salutary and medicinal, melting apparent surfaces away, and displaying the infinite which was hid" ("Marriage" plate 14). Just as Oothoon's rape is meant to unlock the chains of virginal modesty, these "corrosives" melt obscuring surfaces away (the hymen in Oothoon's case) to reveal the "infinite which was hid." Both images gain scientific traction from the medical logic of inoculation in which the corrosive, the violent, and the diseased paradoxically prove "salutary and medicinal."

4 Keats and the End of Disease

1 Since my focus remains literary, I defer to biographers and historians of science for accounts of their radical (and frequently outrageous) theories and experiments. For Priestley's experiments, see Robert E. Schofield's wonderfully thorough biography (227–72). Mike Jay remains my authority for Beddoes, and Jan Golinski, Lynn Hunt, and Margaret Jacob's work on Davy more than suffices to complete the scientific context for my literary argument.

2 For contemporary accounts of Keats's medical career in some of the most comprehensive and stunningly detailed biographies, see Bate (23–83), Barnard (*John Keats* 1–14), and Motion (45–8). Hermione de Almeida even dedicates a full-length study on the relationship between Keats and medicine. And for a concise summary of the most hotly disputed biographical aspects of Keats's medical training, see Barnard ("The Busy Time" 199–218).

3 Derrida's notion of non-binary logic is useful here, an idea that he articulates through the medical metaphor of Plato's *pharmakon*. He argues that "dissemination sets up a pharmacy in which it is no longer possible to count by ones, by twos, or by threes; in which everything starts with the dyad. The dual opposition (remedy/poison …) organizes a conflictual, hierarchically structured field which can neither be reduced to unity, nor dialectically sublated or internalized into a third term" (20). His example "remedy" and "poison" finds its biological proof in the success of vaccination in which smallpox functions as a regulator of both health and disease.

4 I yield to the already robust treatments of the vitality debates. For a representative study, see Sharon Ruston's *Shelley and Vitality* (2005), particularly the first chapter on Abernethy and Lawrence (24–73). Marilyn Butler's discussion of *Frankenstein* and radical science is also helpful in historicizing early nineteenth-century scientific arguments (302–13).

5 See "Penetrale." Def. 1. *Oxford English Dictionary Online*, Oxford UP, n.d. Web. 13 July 2013.

6 For my discussion of Darwin's use of the architectural metaphor, see the "Mansion of Twenty-Four Apartments" section of the second chapter.

7 Hazlitt's influence on the idea of negative capability has already been well documented. Walter Jackson Bate explains that "the immediate suggestions [of negative capability] have come to Keats from Wordsworth but are further substantiated by what he has been reading of Hazlitt" (239). Hazlitt's philosophical criticism, a precursor to Keats's idea of negative capability, is "confidence in the imaginative act – an act whereby sensations, intuitions, and judgments are not necessarily retained in the memory as separate particles of knowledge to be consulted one by one, but can be coalesced and transformed into a readiness of response that is objectively receptive to the concrete process of nature and indeed actively participates in it" (Bate 239).

8 This cosmopolitan dimension of inoculation will be developed further in my fifth chapter's treatment of Mary Shelley's *The Last Man* (1826).

9 Unless otherwise indicated, citations of the poem come from the earlier manuscript version of the poem.

10 Mary Shelley's narrator in *The Last Man* (1826), for example, is certainly aware of the connection between climate and contagion: "Winter was hailed, a general and never-failing physician. The embrowning woods, and swollen rivers, the evening mists, and morning frosts, were welcomed with gratitude. The effects of purifying cold were immediately felt; and the lists of mortality abroad were curtailed each week. Many of our visitors left us: those whose homes were far in the south, fled delightedly from our northern winter, and sought their native land, secure of plenty even after their fearful visitation. We breathed again. What the coming summer would bring, we knew not; but the present months were our own, and our hopes of a cessation of pestilence were high" (*The Last Man* 237–8).

11 Alan Bewell, for example, immediately assumes that the knight's "wasted body and pallid face flushed with fever reveal that he is suffering from consumption" (*Colonial Disease* 187). In this reading, the lily on the brow, the damp fever, and the fading rose are all symptoms of the same disease.

12 In Aristotelian logic, syllogistic deduction has three parts: a major premise, a minor premise, and a conclusion. For example, from the premises "All humans are mortal" (major) and "You are human" (minor) one can deduce "You are mortal" (conclusion). In Keats's poem, the first speaker's three stanzas dully recapitulate this Classical syllogism.

13 McGann says the *Indicator* version is self-consciously ironic (*Beauty of Inflections* 25–65). The change from knight to the archaic "wight" is meant to convey the interlocutor's conservative dependence on precedence and old knowledge.

14 Of the abandoned *Hyperion*, Keats explains that "there were too many Miltonic inversions in it – Miltonic verse cannot be written but in an artful, or rather, artist's humour. I wish to give myself up to other sensations" (*Letters* 272).

15 If Agamben's book had been written more recently, the more familiar example would probably be the controversial case of Terri Schiavo.

16 For an example of such a correlation, see Alter and Carmichael (114–32). The article is also a useful elaboration on the history of the ICD.

17 Canguilhem's work on the history of pathology has become foundational in discussions in medical anthropology. See especially his discussion of "distinguishing anomaly from the pathological state" (181). For some important echoes of this study, see Foucault's *Birth of the Clinic*, especially his shifting definitions of "spaces" and "classes" (*Clinic* 3–21).

18 Tobin Siebers, for example, in his seminal *Disability Theory* (2008), fears that we have not gone far enough in dismantling ableism. "How many books and essays have been written in the last ten years," he asks, "whose authors are content with the conclusion that x, y, or z is socially constructed, as if the conclusion itself were a victory over oppression?" (32).

19 Here, I refer to Foucault's famous description of the clinical gaze. He explains, "The gaze is passively linked to the primary passivity that dedicates it to the endless task of absorbing experience in its entirety, and of mastering it" (*Clinic* xiv).

20 For more on the distinction between the plague victim and the leper, see Foucault (*Discipline* 195–209; *Abnormal* 31–54).

21 Esposito's translator, Timothy Campbell, describes the trilogy as a philosophical genealogy of modern biopolitics. Esposito begins with society's inside (*Communitas*), its outside (*Immunitas*), and the politicization of life itself (*Bíos*).

22 Much has been made of the former paradigm beyond the Romantic period. For a representative study of such a rhetoric of bodily self-defence, see Cohen, especially his reliance on the central example of Metchnikoff's definition of biological immunity and its reliance on metaphors of intrusion and defence (1–2).

23 Especially relevant is Amanda Jo Goldstein's illuminating essay on William Blake (*Systems of Life* 162–200).

24 For the full anecdote, see Charon (3–6).

25 In their influential article, "Narrative Based Medicine: Why Study Narrative?," Tricia Greenhalgh and Brian Hurwitz appeal to a lost "oral tradition of myths and legends" (50) to make their case for narrative in medicine. However, as this chapter demonstrates, the period of Romantic medicine offers a more contemporary and concrete reference point from which to build a theory of narrative medicine.

5 Shelley and Romantic Immunity

1 I use the standard definition of mathematical induction: "The principle of mathematical induction states that if $P(n)$ is a proposition defined for each n in **N**, then $\{P(1)$

& $[P(\mathrm{n}) \rightarrow P(n + 1)]\} \rightarrow (n)P(n)$" (Royden 7). A proposition, in other words, is true *in general* if it is established for just two specific cases: (1) the base case $P(1)$ must be true and (2) assuming that the case $P(n)$ is true, then its successor $P(n + 1)$ must also be true. If a Romantic disease discourse emblematized by the success of vaccination is the proposition in question, Keats has proven its results in the base case of individual health, and the second inductive step belongs to Shelley's apocalyptic novel.

2   For the most influential readings of this scene as inoculation, see Mellor ("Introduction" xxiv) and Bewell (*Colonial Disease* 313–14). For a more sceptical reading, see Melville (825–46).

3   See her 10 March 2017 *New York Times* essay "Margaret Atwood on What 'The Handmaid's Tale' Means in the Age of Trump."

4   Unless otherwise stated, references to *The Last Man* come from the 1998 Oxford World Classics edition and will be cited parenthetically.

5   Throughout, I will use "cosmopolitan" in the Kantian sense. See Kant's "Idea for a Universal History with a Cosmopolitan Purpose" and "Perpetual Peace: A Philosophical Sketch." In these two pieces, Kant explains the paradox of man's "unsocial sociability" (*Universal History* 44). The fourth thesis of "Idea for a Universal History" claims that "The means employed by Nature to bring about the development of all the capacities of men is their antagonism in society, so far as this is, in the end, the cause of a lawful order among men" ("Universal History" 44). The cosmopolitan end of history, then, is the slow, dialectical development of moral laws through various antagonisms between men.

6   Paley even makes the strong claim that "Ultimately *The Last Man* is a repudiation of what might simplistically be termed the Romantic ethos as represented, for example, in the poetics and politics of Percy Bysshe Shelley" ("Apocalypse" 111). This paper references four essays (including Paley's) from the important collection *The Other Mary Shelley: Beyond Frankenstein*: Paley ("Apocalypse" 107–23), O'Sullivan (140–58), Johnson (258–66), and Fisch (267–86).

7   Johnson explains that "The story of *The Last Man* is in the last analysis the story of modern Western man torn between mourning and deconstruction" (265). Mellor proclaims *The Last Man* "the first text to base itself on the philosophical concept we now call Deconstruction" ("Introduction" xxii). Fisch expands on the novel's politics of deconstruction: "The question of the politics of the novel might be read also as a parable of deconstruction" (278).

8   "Ambivalence" is indeed the watchword here. See Barbara Jane O'Sullivan's discussion of Shelley's "ambivalence about female self-assertion" (155) in "Beatrice in *Valperga*." See also "the ambivalence that had begun to cloud her [Mary's] feelings about Percy" in Poovey (149). Even Paley moves inexplicably from a rejection to mere "ambivalence toward millenarianism" ("Apocalypse" 117). Shelley's almost universally acknowledged ambivalence in *The Last Man* should cast suspicions on purely nihilistic or anti-political readings of the novel. At the same time, though, mere ambivalence is not enough to reclaim a politics of possibility or a compensatory poetics from Shelley's apocalypse.

9 Charlotte Sussman foregrounds the novel's concerns with cosmopolitanism and over-population. She articulates an important paradox in Shelley's narrative: "Although *The Last Man* is named for the ultimate solitary individual, Mary Shelley's novel devotes much of its energy to representing human aggregates, to imagining populations" (286). Through an examination of Shelley's models of companionship – ungendered, androgynous, cosmopolitan, and cross-species – I will demonstrate the redemptive viability of these "human aggregates."

10 Here, Adam asks the archangel Michael whether "Famine and anguish will at last consume" (*Paradise Lost* XI.778) and "whether here the race of Man will end" (XI.786). Michael's famous answer in which he foretells the Son's redemptive sacrifice – "One man except" (XI.808) – is notably absent. Shelley's novel has no recourse to Michael's reasoned reassurance, and Adam's question remains open-ended.

11 In addition to Veeder's discussion of androgyny, see William Patrick Day's *In the Circles of Fear and Desire* where he claims that "Central to the treatment of these [Gothic] themes are the problem of sexuality, the relation of sexuality to pleasure and identity, and the possibilities and problems of androgyny as a response to the concept of identity and family that dominated nineteenth-century middle-class life" (5).

12 Mellor offers an excellent and thorough history that cogently connects plot to biography (*Mary Shelley* 141–68).

13 The complicated history of "Lastness," including legal battles, bad reviews, and charges of plagiarism, is ably summarized in Paley's piece ("Apocalypse" 107–9). In Mellor's introduction to *The Last Man*, she hints at a corresponding concern with "firstness" when she suggests, "By fragmenting chronology, Mary Shelley may be writing not so much 'the end of the world' as the possibility of alternative beginnings" ("Introduction" xxiv).

14 Alan Bewell reads Evadne as "a dangerous moral contagion that is undermining British society" and a figure that "emblematizes their [the East and the West's] epidemiological link" (*Colonial Disease* 299) to illustrate his argument about the connection between plague and colonialism.

15 Evadne makes appearances in Euripides's *The Suppliants*, Virgil's *Aeneid*, Beaumont and Fletcher's *The Maid's Tragedy* (1619), and Richard Sheil's *Evadne; or, The Statue* (1819). See the explanatory note about Evadne in Anne McWhir's edition of the novel.

16 For a more detailed discussion of the play's stage history, see T.W. Craik's introduction to *The Maid's Tragedy* (26–33). See also the short passages from *The Maid's Tragedy* in Charles Lamb's *Specimens*.

17 Several studies of *Frankenstein* hinge upon the good scientist/bad scientist dichotomy of the novel. Any recent account of *Frankenstein* will likely include a discussion of Shelley's mostly positive interest in science.

18 Contrast Beatrice's vengeful curse against Count Cenci with Prometheus's renunciation of his curse against Jupiter in the very first speech of the poem: "The curse / Once

breathed on thee I would recall" (I.58–9). See both pieces in the Norton edition of *Shelley's Poetry and Prose* ("Prometheus Unbound" 202–86; "The Cenci" 138–202).

19 Many have noted the social potential of Verney's inoculation. Mellor suggests "If one were forced to embrace the Other rather than permitted to define it exclusively as 'foreign' and 'diseased,' one might escape this socially constructed plague" ("Introduction" xxiv). Similarly, Bewell concludes his chapter on *The Last Man* by suggesting that "biological diversity – the 'foreignness' – that caused so much pain and suffering in the colonial world might also hold within it something that will preserve at least some of us somewhere from the coming plague that Shelley prophesies" (*Colonial Disease* 313–14). More recently, Peter Melville offers a medically informed corrective to these readings of Verney's inoculation (825–46). No one, though, has taken into account Evadne's earlier inoculation, which could account for the unnecessarily tentative conclusions about the redemptive possibility of inoculation.

20 Melville corrects the silence on Alfred's familial presence in this scene, but he also misreads Verney's "forcible exclusion of all those outside the family circle" as a reason to reject the redemptive possibility of his encounter with the "negro half clad" (837).

21 For two representative studies about eighteenth-century notions of race and species, see Rawson (92–182) and Brown (*Fables of Modernity* 221–66).

22 This significant echo of Verney's earlier cosmopolitan embrace seems to have escaped critical notice. Peter Melville, for example, rejects Verney's inoculating embrace of the diseased man partially because he misses Shelley's stunning recapitulation of the scene at the novel's conclusion (835).

23 For an insightful look at Shelley's species discourse, see Cynthia Schoolar Williams's article on the novel's "bestiary" (138–48). She argues, as I do, for a destabilizing discourse of species that challenges humanistic ideologies and categories.

24 See Anne McWhir's article for relevant nineteenth-century debates about contagion (23–38).

25 For a fuller account of Godwin and Percy Shelley's belief in the social construction of disease, see Bewell's chapter on Percy Shelley's "revolutionary climatology" (*Colonial Disease* 205–41).

26 In general, Shelley's "future" is quite similar to her nineteenth-century present. She describes a "sailing balloon," one of the only technological advances in *The Last Man*: "The machine obeyed the slightest motion of the helm; and, the wind blowing steadily, there was no let or obstacle to our course. Such was the power of man over the elements; a power long sought, and lately won" (71).

27 For an interesting take on Shelley's treatment of animals, see Cynthia Williams (138–48).

28 We know that Shelley was quite anxious about the disfiguring scars of smallpox. In her 11 April 1828 journal entry, Shelley narrates her own experience with the disease: "I depart for Paris sick at heart yet pining to see my Friend – There was a reason for my depression – I was sickening of the small pox – I was confined to my bed the moment I arrived in Paris – The nature of my disorder was concealed from me till my

convalescence – & I am so easily duped – Health – buoyant & bright succeeded to my illness – The Parisians were very amiable & a monster to look at as I was – I tried to be agreeable to compensate to them" (*Journals* 507–8).

29 For a history of Jenner's struggle for legitimacy and his subsequent elevation to national hero, see Fulford and Lee (139–65).

30 The creature's body has also been variously associated with, just to name a few, imperial critique, class warfare, and racial science. For these compelling arguments, see Spivak (243–61), Moretti (83–108), and Mellor ("Yellow Peril" 1–28).

31 For some useful close readings of Godwin and Percy Shelley in this respect, see Bewell's chapter on Percy Shelley (*Colonial Disease* 205–41).

32 For example, Paley takes "the failure of the imagination" as the novel's theme. He opposes Mary Shelley's pessimism to Percy Shelley's belief that "imagination is a creative and even a redemptive agency" ("Introduction" xi).

33 See McGann's explanation of "Romantic Ideology" in his introduction (*The Romantic Ideology* 1–14).

34 For biographical correspondences concerning similar amorous entanglements in the Shelley circle, see Mellor's *Mary Shelley*.

35 Shelley may have had Torquato Tasso's epic woman warrior Clorinda in mind when she pits the heterosexual love story against Evadne's failed androgynous ideal. Like Clorinda, Evadne eventually casts off her characteristic hybridity in favour of amorous sacrifice.

6 The Case of Sherlock Holmes

1 The entire Doyle-Koch anecdote is recounted in more detail in Howard Markel's short article "Medical Detectives" in *The New England Journal of Medicine* (2426–8).

2 See "Case, *N.(1)*." Def. 8b. *Oxford English Dictionary Online*, Oxford UP, n.d. Web. 13 July 2013.

3 For my discussion of Esposito's use of immunity, see chapter 4. Vanessa Lemm's answer to Esposito via Nietzsche's dual conception of *Einverleibung* (incorporation) neatly encapsulates the semantic shifts of immunity between a diversity-increasing cosmopolitanism to an exclusionary eugenic principle: "Esposito raises the question of whether it is possible to preserve life by means of immunization without thereby destroying itself. This article argues that the idea of *Einverleibung* in Nietzsche understood as a creative transformation offers an answer to the question posed by Esposito. It moreover points to a different politics of immunity, where immunity does not name the including exclusion of the other, but the openness of life to the horizon of justice and community" (3).

4 See Stephen Jay Gould's *Ever Since Darwin: Reflections in Natural History* (1973) for a representative study of Darwin's legacies.

5 Holmes may have been thinking about the passage in *Origin of Species* in which Darwin uses the example of Wolfgang Amadeus Mozart's natural genius to explain the idea of humanity's instinctive musicality (190).

6 In the preface to *Culture and Anarchy* (1875), Matthew Arnold traces out this disciplinary binary. He mentions a "brilliant and distinguished votary of the natural sciences" (*Culture and Anarchy* 3), a clear allusion to his agnostic interlocutor, Thomas Huxley. Throughout their careers, Arnold and Huxley would debate the merits of literary and scientific educations.

7 Huxley's ardent advocacy of Darwin's theory of natural selection earned him the appropriately bestial nickname.

8 For Cohen's historicization of the defensive body, see my discussion in chapter 4. For my discussion of Shelley's cosmopolitanism, see chapter 5.

9 For a discussion of this parody, see the first chapter on Erasmus Darwin and his hostile reception.

10 This recent result can be found on the *Guinness World Record* website ("Sherlock Holmes Awarded Title for Most Portrayed Literary Human Character in Film & TV").

11 For Data's processing speed, see the episode "The Measure of a Man."

12 In *The Ghost Map* (2006), Steven Johnson casts Dr. John Snow as a kind of Holmesian "investigator," armed with scientific deduction and empirical method (57–80).

Conclusion

1 For more information on the CIA's staged vaccination drive, see the recent *New Yorker* article (Specter, "The C.I.A., Vaccines, and Bin Laden"). According to an article from *Salon*, the rise of vaccine refusal extends also to the super-rich and educated (Seitz-Wald). The story about the measles outbreak in Texas was reported in *The Wall Street Journal* (Zimmerman and McKay).

2 For a comprehensive look at modern strategies of health activism, see Glenn Laverack's book *Health Activism: Foundations and Strategies*.

3 The origins of human smallpox are disputed.

Works Cited

Ackerknecht, Erwin H. *A Short History of Medicine*. Johns Hopkins UP, 1982.

Agamben, Giorgio. *Homo Sacer: Sovereign Power and Bare Life*. Stanford UP, 1998.

Allard, James Robert. *Romanticism, Medicine, and the Poet's Body*. Ashgate, 2007.

Alter, George C., and Ann G. Carmichael. "Classifying the Dead: Toward a History of the Registration of Causes of Death." *Journal of the History of Medicine and Allied Sciences*, vol. 54, no. 2, 1999, pp. 114–32.

Arnold, Matthew. *Culture and Anarchy*, edited by Jane Garnett, Oxford UP, 2009.

– "Dover Beach." *Dover Beach and Other Poems*, Dover Publications, 1994, p. 86.

Atwood, Margaret. "Margaret Atwood on What 'The Handmaid's Tale' Means in the Age of Trump." *The New York Times*, 10 March 2017. https://www.nytimes.com /2017/03/10/books/review/margaret-atwood-handmaids-tale-age-of-trump.html.

Ault, Donald. *Visionary Physics: Blake's Response to Newton*. U of Chicago P, 1976.

Barnard, John. "'The Busy Time': Keats's Duties at Guy's Hospital from Autumn 1816 to March 1817." *Romanticism*, vol. 13, no. 3, 2007, pp. 199–218.

– *John Keats*. Cambridge UP, 1987.

Barney, Richard A., and Warren Montag. "Introduction." *Systems of Life: Biopolitics, Economics, and Literature on the Cusp of Modernity*, edited by Barney and Montag, Fordham UP, 2018, pp. 1–33.

Baron, John. *The Life of Edward Jenner, M.D., LL.D., F.R.S., Physician Extraordinary to the King, &c. &c. with Illustrations of His Doctrines, and Selections from His Correspondence*. London, 1827. *Google Books*, http://books.google.com/books?id=q_g5AAAAcAAJ &printsec=frontcover#v=onepage&q&f=false.

Bate, Walter Jackson. *John Keats*. Harvard UP, 1963.

Baxby, Derrick. "Two Hundred Years of Vaccination." *Current Biology*, vol. 6, no. 7, 1996, pp. 769–72.

Beer, Gillian. *Open Fields: Science in Cultural Encounter*. Oxford UP, 1996.

Bennett, Andrew. *Keats, Narrative and Audience: The Posthumous Life of Writing*. Cambridge UP, 1994.

Bérubé, Michael. *Life as We Know It: A Father, a Family, and an Exceptional Child*. Vintage Books, 1998.

Bewell, Alan. "Erasmus Darwin's Cosmopolitan Nature." *ELH*, vol. 76, no. 1, spring 2009, pp. 19–48.

– *Romanticism and Colonial Disease*. Johns Hopkins UP, 1999.

Bichat, Xavier. *Œuvres Chirurgicales de Desault*. Paris, Magasin de Librairie, rue du Bouloi, No. 56. 1798–9. *Google Books*, https://www.google.com/books/edition /Oeuvres_chirurgicales_de_P_J_Desault_ou_/ubt7PreQseMC?hl=en&gbpv=1.

Birch, John. *Considerations on the Efficacy of Electricity in Removing Female Obstructions*. London, 1780. *Google Books*, https://www.google.com/books/edition/Considerations _on_the_Efficacy_of_Electr/ADWtgoB1uQwC?hl=en&gbpv=0.

– "Serious Reasons for Uniformly Objecting to the Practice of Vaccination: In Answer to the Report of the Jennerian Society, &c." London, 1806. https://curiosity .lib.harvard.edu/contagion/catalog/36-990060173990203941.

Blake, William. "Auguries of Innocence." *The Pickering Manuscript*, 1807. The William Blake Archive, Morgan Library and Museum, http://www.blakearchive.org/copy /bb126.1?descId=bb126.1.ms.13.

– "The Book of Thel." *William Blake: The Complete Illuminated Books*, edited by David Bindman, Thames & Hudson, 2001, pp. 98–105.

– "The Chimney Sweeper." *William Blake: The Complete Illuminated Books*, edited by David Bindman, Thames & Hudson, 2001, p. 54.

– "The Clod & the Pebble." *William Blake: The Complete Illuminated Books*, edited by David Bindman, Thames & Hudson, 2001, p. 74.

– "Europe: A Prophecy." *William Blake: The Complete Illuminated Books*, edited by David Bindman, Thames & Hudson, 2001, pp. 173–91.

– "Holy Thursday." *William Blake: The Complete Illuminated Books*, edited by David Bindman, Thames & Hudson, 2001, p. 61.

– "Jerusalem The Emanation of the Giant Albion." *William Blake: The Complete Illuminated Books*, edited by David Bindman, Thames & Hudson, 2001, pp. 297–397.

– "Laocoön." *William Blake: The Complete Illuminated Books*, edited by David Bindman, Thames & Hudson, 2001, p. 403.

– *The Letters of William Blake*. Edited by Geoffrey Keynes, Macmillan Company, 1956.

– "The Little Black Boy." *William Blake: The Complete Illuminated Books*, edited by David Bindman, Thames & Hudson, 2001, pp. 51–2.

– "London." *William Blake: The Complete Illuminated Books*, edited by David Bindman, Thames & Hudson, 2001, p. 88.

– "The Marriage of Heaven and Hell." *William Blake: The Complete Illuminated Books*, edited by David Bindman, Thames & Hudson, 2001, pp. 106–33.

– "Milton." *William Blake: The Complete Illuminated Books*, edited by David Bindman, Thames & Hudson, 2001, pp. 245–96.

– "The Sick Rose." *William Blake: The Complete Illuminated Books*, edited by David Bindman, Thames & Hudson, 2001, p. 81.

– "The Song of Los." *William Blake: The Complete Illuminated Books*, edited by David Bindman, Thames & Hudson, 2001, pp. 193–201.

- "There Is No Natural Religion." *The Complete Poetry & Prose of William Blake*, edited by David V. Erdman, Anchor Books, 1997, pp. 2–3.
- "Visions of the Daughters of Albion." *William Blake: The Complete Illuminated Books*, edited by David Bindman, Thames & Hudson, 2001, pp. 142–52.

Bliss, Jonathan. Jonathan Bliss Notebook, 1723–1724. Los Angeles County Medical Association Collection, Huntington Library, HM 74094.

Bloomfield, Robert. *Good Tidings; or, News From the Farm, A Poem*. Parnassian Press, 1804.

Blunt, Wilfrid. *Linnaeus: The Compleat Naturalist*. Princeton UP, 2002.

Broglio, Ron. *Technologies of the Picturesque: British Art, Poetry, and Instruments, 1750–1830*. Bucknell UP, 2008.

Brooks, Robin. *The Portland Vase: The Extraordinary Odyssey of a Mysterious Roman Treasure*. HarperCollins Publishers, 2004.

Brown, John. *Elementa Medicinæ*. BiblioBazaar, LLC, 2009.

Brown, John, and Thomas Beddoes. "The Elements of Medicine of John Brown, M.D." *Romanticism and Science, 1773–1833*, edited by Tim Fulford, vol. 1, Routledge, 2002, pp. 81–98.

Brown, Laura. *Fables of Modernity: Literature and Culture in the English Eighteenth Century*. Cornell UP, 2001.

Brunton, Deborah. *The Politics of Vaccination: Practice and Policy in England, Wales, Ireland, and Scotland, 1800–1874*. U of Rochester P, 2008.

Burke, Edmund. *Reflections on the Revolution in France*. Edited by J.C.D. Clark, Stanford UP, 2001,

Butler, Marilyn, "Frankenstein and Radical Science." *Frankenstein; or, The Modern Prometheus*, edited by Butler, Oxford UP, 1998, pp. 302–13.

Canguilhem, Georges. *The Normal and the Pathological*. Zone Books, 1991.

Charon, Rita, et al., editors. *The Principles and Practice of Narrative Medicine*. Oxford UP, 2017.

Clarke, Susan A. "Royalists Write the Death of Lord Hastings: Post-Regicide Funerary Propaganda." *Parergon*, vol. 22, no. 2, 2005, pp. 113–30.

Cohen, Ed. *A Body Worth Defending: Immunity, Biopolitics, and the Apotheosis of the Modern Body*. Duke UP, 2009.

Coleridge, Samuel Taylor. *Letters of Samuel Taylor Coleridge*. Edited by Ernest Hartley Coleridge. Vol. 1, New York, 1895. *Google Books*, https://www.google.com/books/edition/Letters_of_Samuel_Taylor_Coleridge/YikLAAAAYAAJ?hl=en&gbpv=0.

Cory, Herbert E. "Spenser, Thomson, and Romanticism." *PMLA*, vol. 26, no. 1, 1911, pp. 51–91.

Cox, Stephen. *Love and Logic: The Evolution of Blake's Thought*. U of Michigan P, 1992.

Craciun, Adriana. *British Women Writers and the French Revolution: Citizens of the World*. Palgrave Macmillan, 2005.

Craik, T.W. "Introduction." *The Maid's Tragedy: Beaumont and Fletcher*, edited by Craik, Manchester UP, 1999.

Cullen, William. *Nosology; or, A Systematic Arrangement of Diseases by Classes, Orders, Genera, and Species.* C. Stewart and Co., 1800, http://books.google.com/books ?id=3IgUAAAAQAAJ&printsec=frontcover#v=onepage&q&f=false.

– "Of the Hysteria, or the Hysteric Disease." *Practice of Physic.* Edinburgh, 1816. *Google Books,* http://books.google.com/books?id=_5_y9ezzNucC&lpg=PA153&ots =5PqhcsGj7t&dq=william%20cullen%20hysteria&pg=PA153#v=onepage&q&f=false.

Curran, Stuart. "Introduction." *The Poems of Charlotte Smith*, edited by Stuart Curran, Oxford UP, 1993.

Damon, S. Foster. *A Blake Dictionary: The Ideas and Symbols of William Blake.* Brown UP, 1988.

Darwin, Charles. *On the Origin of Species by Means of Natural Selection; or, The Preservation of Favoured Races in the Struggle for Life.* Edited by William Bynum, Penguin Classics, 2009.

Darwin, Erasmus. "The Botanic Garden." *Eighteenth Century Collections Online*, 1798.

– *The Collected Letters of Erasmus Darwin.* Edited by Desmond King-Hele, Cambridge UP, 2007.

– *The Temple of Nature: A Romantic Circles Electronic Edition.* Edited by Martin Priestman, e-book ed., U of Colorado Boulder P, 2006, http://www.rc.umd.edu /editions/darwin_temple/.

Davenport, Romola J., et al. "Urban Inoculation and the Decline of Smallpox Mortality in Eighteenth-century Cities – a Reply to Razzell." *The Economic History Review*, vol. 69, no. 1, 2016, pp. 188–214.

Day, William Patrick. *In the Circles of Fear and Desire: A Study of Gothic Fantasy.* U of Chicago P, 1985.

de Almeida, Hermione. *Romantic Medicine and John Keats.* Oxford UP, 1991.

Defoe, Daniel. *Robinson Crusoe.* Penguin, 2001.

Derrida, Jacques. *Dissemination.* Translated by Barbara Johnson, Continuum, 2004.

Dickens, Charles. *Bleak House.* Edited by Stephen Gill, Oxford UP, 2008.

– *The Household Words Almanac.* London, 1856. *Google Books,* http://books.google.com /books?id=Zoh--ALcrdMC&lpg=PA10&ots=NdENW1Q8im&dq=quadrupedan %20sympathy&pg=PA1#v=onepage&q=quadrupedan&f=false.

Di Leo, Jeffrey R., and Peter Hitchcock, editors. "Biotheory: An Introduction." *Biotheory: Life and Death under Capitalism*, Routledge, 2020, pp. 1–20.

Donne, John. "Death Be Not Proud." *John Donne: The Complete English Poems*, edited by A.J. Smith, Penguin, 1996, p. 313.

Doyle, Arthur Conan. "Compulsory Vaccination." *Round the Red Lamp and Other Medical Writings,* edited by Robert Darby, e-book ed., Valancourt Books, 2007, pp. 6124–255.

– *Memories and Adventures.* Cambridge UP, 2012.

– "The Sign of Four." *Sherlock Holmes: The Complete Novels and Stories.* Vol. 1, Bantam Dell, 2003, pp. 121–236.

– "A Study in Scarlet." *Sherlock Holmes: The Complete Novels and Stories.* Vol. 1, Bantam Dell, 2003, pp. 1–120.

Dryden, John. "Upon the Death of Lord Hastings." *Selected Poems*, Penguin Classics, 2002.

Eaves, Morris, et al. "Introduction." *The Pickering Manuscript*. Blake Archive, Morgan Library and Museum.

Eberle, Roxanne. *Chastity and Transgression in Women's Writing, 1792–1897: Interrupting the Harlot's Progress*. Palgrave Macmillan, 2002.

Erdman, David V. *Blake, Prophet Against Empire: A Poet's Interpretation of the History of His Own Times*. Princeton UP, 1954.

Esposito, Roberto. *Bíos: Biopolitics and Philosophy*. Translated by Timothy C. Campbell, U of Minnesota P, 2008.

– *Communitas: The Origin and Destiny of Community*. Translated by Timothy C. Campbell, Stanford UP, 2009.

– *Immunitas: The Protection and Negation of Life*. Translated by Zakiya Hanafi, Polity Press, 2011.

Fanon, Frantz. *The Wretched of the Earth*. Translated by Richard Philcox, Grove Press, 2004.

Ferber, Michael. *The Social Vision of William Blake*. Princeton UP, 1985.

Filmer, Robert. *Patriarcha and Other Writings*. Edited by Jóhann P. Sommerville, Cambridge UP, 1991.

Fisch, Audrey A. "Plaguing Politics: AIDS, Deconstruction, and *The Last Man*." *The Other Mary Shelley: Beyond Frankenstein*, edited by Audrey A. Fisch et al., Oxford UP, 1993, pp. 267–86.

Fissell, Mary E. *Patients, Power, and the Poor in Eighteenth-Century Bristol*. Cambridge UP, 1991.

Fogel, Aaron. "Wordsworth's 'We Are Seven' and Crabbe's 'The Parish Register': Poetry and Anti-Census." *Studies in Romanticism*, vol. 48, no. 1, 2009, pp. 23–65.

Foucault, Michel. *Abnormal: Lectures at the College de France, 1974-1975*. Edited by Valerio Marchetti and Antonella Salomoni, Picador, 2003.

– *The Birth of Biopolitics: Lectures at the Collège de France, 1978–1979*. Edited by Michel Senellart et al., translated by Graham Burchell, Picador, 2008.

– *The Birth of the Clinic: An Archaeology of Medical Perception*. Translated by Alan Sheridan, Vintage Books, 1994.

– *Discipline and Punish: The Birth of the Prison*. Vintage Books, 1995.

– *The History of Sexuality Vol. 1: An Introduction*. Translated by Robert Hurley, Vintage Books, 1990. 4 vols.

– *Security, Territory, Population: Lectures at the Collège de France 1977–1978*. Edited by Michel Senellart et al., translated by Graham Burchell, Picador, 2009.

– *Society Must Be Defended: Lectures at the Collège de France 1975–1976*. Edited by Mauro Bertani et al., translated by David Macey, Picador, 2003.

Frye, Northrop. *Fearful Symmetry: A Study of William Blake*. Princeton, NJ: Princeton UP, 1947.

Fulford, Tim, and Debbie Lee. "The Jenneration of Disease: Vaccination, Romanticism, and Revolution." *Studies in Romanticism*, vol. 39, no. 1, spring 2000, pp. 139–65.

Fuller, Thomas. *Pharmacopoèia Extemporanea*. London, 1761, http://find.galegroup.com/ecco/infomark.do?&contentSet=ECCOArticles&type=multipage&tabID=T001&prodId=ECCO&docId=CW3308242569&source=gale&userGroupName=uclosangeles&version=1.0&docLevel=FASCIMILE.

Garland-Thomson, Rosemarie. "Eugenics." *Keywords for Disability Studies*, edited by Rachel Adams et al., New York UP, 2015, pp. 74–9.

Gigante, Denise. *Life: Organic Form and Romanticism*. Yale UP, 2009.

Gilbert, Sandra M., and Susan Gubar. *The Madwoman in the Attic: The Woman Writer and the Nineteenth-Century Literary Imagination*. Yale UP, 2000.

Gillam, Stephen. "The Reappearance of the Sick Man: A Landmark Publication Revisited." *British Journal of General Practice*, vol. 66, no. 653, 2016, pp. 616–17.

Ginsburg, Faye, and Rayna Rapp. "Family." *Keywords for Disability Studies*, edited by Rachel Adams et al., New York UP, 2015, pp. 81–4.

Glass, Bentley. "Eighteenth-Century Concepts of the Origins of Species." *Proceedings of the American Philosophical Society*, vol. 104, no. 2, 1960, pp. 227–34.

Goellnicht, Donald C. *The Poet-Physician: Keats and Medical Science*. U of Pittsburgh P, 1984.

Goldstein, Amanda Jo. "William Blake and the Time of Ontogeny." *Systems of Life: Biopolitics, Economics, and Literature at the Cusp of Modernity*, edited by Richard A. Barney and Warren Montag, Fordham UP, 2018, pp. 162–200.

Golinski, Jan. *Science as Public Culture: Chemistry and Enlightenment in Britain, 1760–1820*. Cambridge UP, 1999.

Gould, Stephen Jay. *Ever Since Darwin: Reflections in Natural History*. W.W. Norton & Company, 1992.

Green, Matthew. "Blake, Darwin and the Promiscuity of Knowing: Rethinking Blake's Relationship to the Midlands Enlightenment." *British Journal for Eighteenth-Century Studies*, vol. 30, no. 2, 2007, pp. 193–208.

Greenhalgh, Tricia and Brian Hurwitz. "Narrative Based Medicine: Why Study Narrative?" *British Medical Journal*, vol. 318, no. 7175, 1999, pp. 48–50. https://doi.org/10.1136/bmj.318.7175.48.

Griffiths, Devin. "The Intuitions of Analogy in Erasmus Darwin's Poetics." *SEL: Studies in English Literature 1500–1900*, vol. 51, no. 3, 2011, pp. 645–65.

Grinnell, George. *The Age of Hypochondria: Interpreting Romantic Health and Illness*. Palgrave Macmillan, 2010.

Hardt, Michael, and Antonio Negri. *Commonwealth*. Harvard UP, 2009.

Harris, Stuart. *Erasmus Darwin's Enlightenment Epic*. Harris, 2002.

Harris, Susan Cannon. "Pathological Possibilities: Contagion and Empire in Doyle's Sherlock Holmes Stories." *Victorian Literature and Culture*, vol. 31, no. 2, 2003, pp. 447–66.

Hartman, Geoffrey H. *Wordsworth's Poetry 1787–1814*. Yale UP, 1967.

Harvey, William. "De Motu Cordis." *The Anatomical Exercises: De Motu Cordis and De Circulatione Sanguinus in English Translation*, edited by Geoffrey Keynes, Dover, 1995.

Haslam, Fiona. *From Hogarth to Rowlandson: Medicine in Art in Eighteenth-Century Britain.* Liverpool UP, 1996.

Hassler, Donald M. *The Comedian as the Letter D: Erasmus Darwin's Comic Materialism.* Martinus Nijhoff, 1973.

Homans, Margaret. "Keats Reading Women, Women Reading Keats." *Studies in Romanticism*, vol. 29, no. 3, fall 1990, pp. 341–70.

Horowitz, Tamara, and Allen A. Janis. "Introduction." *Scientific Failure*, edited by Horowitz and Janis, Rowman & Littlefield Publishers, Inc., 1994, pp. 1–12.

Hunt, Lynn, and Margaret Jacob. "The Affective Revolution in 1790s Britain." *Eighteenth-Century Studies*, vol. 34, no. 4, summer 2001, pp. 491–521.

Hunter, J. Paul. "Formalism and History: Binarism and the Anglophone Couplet." *MLQ: Modern Language Quarterly*, vol. 61, no. 1, 2000, pp. 109–29.

Jacob, François. "Evolution and Tinkering." *Science*, vol. 196, no. 4295, 1977, pp. 1161–6.

Jameson, Fredric. *The Political Unconscious: Narrative as a Socially Symbolic Act.* Cornell UP, 1982.

Jay, Mike. *The Atmosphere of Heaven: The Unnatural Experiments of Dr. Beddoes and His Sons of Genius.* Yale UP, 2009.

Jenner, Edward. *An Inquiry into the Causes and Effects of the Variolæ Vaccinæ.* London, 1798, *Google Books*, http://books.google.com/books?id=tj3h3ZA0ppAC&printsec =frontcover#v=onepage&q&f=false.

– Letter to William Clement. 19 December 1807. Huntington Library, HM 74097.

Jewson, N.D. "The Disappearance of the Sick-Man from Medical Cosmology, 1770–1870." *Sociology*, vol. 10, no. 2, 1976, pp. 225–44.

Johnson, Barbara. "The Last Man." *The Other Mary Shelley: Beyond Frankenstein*, edited by Audrey A. Fisch et al., Oxford UP, 1993, pp. 258–66.

Johnson, Samuel. "Dryden." *The Lives of the Poets: A Selection*, edited by Roger Lonsdale and John Mullan, Oxford UP, 2009.

Johnson, Steven. *The Ghost Map: The Story of London's Most Terrifying Epidemic – and How It Changed Science, Cities, and the Modern World.* Riverhead Books, 2006.

Journals of the House of Commons. United Kingdom, H.M. Stationery Office, 1803. *Google Books*, https://www.google.com/books/edition/Journals_of_the_House_of_Commons/ XgdDAAAAcAAJ?hl=en&gbpv=0.

Kant, Immanuel. "Idea for a Universal History with a Cosmopolitan Purpose." *Kant: Political Writings*, edited by H.S. Reiss, Cambridge UP, 1991, pp. 41–53.

– "Perpetual Peace: A Philosophical Sketch." *Kant: Political Writings*, edited by H.S. Reiss Cambridge UP, 1991, pp. 93–130.

Keats, John. "The Fall of Hyperion." *Keats's Poetry and Prose*, edited by Jeffrey N. Cox, W.W. Norton & Company, 2008, pp. 497–510.

– "Hyperion." *Keats's Poetry and Prose*, edited by Jeffrey N. Cox, W.W. Norton & Company, 2008, pp. 475–95.

- "La Belle Dame Sans Merci." *John Keats: The Major Works*, edited by Elizabeth Cook, Oxford UP, 2009, pp. 273–4.
- "Lamia." *Keats's Poetry and Prose*, edited by Jeffrey N. Cox, W.W. Norton & Company, 2008, pp. 412–29.
- "Ode on a Grecian Urn." *John Keats: The Major Works*, edited by Elizabeth Cook, Oxford UP, 2009, pp. 288–9.
- "Ode to a Nightingale." *John Keats: The Major Works*, edited by Elizabeth Cook, Oxford UP, 2009, pp. 285–8.
- "On First Looking into Chapman's Homer." *John Keats: The Complete Poems*, 3rd ed., Penguin, 1988, p. 72.
- *Selected Letters*. Edited by Robert Gittings and Jon Mee, Oxford UP, 2002.
- "Sleep and Poetry." *Keats's Poetry and Prose*, edited by Jeffery N. Cox, W.W. Norton & Company, 2008, pp. 58–68.
- "This Living Hand, Now Warm and Capable." *John Keats: The Major Works*, edited by Elizabeth Cook, Oxford UP, 2009, p. 331.
- Kelley, Theresa M. "Romantic Nature Bites Back: Adorno and Romantic Natural History." *European Romantic Review*, vol. 15, no. 2, 2004, pp. 193–203.
- Kidd, Michael, editor. "Case Report Criteria." *Journal of Medical Case Reports*, https://jmedicalcasereports.biomedcentral.com/submission-guidelines/preparing-your-manuscript/case-report.
- King-Hele, Desmond. "Disenchanted Darwinians: Wordsworth, Coleridge, Blake." *Wordsworth Circle*, vol. 25, no. 2, 1994, pp. 114–18.
- *Doctor of Revolution: The Life and Genius of Erasmus Darwin*. Faber & Faber, 1977.
- *Erasmus Darwin*. St. Martin's Press, 1963.
- Kislev, Mordechai E., et al. "Early Domesticated Fig in the Jordan Valley." *Science*, vol. 312, no. 5778, 2006, pp. 1372–4.
- Lawlor, Clark. *Consumption and Literature: The Making of the Romantic Disease*. Palgrave, 2008.
- Lemke, Thomas. *Biopolitics: An Advanced Introduction*. Translated by Eric Frederick Trump, New York UP, 2011.
- Lemm, Vanessa. "Nietzsche, *Einverleibung* and the Politics of Immunity." *International Journal of Philosophical Studies*, vol. 21, no. 1, 25 February 2013, pp. 3–19.
- Levinson, Marjorie. *The Romantic Fragment Poem: A Critique of a Form*. U of North Carolina P, 1986.
- Levitt, Annette S. "Comus, Cloud, and Thel's Unacted Desires." *Colby Quarterly*, vol. 14, no. 2, 1978, pp. 72–83.
- Liebow, Ely M. *Dr. Joe Bell: Model for Sherlock Holmes*. Popular Press, 1982.
- List, Julia. "Sometimes a Stamen Is Only a Stamen: Sexuality, Women and Darwin's *Loves of the Plants*." *Nineteenth-Century Contexts*, vol. 32, no. 3, 2010, pp. 199–218.
- Locke, John. *An Essay Concerning Human Understanding*. Edited by Peter H. Nidditch, Oxford UP, 1979.
- "The Loves of the Triangles." *Poetry of the Anti-Jacobin*. London, 1800, pp. 108–41. *Google Books*, ttps://www.google.com/books/edition/Poetry_of_the_Anti_Jacobin/kExmj5-0abgC?hl=en&gbpv=0.

Loxley, James. *Royalism and Poetry in the English Civil Wars*. Palgrave Macmillan, 1997.

Lucas, J.R. "Wilberforce and Huxley: A Legendary Encounter." *The Historical Journal*, vol. 22, no. 2, June 1979, pp. 313–30.

Lussier, Mark. "Blake and Science Studies." *Palgrave Advances in William Blake Studies*, edited by Nicholas M. Williams, Palgrave Macmillan, 2006, pp. 186–213.

– "Scientific Objects and Blake's Objections to Science." *The Wordsworth Circle*, vol. 39, no. 3, 2008, pp. 120–2.

Maines, Rachel P. *The Technology of Orgasm: "Hysteria," the Vibrator, and Women's Sexual Satisfaction*. Johns Hopkins UP, 2001.

Makdisi, Saree. *William Blake and the Impossible History of the 1790s*. U of Chicago P, 2003.

Malthus, T. R. *An Essay on the Principle of Population, or, A View of Its Past and Present Effects on Human Happiness : With an Inquiry into Our Prospects Respecting the Future Removal or Mitigation of the Evils Which It Occasions*. Cambridge UP, 1992.

Markel, Howard. "The Medical Detectives." *New England Journal of Medicine*, vol. 353, no. 23, 8 December 2005, pp. 2426–8.

McGann, Jerome J. *The Beauty of Inflections: Literary Investigations in Historical Method and Theory*. Clarendon Press, 1988.

– *The Romantic Ideology: A Critical Investigation*. U of Chicago P, 1983.

McWhir, Anne. "Mary Shelley's Anti-Contagionism: *The Last Man* as 'Fatal Narrative.'" *Mosaic: An Interdisciplinary Critical Journal*, vol. 35, no. 2, June 2002, pp. 23–38.

"The Measure of a Man." *Star Trek: The Next Generation*, created by Melinda Snodgrass, season 2, episode 9, CBS, 13 February 1989.

Mee, Jon. *Conversable Worlds: Literature, Contention, and Community 1762–1830*. Oxford UP, 2011.

Mellor, Anne K. *Blake's Human Form Divine*. U of California P, 1974.

– "Blake's Portrayal of Women." *Blake: An Illustrated Quarterly*, vol. 16, no. 3, 1983, pp. 148–55.

– "*Frankenstein*, Racial Science, and the Yellow Peril." *Nineteenth-Century Contexts*, vol. 23, no. 1, 2001, pp. 1–28.

– "Introduction." *The Last Man*, edited by Hugh J. Luke Jr., U of Nebraska P, 1993, pp. vii–xxvi, http://www.loc.gov/catdir/enhancements/fy0727/92041933-b.html.

– *Mary Shelley: Her Life, Her Fiction, Her Monsters*. Routledge, 1988.

– *Romanticism & Gender*. Routledge, 1993.

– "Sex, Violence, and Slavery: Blake and Wollstonecraft." *The Huntington Library Quarterly*, vol. 58, no. 3/4, 1995, pp. 345–70.

Melville, Peter. "The Problem of Immunity in *The Last Man*." *SEL Studies in English Literature 1500–1900*, vol. 47, no. 4, autumn 2007, pp. 825–46. https://doi .org/10.1353/sel.2007.0042.

Meyer, Nicholas. *Star Trek II: The Wrath of Khan*. Paramount Pictures, 1982.

Milton, John. "Areopagitica." *John Milton: Complete Poems and Major Prose*, edited by Merritt Yerkes Hughes, Hackett Publishing Company, Inc., 2003, pp. 716–49.

– "A Mask (Comus)." *John Milton: Complete Poems and Major Prose*, edited by Merritt Yerkes Hughes, Hackett Publishing Company, Inc., 2003, pp. 86–113.

– *Paradise Lost. John Milton: Complete Poems and Major Prose*, edited by Merritt Yerkes Hughes, Hackett Publishing Company, Inc., 2003, pp. 173–470.

Montagu, Mary Wortley. "Saturday. The Small-Pox." *Six Town Eclogues*. London, 1747. *Google Books*, https://www.google.com/books/edition/Six_Town_Eclogues _With_Some_Other_Poems/m6tYAAAAcAAJ?hl=en&gbpv=0.

– *Turkish Embassy Letters*. Edited by Anita Desai, Virago Press, 1994.

Moretti, Franco. *Signs Taken for Wonders*. Translated by Susan Fischer et al. Verso, 1988.

Motion, Andrew. *Keats*. U of Chicago P, 1997.

Moylan, Christopher. "T.L. Beddoes, Romantic Medicine, and the Advent of Therapeutic Theater." *Studia Neophilologica*, vol. 63, no. 2, 1991, pp. 181–8.

Nealon, Jeffrey. *Foucault Beyond Foucault: Power and Its Intensifications since 1984*. Stanford UP, 2007.

Nettleton, Sarah. "The Emergence of E-Scaped Medicine?" *Sociology*, vol. 38, no. 4, 2004, pp. 661–79. https://doi.org/10.1177/0038038504045857.

Nettleton, Sarah, and Roger Burrows. "E-Scaped Medicine?: Information, Reflexivity and Health." *Critical Social Policy*, vol. 23, no. 2, 2003, pp. 165–85. https://doi.org/10.1177 %2F0261018303023002003.

Nussbaum, Felicity. *The Limits of the Human: Fictions of Anomaly, Race, and Gender in the Long Eighteenth Century*. Cambridge UP, 2003.

O'Sullivan, Barbara Jane. "Beatrice in *Valperga*: A New Cassandra." *The Other Mary Shelley: Beyond Frankenstein*, edited by Audrey A. Fisch et al., Oxford UP, 1993, pp. 140–58.

Otis, Laura. *Membranes: Metaphors of Invasion in Nineteenth-Century Literature, Science, and Politics*. Johns Hopkins UP, 1999.

Palacio, Jean de. *Mary Shelley dans son œuvre; Contribution aux études shelleyennes*. Klincksieck, 1969.

Paley, Morton D. *Energy and the Imagination: A Study of the Development of Blake's Thought*. Clarendon Press, 1970.

– "Introduction." *The Last Man*, Oxford UP, 1998, pp. vii–xxiii. http://www.loc.gov /catdir/enhancements/fy0604/98207341-d.html.

– "The Last Man: Apocalypse without Millennium." *The Other Mary Shelley: Beyond Frankenstein*, edited by Audrey A. Fisch et al., Oxford UP, 1993, pp. 107–23.

Pamboukian, Sylvia A. *Doctoring the Novel: Medicine and Quackery from Shelley to Doyle*. Ohio UP, 2012.

Park, Alice. "Scientists Gone Rogue." *Time: Health & Family*, 12 January 2012, http:// healthland.time.com/2012/01/13/great-science-frauds/.

Percival, Thomas. *Medical Ethics; or, A Code of Institutes and Precepts, Adapted to the Professional Conduct of Physicians and Surgeons*. London, 1803.

Peterfreund, Stuart. *William Blake in a Newtonian World: Essays on Literature as Art and Science*. U of Oklahoma P, 1998.

Poovey, Mary. *The Proper Lady and the Woman Writer: Ideology as Style in the Works of Mary Wollstonecraft, Mary Shelley, and Jane Austen*. U of Chicago P, 1984.

Porter, Roy. *Bodies Politic: Disease, Death, and Doctors in Britain, 1650–1900*. Cornell UP, 2001. *Google Books*, https://books.google.com/books?id=dFU_FrtSCr4C.

– *The Greatest Benefit to Mankind: A Medical History of Humanity*. W.W. Norton & Company, Inc., 1999.

– "The Patient's View: Doing Medical History from Below." *Theory and Society*, vol. 14, no. 2, March 1985, pp. 175–98.

Rawson, Claude Julien. *God, Gulliver, and Genocide: Barbarism and the European Imagination, 1492–1945*. Oxford UP, 2001.

Richardson, Alan. *British Romanticism and the Science of the Mind*. Cambridge UP, 2005.

Richardson, Ruth. *Death, Dissection and the Destitute*. U of Chicago P, 2001.

Robbins, Hollis. "'We Are Seven' and the First British Census." *English Language Notes*, vol. 48, no. 2, 2010, pp. 201–13.

Roe, Nicholas. *John Keats and the Culture of Dissent*. Oxford UP, 1999.

Royden, H. L. *Real Analysis*. 3rd ed., Prentice Hall, 2011.

Ruston, Sharon. *Shelley and Vitality*. Palgrave Macmillan, 2005.

Saler, Michael. *As If: Modern Enchantment and the Literary Prehistory of Virtual Reality*. Oxford UP, 2012.

Schofield, Robert E. *The Enlightenment of Joseph Priestley: A Study of His Life and Work from 1733 to 1773*. Illustrated edition, Pennsylvania State UP, 1997.

Schott, G.D. "William Blake's *Milton*, John Birch's 'Electrical Magic,' and the 'falling star.'" *The Lancet*, vol. 362, no. 9401, 2003, pp. 2114–16.

Schwartz, Janelle. *Worm Work: Recasting Romanticism*. U of Minnesota P, 2012.

Seitz-Wald, Alex. "What's with Rich People Hating Vaccines?" *Salon*, 14 August 2013, http://www.salon.com/2013/08/14/whats_with_rich_people_hating_vaccines.

Sha, Richard. *Perverse Romanticism: Aesthetics and Sexuality in Britain, 1750–1832*. Johns Hopkins UP, 2008.

Shakespeare, William. *Hamlet*. 2nd ed., W.W. Norton & Company, Inc., 1992.

– *Henry V*. Edited by John Russell Brown, Signet Classic, 1998.

Sheil, Richard Lalor. *Evadne; or, The Statue*. Boston, 1824. *Google Books*, https://www.google.com/books/edition/Evadne_Or_The_Statue/wpREAQAAMAAJ?hl=en&gbpv=1.

Shelley, Mary Wollstonecraft. *Frankenstein*. Edited by J. Paul Hunter, 2nd ed., W.W. Norton & Company, 2012.

– *The Journals of Mary Shelley*. Edited by Paula R. Feldman and Diana Scott-Kilvert, Johns Hopkins UP, 1995.

– *The Last Man*. Oxford UP, 1998. http://www.loc.gov/catdir/enhancements/fy0604/98207341-d.html.

Shelley, Percy Bysshe. "The Cenci." *Shelley's Poetry and Prose*, edited by Donald H. Reiman and Neil Fraistat, W.W. Norton & Company, 2002, pp. 138–202.

– "Prometheus Unbound." *Shelley's Poetry and Prose*, edited by Donald H. Reiman and Neil Fraistat, W.W. Norton & Company, 2002, pp. 202–86.

"Sherlock Holmes Awarded Title for Most Portrayed Literary Human Character in Film & TV." *Guinness World Records*, 14 May 2012, http://www.guinnessworldrecords.com

/news/2012/5/sherlock-holmes-awarded-title-for-most-portrayed-literary-human
-character-in-film-tv-41743/.

Shuttleton, David E. *Smallpox and the Literary Imagination, 1660–1820.* Cambridge UP,
2007.

Siebers, Tobin. *Disability Theory.* U of Michigan P, 2008.

Simpson, David. *Irony and Authority in Romantic Poetry.* Palgrave Macmillan, 1979.

Smith, Charlotte Turner. "The Emigrants." *The Poems of Charlotte Smith,* edited by Stuart
Curran, Oxford UP, 1993, pp. 131–66.

Snow, C.P. *The Two Cultures.* Cambridge UP, 1998.

Snyder, Robert Lance. "Apocalypse and Indeterminacy in Mary Shelley's *The Last Man.*"
Studies in Romanticism, vol. 17, no. 4, fall 1978, pp. 435–52.

Sontag, Susan. *Illness as Metaphor and AIDS and Its Metaphors.* Picador, 1989.

Specter, Michael. "The C.I.A., Vaccines, and Bin Laden." *The New Yorker,* 12 July 2011,
http://www.newyorker.com/online/blogs/newsdesk/2011/07/the-cia-vaccines-and-bin
-laden.html.

– *Denialism: How Irrational Thinking Hinders Scientific Progress, Harms the Planet, and
Threatens Our Lives.* Penguin Press, 2009.

Spivak, Gayatri Chakravorty. "Three Women's Texts and Critique of Imperialism." *Critical
Inquiry,* vol. 12, no. 1, 1985, pp. 243–61.

Spratt, Hartley S. "Mary Shelley's Last Men: The Truth of Dreams." *Studies in the Novel,*
vol. 7, no. 4, winter 1975, pp. 526–37.

Sterrenburg, Lee. "The Last Man: Anatomy of Failed Revolutions." *Nineteenth-Century
Fiction,* vol. 33, no. 3 December 1978, pp. 324–47.

Sussman, Charlotte. "'Islanded in the World': Cultural Memory and Human Mobility in
The Last Man." *PMLA,* vol. 118, no. 2, March 2003, pp. 286–301.

Swann, Karen. "Harassing the Muse." *Romanticism and Feminism,* edited by Anne K.
Mellor, Indiana UP, 1988, pp. 81–92.

Swift, Jonathan. "The Battle of the Books." *Jonathan Swift: Major Works,* edited by Angus
Ross and David Woolley, Oxford UP, 2008, pp. 1–22.

Tannenbaum, Leslie. *Biblical Tradition in Blake's Early Prophecies: The Great Code of Art.*
Princeton UP, 1982.

Teute, Fredrika J. "The Loves of the Plants; or, the Cross-Fertilization of Science and
Desire at the End of the Eighteenth Century." *The Huntington Library Quarterly,* vol.
63, no. 3, 2000, pp. 319–45.

Thomas, Keith. *Religion and the Decline of Magic.* Oxford UP, 1997.

Thompson, E.P. *The Making of the English Working Class.* Vintage, 1966.

Tsianos, George I., et al. "Pyosalpinx as a Sequela of Labial Fusion in a Post-Menopausal
Woman: A Case Report." *Journal of Medical Case Reports,* vol. 5, no. 546, November
2011. https://doi.org/10.1186/1752-1947-5-546.

Uglow, Jennifer S. *The Lunar Men: The Friends Who Made the Future, 1730–1810.* Faber
& Faber, 2002.

Van Dine, S.S. "Twenty Rules for Writing Detective Stories." *The Art of the Mystery Story: A Collection of Critical Essays*, edited by Howard Haycraft, Biblo and Tannen, 1976, pp. 189–93.

Veeder, William R. *Mary Shelley & Frankenstein: The Fate of Androgyny*. U of Chicago P, 1988.

Viscomi, Joseph. *Blake and the Idea of the Book*. Princeton UP, 1993.

Wakefield, A.J., et al. "Ileal-Lymphoid-Nodular Hyperplasia, Non-Specific Colitis, and Pervasive Developmental Disorder in Children." *Lancet*, vol. 351, no. 9103, 1998, pp. 637–41. https://doi.org/10.1016/S0140-6736(97)11096-0. Retraction in: *Lancet*, vol. 375, no. 9713, 2010, p. 445. Erratum in: *Lancet*, vol. 363, no. 9411, 2004, p. 750.

Wallace, Alfred Russel. *The Wonderful Century: Its Success and Its Failures*. London, 1899. *Google Books*, http://books.google.com/books?id=gykMAAAAIAAJ&dq=alfred %20russel%20wallace%20wonderful%20century&pg=PP1#v=onepage&q&f=false.

Welch, Dennis M. "Essence, Gender, Race: William Blake's *Visions of the Daughters of Albion*." *Studies in Romanticism*, vol. 49, no. 1, 2010, pp. 105–31.

Williams, Cynthia Schoolar. "Mary Shelley's Bestiary: *The Last Man* and the Discourse of Species." *Literature Compass*, vol. 3, no. 2, March 2006, pp. 138–48.

Williams, Elizabeth A. *A Cultural History of Medical Vitalism in Enlightenment Montpellier*. Ashgate, 2003.

Wolfson, Susan J. *Borderlines: The Shiftings of Gender in British Romanticism*. Stanford UP, 2006.

– "Late Lyrics." *The Cambridge Companion to Keats*, edited by Wolfson, Cambridge UP, 2001, pp. 102–19.

– *The Questioning Presence: Wordsworth, Keats, and the Interrogative Mode in Romantic Poetry*. Cornell UP, 1986.

Wollstonecraft, Mary. *Vindication of the Rights of Woman and The Wrongs of Woman; or, Maria*. Edited by Anne Mellor and Noelle Chao, Longman, 2006.

Woodville, William. *Medical Botany: Containing Systematic and General Descriptions, With Plates of All the Medicinal Plants Indigenous and Exotic Comprehended in the Catalogues of the Materia Medica*. London, 1810. *Google Books*, http://books.google.com/books ?id=ioMfAAAAYAAJ&printsec=frontcover#v=onepage&q&f=false.

Wordsworth, William. "Expostulation and Reply." *William Wordsworth: The Major Works*, edited by Stephen Gill, Oxford UP, 2008, pp. 129–30.

– "The Idiot Boy." *William Wordsworth: The Major Works*, edited by Stephen Gill, Oxford UP World's Classics, 2008, pp. 67–80.

– "Lines Written a Few Miles above Tintern Abbey." *William Wordsworth: The Major Works*, edited by Stephen Gill, Oxford UP, 2008, pp. 131–5.

– "Preface to *Lyrical Ballads* (1802)." *William Wordsworth: The Major Works*, edited by Stephen Gill, Oxford UP, 2008, pp. 595–615.

– "The Tables Turned; an Evening Scene, on the Same Subject." *William Wordsworth: The Major Works*, edited by Stephen Gill, Oxford UP, 2008, pp. 130–1.

– "We Are Seven." *William Wordsworth: The Major Works*, edited by Stephen Gill, Oxford UP, 2008, pp. 83–5.

Wrigley, E.A., and R.S. Schofield. *The Population History of England 1541–1871*. Cambridge UP, 1989.

Yanoff, K.L., and F.D. Burg. "Types of Medical Writing and Teaching of Writing in U.S. Medical Schools." *Academic Medicine*, vol. 63, no. 1, 1988, https://journals.lww.com /academicmedicine/Fulltext/1988/01000/Types_of_medical_writing_and _teaching_of_writing.6.aspx.

Youngquist, Paul. "Accidental Histories: Fieldwork Among the Maroons of Jamaica." *Theorizing Fieldwork in the Humanities: Methods, Reflections, and Approaches to the Global South*, edited by Shalini Puri and Debra A. Castillo, Palgrave Macmillan, 2016, pp. 213–34.

– *Monstrosities: Bodies and British Romanticism*. U of Minnesota P, 2003.

Zimmerman, Ann, and Betsy McKay. "Texas Church Is Center of Measles Outbreak." *The Wall Street Journal*, 27 August 2013, http://online.wsj.com/article/SB1000142412 7887324906304579039330555205364.

Index

Abbot, Charles, 43
Abernethy, John, 21, 188, 208n6, 220n4
Ackerknecht, Erwin H., 209n16
Adanson, Michel, 61, 75, 77, 80
Agamben, Giorgio, 52–5, 145–7, 207n3, 213n18, 221n15
Allard, James Robert, 21, 208nn6, 8, 210n17
Alter, George C., 221n16
Anatomy Act (1832), 48–53
anti-vaccination, 4, 23, 25, 27–31, 37, 38, 154, 173, 195, 199–200, 205; anti-vaxxer, 4, 26, 27, 35, 36, 38, 200–2; conspiracy theories, 23, 26–7, 37; denialism, 9, 23, 26–7, 60, 205; vaccine hesitancy, ix, 111, 118, 199
Arabian Nights' Entertainments, 134–5
Arnold, Matthew, 187–97, 226n6
Atwood, Margaret, 155, 222n3
Ault, Donald, 218n13

Bacon, Francis, 87, 110,
Barnard, John, 219n2
Barney, Richard A., 5, 149, 208n3
Baron, John, 6–7, 84–5
Bate, Walter Jackson, 130, 219n2, 220n7
Baxby, Derrick, 8, 10
Beddoes, Thomas, 32, 124, 219n1

Beddoes, Thomas Lovell, 21, 208n6
Beer, Gillian, 188–9
Bennett, Andrew, 136
Bentham, Jeremy, 133
Bérubé, Michael, 212n17
Bewell, Alan, 21, 37, 68, 136, 161, 168–9, 171, 176, 208n8, 213n5, 214n10, 216nn22, 24, 220n11, 222n2, 223n14, 224nn19, 25, 225n31
Bichat, Xavier, 21–5, 28–9, 60
bioethics, 29, 32, 59, 145–6, 151, 173, 198
biopolitics, 3–5, 9–10, 20–9, 34, 38–55, 145–51, 177, 187, 195–7, 201–5, 207nn1, 3, 208n5, 211n4, 221n21
biopower, 4, 16–37, 38–55, 59–64, 123, 145–51, 181–205, 207n1, 208n5, 210–11n21, 211n4, 212n9, 213n17
biotheory, 4–5
Birch, John, 30–2, 35, 68–9, 88–9, 109–10, 115, 118
Blake, William, 5–6, 30, 34–6, 64, 68–9, 86–8, 147, 149, 184, 186, 197, 199, 200, 201, 217nn2–3, 7, 10, 218nn13–14, 218nn17–18, 219n22, 221n23; "Auguries of Innocence," 96–7, 217n11, 218n14; "The Book

of Thel," 92–6, 97, 99–100, 115,
217n9; "The Chimney Sweeper," 113;
"The Clod & the Pebble," 96, 114;
"Europe," 218n21; "Holy Thursday,"
113; "Jerusalem," 87–8; "Laocoön," 87;
"The Little Black Boy," 113; "London,"
69, 86; "The Marriage of Heaven and
Hell," 92, 97, 99, 113–14, 219n23;
"Milton," 87; "The Sick Rose," 92,
96, 97–9, 113–15; "The Song of
Los," 218n21; "There Is No Natural
Religion," 118–19; "Visions of the
Daughters of Albion," 35–6, 50, 92,
94, 96–101, 103–11, 111–15, 118,
212n16, 217n12, 218nn17, 19, 21,
219nn22–3
Bliss, Jonathan, 12–14, 21
Bloomfield, Robert, 22, 66–8, 111, 139
Blunt, Wilfrid, 71, 213n6
Boulton, Matthew, 87, 88, 213n5
Broglio, Ron, 209n14
Brooks, Robin, 217n1
Brown, John, 21, 33, 127, 208n7,
216n25
Brown, Laura, 224n21
Brunton, Deborah, 209n11
Burke, Edmund, 20–1, 30, 62, 66–70,
74, 81, 82, 84, 111, 119, 153, 163,
208n8, 213n3, 215n15
Butler, Marilyn, 220n4
Butts, Thomas, 92, 117
Byron, George Gordon, 158, 160, 192, 204

Canguilhem, Georges, 32, 132, 147–8,
221n17
Carlyle, Thomas, 190–2
Carmichael, Ann G., 221n16
case study, 10–17, 34, 36, 40, 42, 48,
50–3, 55, 59–60, 146, 151, 184–5,
196–7, 200–1, 225n2
census, 16, 40–51, 54, 59, 200–1,
211nn6–7, 212n12

Charon, Rita, 150, 209n13, 221n24
Clarke, Susan A., 214n7
Clement, William, 16, 18–19, 213n1
Cohen, Ed, 150–1, 193, 221n22, 226n8
Coleridge, Samuel Taylor, 22, 63, 71, 78,
79, 215n16
colonialism, 21, 30, 84, 166–7, 168–9,
171, 182, 208n8, 223n14, 224n19.
See also imperialism
consumption, 125–30, 134, 137–8,
149–50, 183–4, 220n11
Cory, Herbert, 204
conservatism, 22–3, 55, 65–9, 71, 84,
89, 108–10, 118–19, 152, 156, 163,
166, 176–7, 208n8, 209n11, 214n9,
220n13
Cooper, Astley, 124
cosmopolitanism, 35, 45, 48, 52–3,
61, 63–4, 68, 81, 82, 84, 86, 88, 96,
109–11, 113–14, 119, 123, 152–3,
156, 158, 164–8, 169–73, 174–7, 185,
193, 197, 213n5, 214n10, 216nn22,
24, 220n8, 222n5, 223n9, 224n22,
225n3, 226n8
COVID-19, ix, 3, 5, 9, 16, 23, 25–6, 31,
111, 118, 199, 205
cowpox, 8, 11, 14–24, 59, 64–6, 82, 124,
147, 153, 170–3, 200–3
Cox, Stephen, 101
Craciun, Adriana, 218n19
Craik, T.W., 223n16
Cruikshank, Isaac, 9
Cullen, William, 21, 33, 127, 137–8,
208n7, 216n25
Curran, Stuart, 212n10

Damon, S. Foster, 92
Darwin, Charles, 28, 61–2, 74, 187–9,
191–2, 215n15, 216n23
Darwin, Erasmus, 5, 6, 34, 35, 36,
60–70, 123, 183, 194, 210n17,
215n15, 226n9; The Loves of the Plants,

35, 60–5, 69–81, 86–91, 95, 99,
101–2, 106, 133, 194, 215n13,
216n25; *The Temple of Nature*, 63–4,
81–5, 109, 216nn23, 25
Davenport, Romola J., 14
Davis, Lennard J., 214n12
Day, William Patrick, 223n11
de Almeida, Hermione, 9, 21, 25, 127,
129, 135, 208n8, 210nn17–18, 219n2
Defoe, Daniel, 166–7
Derrida, Jacques, 219n3
detection, 12, 182–6, 186–90, 193–4,
197, 202–3
diagnosis, 28–9, 33, 36, 38–40, 42,
49–50, 128, 132, 135–41, 144, 148,
181–2, 185–6, 194, 200, 208n8,
210n19. *See also* DSM
Dickens, Charles, 27–31, 181–2
Di Leo, Jeffrey R., 4
Dimsdale, Thomas, 8–11
disability studies, 20, 51–2, 147–8, 151,
212n17, 213n20, 221n18
Donne, John, 141
Down's Syndrome, 52, 147, 148, 212n17
Doyle, Arthur Conan, 5, 36, 182–5,
195–8, 199, 202, 225n1; "The Sign
of Four," 193–4, 202; "A Study in
Scarlet," 183, 184, 185–93, 194, 196,
197, 202
Dryden, John, 65–8, 109, 111, 138,
213n4, 214nn8, 12
DSM, 147–8

Eaves, Morris, 97
Eberle, Roxanne, 102
English Civil War, 54, 66–7, 214n7
Enlightenment, 6, 8–9, 11, 25, 29–30,
33, 69, 71–5, 80–1, 82, 84, 86–9, 100,
106–8, 110, 119, 124–5, 129, 134,
151, 189, 207n3, 209n16, 210n18,
216n17, 217n3, 218n13
Erdman, David V., 218n17

Esposito, Roberto, 148–51, 187, 207n3,
221n21, 225n3
eugenics, 32, 48, 51–2, 53, 147, 148,
149, 212n17, 225n3
evolution, 28, 61–4, 74–5, 81, 82, 84,
86, 187–93, 197, 201, 213n2, 215n15,
216nn20, 23, 25

faith, 82, 95, 170, 187, 199. *See also*
religion
Fanon, Frantz, 84, 111
Ferber, Michael, 217n12
Filmer, Robert, 54
Fisch, Audrey, 157–8, 222nn6–7
Fissell, Mary, 10, 59–60
Fogel, Aaron, 41–3, 211n6
Foucault, Michel, 4, 21–2, 28–31, 33,
36, 132, 147–8, 207nn1, 3, 210n21;
Abnormal, 221n20; *The Birth of
Biopolitics*, 29, 207n1; *The Birth of the
Clinic*, 21, 28, 31, 59–60, 136, 199,
221nn17, 19; *Discipline and Punish*,
45, 212n9, 221n20; *The History
of Sexuality*, 145–6, 148; *Security,
Territory, Population*, 221n4; *Society
Must Be Defended*, 45–6, 48, 51–2
Frost, Robert, 43
Frye, Northrop, 217n8
Fulford, Tim, 22–3, 209n11, 214n9,
225n29
Fuller, Thomas, 130, 134

Garland-Thomson, Rosemarie, 51–2
gender, 46, 62, 67–8, 138, 153, 158–62,
164, 171, 176, 199, 223n9
Gigante, Denise, 21, 129, 137, 208n6
Gilbert, Sandra M., 157–8
Gillam, Stephen, 60
Gillray, James, 23–5
Ginsburg, Faye, 52
Glass, Bentley, 74–5
Goellnicht, Donald C., 126–7, 213n3

Goldstein, Amanda Jo, 221n23
Golinski, Jan, 210n17, 219n1
Gould, Stephen Jay, 188, 225n4
Graham, James, 32
Green, Matthew, 88
Greenhalgh, Tricia, 221n25
Griffiths, Devin, 213n5
Grinnell, George, 33, 210n19
Gubar, Susan, 157–8

Hamilton, William, 86–7
Hardt, Michael, 4, 207n2
Harris, Stuart, 72, 216n17
Harris, Susan Cannon, 185, 189
Hartman, Geoffrey H., 41, 211n3
Harvey, William, 129, 132
Haslam, Fiona, 209n14
Hassler, Donald M., 72, 216n17
Hatty, James, 210n17
Hatty, Suzanne E., 210n17
Hays, Mary, 102
Hitchcock, Peter, 4
Holmes, Sherlock, 182–3, 185–6, 189–94,
    195–7, 202, 225n5, 226nn10, 12
Homans, Margaret, 138
Horowitz, Tamara, 209n15
human flourishing, 5, 14, 20, 46, 52,
    149, 201, 212n17
Hunt, Lynn, 210n17, 219n1
Hunter, John, 6–8, 25, 208n6
Hunter, J. Paul, 72–3
Hurwitz, Brian, 221n25
Huxley, Thomas Henry, 187, 188–93,
    216n23, 226nn6–7

illness narrative, 3–5, 11–12, 26–7, 30–1,
    34–7, 40, 42–3, 45, 51, 60, 64, 106,
    110, 111, 113–15, 118–19, 123–5,
    139–40, 145–51, 152–5, 177, 195,
    197–8, 199–205
immunity, 5, 8, 9, 13, 17, 20, 29, 32,
    34, 62, 80, 82–3, 95, 111, 114, 124,

    128, 134, 144, 148–51, 153, 163–4,
    171–2, 182, 187, 197, 199–201, 204,
    221nn21–2, 225n3
imperialism, 14, 59, 106, 112–13, 169,
    171, 182, 218n17, 225n30. *See also*
    colonialism
inoculation, 5, 8, 10–11, 14, 16–31,
    34–7, 38, 59–64, 65, 66–70, 74,
    76–81, 82–5, 86, 88, 92, 96, 99–102,
    105–11, 113–15, 118–19, 123–4,
    128, 133, 135, 141, 148–9, 150, 153,
    155, 163–5, 168–73, 176–7, 182,
    184, 187, 193, 195, 200–1, 209nn9,
    13, 17, 210n21, 213nn3–4, 214nn8,
    12, 219n23, 220n8, 222n2, 224nn19,
    22; caprification, 75–7, 79, 80, 82, 84,
    99–102, 104, 106–11, 114, 118, 119,
    216n21, 218nn15, 21; contamination,
    17, 20, 24–5, 26, 32, 35, 66–7, 70,
    81, 84, 95, 100–2, 106, 148–50, 153,
    171, 197, 213n3; grafting, 20, 62–5,
    68, 70, 73–4, 80, 82, 88, 153, 170–2;
    vaccination, ix, 3–5, 6, 8–11, 13–16,
    17, 20, 22–3, 25, 27–31, 36–7, 38, 40,
    55, 59, 64, 66–8, 82–5, 86, 88–9, 111,
    115, 118, 123–5, 127–9, 133–5, 139,
    141, 146, 148–51, 153–4, 170–3, 177,
    194–8, 199–205, 209nn11–12, 14,
    16, 210n17, 211n21, 214nn8–9, 12,
    219n3, 222n1, 226n1; variolation, 6,
    8, 13–14, 17, 30, 60, 64, 66–8, 83–4,
    89, 102, 104–6, 110–11, 114, 124,
    134, 153, 172–3, 177, 195

Jacob, François, 61, 64, 213n2
Jacob, Margaret, 210n17, 219n1
Jameson, Fredric, 41, 48, 211n2
Janis, Allen A., 209n15
Jay, Mike, 124
Jenner, Edward, 5–37, 38–40, 42–3, 45,
    55, 59–61, 64, 66, 68, 78, 82–4, 119,
    123, 125, 146, 148, 153, 170–3, 183,

185, 197, 199–202, 208n6, 209n9, 210n17, 213n1, 214n8, 215n12, 225n29

Jewson, Nicholas D., 33–4, 59–60, 210n20

Johnson, Barbara, 157, 222nn6–7

Johnson, Joseph, 86–7

Johnson, Samuel, 65–8, 214n11

Johnson, Steven, 197, 226n12

Kant, Immanuel, 45, 81, 152–3, 164–7, 222n5

Keats, John, 5, 6, 21, 25, 34, 36, 41–2, 48–53, 54–5, 119, 124–35, 145–51, 152, 154, 177, 183, 184, 186, 194, 197, 198, 199, 200, 201–2, 210n18, 212nn11, 15, 213n3, 219n2, 220n7, 222n1; *The Fall of Hyperion*, 126-8, 127, 141–5; *Hyperion*, 126–8, 142–4, 221n14; "La Belle Dame Sans Merci," 36, 42, 48–50, 126, 129–45, 146, 148, 212n14, 220nn9, 11–13; *Lamia*, 109–10, 129, 135; "Ode on Grecian Urn," 50; "Ode to a Nightingale," 50; "On First Looking into Chapman's Homer," 41; "Sleep and Poetry," 123–4; "This Living Hand," 203–5

Kelley, Theresa M., 216n22

King-Hele, Desmond, 63, 215n15, 216n25, 217n3

Kislev, Mordechai E., 218n16

Koch, Robert, 183–5, 188, 196, 225n1

Laverack, Glenn, 226n2

Lawlor, Clark, 149–50

Lawrence, William, 21, 133, 188, 208n6, 220n4

Lee, Debbie, 22–3, 209n11, 214n9, 225n29

Lemke, Thomas, 149

Lemm, Vanessa, 225n3

Levinson, Marjorie, 142

Levitt, Annette S., 217n6

Liebow, Ely M., 183

Linnaeus, 21, 23, 32, 35, 60–5, 69–70, 71–7, 81, 82–5, 88–9, 90–1, 92, 95, 107, 118–19, 123, 127, 184, 201, 213n6, 215n15, 216n25

List, Julia, 213n5

Locke, John, 72–3, 81–2, 87, 97, 105–6, 109–10, 119, 131, 134, 216n18

Loxley, James, 214n7

Lucas, J.R., 188–90, 192

Lussier, Mark, 97, 218nn13–14

Maclean, Ian, 210n17

Maines, Rachel P., 137

Makdisi, Saree, ix, 218n17, 219n22

Malthus, Thomas, 169

Markel, Howard, 225n1

materialism, 21, 133, 154, 190, 194, 196–7, 208nn6–7

McGann, Jerome, 40–2, 174, 211n1, 220n13, 225n33

McWhir, Anne, 168, 223n15, 224n24

medical and health humanities, ix–x, 3–4, 147, 151

Mee, Jon, ix, 130, 212n11, 214n11

Mellor, Anne K., ix, 103–4, 110, 138, 156–7, 161, 164, 176, 211n5, 217n9, 222nn2, 7, 223nn12, 13, 224n19, 225nn30, 34

Melville, Peter, 166, 176, 222n2, 224nn19–20, 22

Milton, John, 72, 92–6, 100–2, 104, 107, 115–19, 131, 142–4, 162, 165, 221n14; "Areopagitica," 92, 95, 102; "Comus," 99, 102, 115–18, 217n6; *Paradise Lost*, 92, 95, 118, 159, 165, 223n10

Montag, Warren, 5, 149

Montagu, Mary Wortley, 8, 20, 22, 26, 60–1, 66, 99–100, 102, 104–7, 109, 118, 134, 153, 170–3, 214n12, 218n19

Moretti, Franco, 225n30
Motion, Andrew, 219n2
Moylan, Christopher, 21

narrative medicine, 147, 150–1, 209n13, 221n25
Nealon, Jeffrey, 212n9
negative capability, 129, 138, 220n7
Negri, Antonio, 4, 207n2
neoliberalism, 4, 5, 48, 52, 207n1
Nettleton, Sarah, 60
Newton, Isaac, 87, 97, 106, 107, 110, 119, 218nn13, 18
Northcote, James, 7
Novalis, 127
Nussbaum, Felicity, ix, 209n9

O'Sullivan, Barbara Jane, 222nn6, 8
Otis, Laura, 182, 189, 193

Palacio, Jean de, 157
Paley, Morton, 156–7, 160, 169, 217n11, 222nn6, 8, 223n13, 225n32
Pamboukian, Sylvia A., 185, 189
Park, Alice, 199
Percival, Thomas, 13–14, 16, 32
Peterfreund, Stuart, 218nn13, 18
Phipps, James, 8
Poovey, Mary, 157, 161, 174, 222n8
Porter, Roy, 10, 12–14, 27–31, 59–60, 125, 209n16
Portland Vase, 86–7, 217n1

Quinlan, Karen Ann, 145–7

radicalism, 5, 16, 20, 23, 25, 28, 36–7, 44, 62–70, 71–2, 81, 82, 84–5, 86, 88–9, 92, 99, 110–11, 114–15, 118–19, 125, 128–9, 151, 152–3, 155–6, 162, 169, 176, 181, 190, 197, 208nn6, 8, 210nn17, 21, 216n22, 218n19, 219nn22–1, 220n4

Rapp, Rayna, 52
Rawson, Claude, 224n21
religion, 36, 189, 212n13, 216n23; Christianity, 23, 170; Mormonism, 184, 186, 192–4, 196–7, 202; Wilberforce-Huxley debate, 188–93. *See also* faith
revolution, 6, 23, 81, 84–5, 86–8, 89, 105, 110–11, 113–15, 119, 157, 197, 224n25; American Revolution, 55, 99, 105, 112; French Revolution, 20, 30, 41–2, 43–8, 52–3, 54–5, 62, 65–6, 67, 69–70, 105, 112, 153, 155, 156, 163, 169, 176, 208n8, 216n22; Industrial Revolution, 49, 87–8, 171, 207n3, 217n4
Richardson, Alan, 125
Richardson, Ruth, 49
Richardson, Samuel, 102
Rickman, John, 43, 45, 49
Robbins, Hollis, 43, 47, 211n7
Roe, Nicholas, 124
Royden, H.L., 221n1
Romantic disease discourse, 31–7, 64, 125, 129, 135, 140–1, 144–5, 146, 148, 150–1, 152, 181–2, 184, 187, 189, 201–2, 215n12, 222n1
Rose, George, 8
Ruston, Sharon, 208n6, 220n4

Saler, Michael, 195–6
Schelling, Friedrich Wilhelm Joseph, 21, 127
Schiavo, Terri, 221n15
Schiller, Friedrich, 21
Schlegel, Friedrich, 21
Schofield, Robert E., 219n1
Schofield, R.S., 212n12
Schott, G.D., 89
Schwartz, Janelle, 217n10
Seitz-Wald, Alex, 226n1
Sha, Richard, 68, 89, 214n10, 218n13

Shakespeare, William, 78–9, 82; *Hamlet*, 79, 195; *Henry V*, 79–80

Sheil, Richard Lalor, 161, 175, 223n15

Shelley, Mary Wollstonecraft, 5, 6, 29–30, 32, 34, 36, 51–2, 54, 119, 149, 152–8, 174–7, 184, 187, 193, 211n5, 223nn11–12, 224n28, 225nn32, 34, 226n8; *Frankenstein*, 32, 51–2, 156, 159, 161–2, 165, 172–3, 174, 176–7, 196, 211n5, 220n4, 223n17, 225n30; *The Last Man*, 29–30, 36, 152–73, 174–7, 181, 201, 211n6, 220nn8, 10, 222nn1–2, 4, 6–8, 223nn9, 12–14, 224nn19–20, 22–4, 26–7, 225nn32, 35

Shelley, Percy Bysshe, 21, 208n6, 211n5; *Alastor*, 149–50, 156, 158–9, 162–3, 169, 173, 177, 222nn6, 8, 224n25, 225nn31–2; *The Cenci*, 162, 223n18; *The Defence of Poetry*, 174; *Prometheus Unbound*, 157, 162–3, 224n18

Shuttleton, David, 11, 65, 66, 138, 214nn9, 12

Siebers, Tobin, 221n18

Simpson, David, 135

slavery, 13, 103–6, 110–13, 218n17

smallpox, 3–205; contagion, 30, 83, 108, 163, 168–9, 171, 172, 181–2, 184, 208n8, 220n10, 223n14, 224n24; compulsion, 5, 16, 25, 28, 36–7, 38, 59, 135, 146, 149, 195, 199–200, 211n21; eradication, 6, 9, 11, 13, 23, 24, 30, 33, 55, 84, 172–3, 200–1, 215n12; history, 3–5, 6, 8–16, 17, 21–4, 25–37, 40, 60, 63, 65, 68–9, 86, 109, 125, 128–9, 138–9, 148, 151, 153–4, 170, 172–3, 176–7, 199–203, 209nn9, 12, 16–17, 210n21, 214n12, 225n29; immunity, 5, 8, 9, 13, 17, 20, 29, 32, 34, 62, 80, 82–3, 95, 111, 114, 124, 128, 134, 144, 148–51, 153, 163–4, 171–2, 182, 187, 197,

199–201, 204, 221nn21–2, 225n3; public health, 9, 16, 26, 59, 67, 123, 147, 195, 200, 204, 208n5; pustules, 11, 14–15, 59, 66, 83, 109, 139, 141, 200–1, 202–3, 214n12; scars, 10, 11, 13, 203, 214n12, 224n28; statistics, 13–14; vaccination, ix, 3–5, 6, 8–11, 13–16, 17, 20, 22–3, 25, 27–31, 36–7, 38, 40, 55, 59, 64, 66–8, 82–5, 86, 88–9, 111, 115, 118, 123–5, 127–9, 133–5, 139, 141, 146, 148–51, 153–4, 170–3, 177, 194–8, 199–205, 209nn11–12, 14, 16, 210n17, 211n21, 214nn8–9, 12, 219n3, 222n1, 226n1; variolation, 6, 8, 13–14, 17, 30, 60, 64, 66–8, 83–4, 89, 102, 104–6, 110–11, 114, 124, 134, 153, 172–3, 177, 195

Smith, Charlotte Turner, 44–8, 51, 212n10

Snow, C.P., 186

Snow, John, 197, 202, 226n12

Snyder, Robert Lance, 157

Sontag, Susan, 3–5, 149–50, 182, 214–15n12

Specter, Michael, 9, 23, 226n1

Spivak, Gayatri Chakravorty, 225n30

Spratt, Hartley S., 157–8

Stanback, Emily, 213

Star Trek, 51, 196

Sterrenburg, Lee, 156

Sussman, Charlotte, 43, 211n6, 223n9

Sutton, Daniel, 8, 11

Swann, Karen, 138

Swift, Jonathan, 190, 211n8

symptom, 3, 11, 28, 40, 53, 124–5, 128, 136–7, 139–41, 145, 220n11

Tannenbaum, Leslie, 219n21

Teute, Fredrika J., 62, 216n22

Thelwall, John, 21, 208n6

Thomas, Keith, 212n13

Thompson, E.P., 10
Tsianos, George I., 11–12

Uglow, Jennifer S., 72, 213n5, 216n17,
    217n4

vaccine-preventable human diseases
    (other than smallpox), ix, 9, 118,
    200–1; cholera, 168, 172, 183, 197,
    202; measles, ix, 83, 118, 148, 173,
    199, 226n1; mumps, 173; polio, 173,
    201; pertussis, 173, 199; rubella, 173;
    tuberculosis, 147, 149–50, 183–4
Van Dine, S.S., 186–7, 193
vitalism, 21, 129, 133–5, 146, 154, 188,
    208nn6–7, 220n4
Veeder, William R., 159, 223n11
Viscomi, Joseph, 115

Wakefield, Andrew, 23, 118, 199, 209n10
Walker, John, 16, 18–19, 59
Wallace, Alfred Russel, 28–31
Watt, James, 87, 88, 213n5
Wedgwood, Josiah, 87, 213n5, 217n1
Welch, Dennis M., 110
Wilberforce, Samuel, 188–93

Williams, Cynthia Schoolar, 224nn23, 27
Williams, Elizabeth A., 208n7
Wolfson, Susan, 44, 138, 204
Wollstonecraft, Mary, 103–5, 112–13,
    161, 208n8, 218n19, 219n22
Woodville, William, 137
Wordsworth, William, 5, 6, 10, 14, 16,
    22, 34–5, 36, 38–40, 40–3, 45–6,
    47–55, 59–61, 63–4, 72, 123, 130–2,
    144, 146, 156, 184–5, 195, 197,
    199–201, 211nn3, 7, 212nn10–11,
    16, 220n7; "Expostulation and
    Reply," 54, 132; "The Idiot Boy," 14,
    16, 54, 197, 213n20; "Lines Written
    a Few Miles above Tintern Abbey,"
    54, 130, 132; "The Mad Mother," 14,
    213n20; "Preface to Lyrical Ballads,"
    44, 46, 53–5, 211n3; "Simon Lee,"
    16; "The Tables Turned," 42; "The
    Thorn," 14, 213n20; "We Are Seven,"
    14, 16, 40–53, 54, 59, 200, 201,
    211n3
Wrigley, E.A., 212n12

Youngquist, Paul, 10, 32